Clinical Procedures

for Physician Assistants

Clinical Procedures

for **Physician Assistants**

Richard W. Dehn, MPA, PA-C
Clinical Professor and Assistant Director
Physician Assistant Program
The University of Iowa College of Medicine
Iowa City, Iowa

David P. Asprey, PhD, PA-C
Associate Professor and Program Director
Physician Assistant Program
The University of Iowa College of Medicine
Iowa City, Iowa

SAUNDERS
An Imprint of Elsevier

SAUNDERS

An Imprint of Elsevier

The Curtis Center
Independence Square West
Philadelphia, Pennsylvania 19106

Library of Congress Cataloging-in-Publication Data

Clinical procedures for physician assistants/[edited by] Richard W. Dehn, David P. Asprey.

p.; cm.

Includes index.

ISBN-13: 978-0-7216-9073-5 ISBN-10: 0-7216-9073-4

1. Physicians' assistants. I. Dehn, Richard. II. Asprey, David P.
   [DNLM: 1. Diagnostic Techniques and Procedures. 2. Physician Assistants.
   WB 141 C6413 2002]

R697.P45 C56 2002

610.73'7—dc21   2001049090

Editor-in-Chief: Andrew Allen
Acquisitions Editor: Shirley Kuhn
Developmental Editor: Helaine Tobin
Project Manager: Agnes Byrne
Manuscript Editor: Jodi Kaye
Production Manager: Peter Faber
Illustration Specialist: Lisa Lambert

Clinical Procedures for Physician Assistants

Permissions may be sought directly from Elsevier's Health Sciences Rights Department in Philadelphia, PA, USA: phone: (+1) 215 239 3804, fax: (+1) 215 239 3805, e-mail: healthpermissions@elsevier.com. You may also complete your request on-line via the Elsevier homepage (http://www.elsevier.com), by selecting 'Customer Support' and then 'Obtaining Permissions'.

ISBN-13: 978-0-7216-9073-5
ISBN-10: 0-7216-9073-4

Printed in the United States of America.

Last digit is the print number: 9   8   7   6   5   4

This book is dedicated to all physician assistants who are learning the science and art of practicing medicine as a physician assistant.

This book is also dedicated to my wife, Elizabeth, and my children Jonathan, Michael, Clare, and Kelley, without whose support I could not have finished this project.

RWD

To my wife, Jill, who has consistently encouraged and supported me each step of the way; without you this accomplishment would not have been possible. To Laura, Nolan, and Caleb for the love, patience, and tolerance you have demonstrated to me at times when Dad "went back to the office."

DPA

Reviewers

Margaret E. Allen, PA-C
Stanford University Medical
School/Foothill College
Palo Alto, California

Kay Arlene Erickson, PA-C
University of Findlay
Findlay, Ohio

Carmen B. Fox, MPA, PA-C
Nova Southeastern University
Ft. Lauderdale, Florida

Patricia A. Francis, MS, PA-C
Medical College of Ohio
Toledo, Ohio

Nancy Freeborne, MPH, PA-C
Physician Assistant Program
George Washington University
Washington, D.C.

**Catherine A. Gillespie,
MPAS, PA-C**
Physician Assistant Program
Gannon University
Erie, Pennsylvania

Elaine E. Grant, MPH, PA-C
Assistant Dean, Yale University School
of Medicine
Dean and Director, Physician Assistant
Program
Yale University School of Medicine
New Haven, Connecticut

Michelle L. Heinan, MS, PA-C
Physician Assistant Program
East Carolina University
Greenville, North Carolina

Sandra Keavy, MPAS, PA-C
University of Detroit Mercy
Detroit, Michigan

Melinda Luce, PA-C
Rocky Mountain College
Billings, Montana

**Amelia Naccarto-Coleman,
MAS, PA-C**
Assistant Professor of Physician
Assistant Education
Western University Health Sciences
Pomona, California

John W. Rafalko, MS, PA-C
Assistant Professor
Physician Assistant Program
Nova Southeastern University
Fort Lauderdale, Florida

Kara N. Roman, MMS, PA-C
Midwestern University
Downers Grove, Illinois

Nancy M. Valentage, MS, RPA-C
Associate Director
Physician Assistant Program
Rochester Institute of Technology
College of Science
Rochester, New York

Pamela Van Bevern, MPAS, PA-C
Assistant Professor
Physician Assistant Program
Saint Louis University
Saint Louis, Missouri

Thomas J. Williams, MHP, PA-C
Physician Assistant Program
Northeastern University
Boston, Massachusetts

Contributors

David P. Asprey, PhD, PA-C
Associate Professor and Program Director, Physician Assistant Program, University of Iowa College of Medicine, Iowa City, Iowa
Documentation

Patrick C. Auth, MS, PA-C
Program Director, Assistant Professor, MCP Hahnemann University College of Nursing and Health Professions, Philadelphia, Pennsylvania
Incision and Drainage of an Abscess

George S. Bottomley, DVM, PA-C
Vice Chair and Academic Coordinator, Assistant Professor, Physician Assistant Studies Program, Massachusetts College of Pharmacy and Health Sciences, Boston, Massachusetts
Incision and Drainage of an Abscess

Darwin Brown, PA-C
Instructor, Physician Assistant Program, University of Nebraska Medical Center, Omaha, Nebraska
Obtaining Blood Cultures; Draining Subungual Hematomas

L. Gail Curtis, BA, PA-C
Assistant Professor, Wake Forest University School of Medicine, Winston-Salem, North Carolina
The Pelvic Examination and Obtaining a Routine Papanicolaou's Smear

Randy Danielsen, MPAS, PA-C
Associate Professor and Chair, Physician Assistant Studies, Arizona School of Health Sciences, Mesa, Arizona
Blood Pressure Measurement

Ellen Davis-Hall, PhD, PA-C
Associate Professor and Academic Coordinator, Physician Assistant Program, University of Nebraska Medical Center, Omaha, Nebraska
Inserting Intravenous Catheters

Richard W. Dehn, MPA, PA-C
Clinical Professor and Assistant Director, Physician Assistant Program, University of Iowa College of Medicine, Iowa City, Iowa
Examination of the Male Genitalia

Michelle DiBaise, MPAS, PA-C
Assistant Professor, University of Nebraska Medical Center, Omaha, Nebraska
Local Anesthesia; Dermatologic Procedures

Roger A. Elliott, MPH, PA-C
Associate Professor and Associate Director, University of Oklahoma Physician Associate Program, University of Oklahoma College of Medicine, Oklahoma City, Oklahoma
Office Pulmonary Function Testing

Sue M. Enns, MHS, PA-C
Assistant Professor, Department of Physician Assistant, College of Health Professions, Wichita State University, Wichita, Kansas
Treating Ingrown Toenails; Anoscopy

Donald R. Frosch, PA-C
Instructor, General Medicine and Research Coordinator, Physician Assistant Program, Finch University of Health Sciences/The Chicago Medical School, North Chicago, Illinois
Casting and Splinting

Kenneth R. Harbert, PhD, CHES, PA-C
Professor and Chair, Department of Physician Assistant Studies, Philadelphia College of Osteopathic Medicine, University of the Sciences in Philadelphia, Philadelphia, Pennsylvania
Venipuncture

Paul C. Hendrix, MHS, PA-C
Surgical Coordinator, Duke University Physician Assistant Program, Durham, North Carolina; Assistant Clinical Professor, Department of Surgery, Duke University Medical Center, Durham, North Carolina
Sterile Technique

Paul F. Jacques, EdM, RPA-C
Assistant Professor and Chair, Physician Assistant Department, Daemen College, Amherst, New York
Wound Dressing Techniques

P. Eugene Jones, PhD, PA-C
Professor and Chair, Department of Physician Assistant Studies, University of Texas Southwestern Medical Center, Dallas, Texas
Cryosurgery

Patricia Kelly, EdD, MHS, PA-C
Associate Professor and Program Director, Physician Assistant Program, Central Michigan University, Mt. Pleasant, Michigan
Clinical Breast Examination

Charles S. King, PA-C
Senior Physician Assistant, Division of Cardiology, Department of Internal Medicine, University of Utah Hospital, Salt Lake City, Utah
Exercise Stress Testing for the Primary Care Provider

Patrick Knott, PhD, PA-C
Associate Professor and Chair, Physician Assistant Department, Finch University of Health Sciences/The Chicago Medical School, North Chicago, Illinois; Co-director, Illinois Bone and Joint Physician Assistant Residency Program, Lutheran General Hospital, Park Ridge, Illinois
Casting and Splinting

Daniel L. McNeill, PhD, PA-C
Professor and Director, Physician Associate Program, University of Oklahoma College of Medicine, Oklahoma City, Oklahoma
Office Pulmonary Function Testing

Robert J. McNellis, MPH, PA-C
Director, Clinical Affairs and Education, American Academy of Physician Assistants, Alexandria, Virginia
Injection Techniques

Dawn Morton-Rias, PD, PA-C
Assistant Professor and Chairperson, Associate Dean for Primary Care, College of Health Related Professions, SUNY Downstate Medical Center Physician Assistant Program, Brooklyn, New York
Flexible Sigmoidoscopy

Richard D. Muma, MPH, PA-C
Acting Chair/Associate Professor, Department of Physician Assistant, College of Health Professions, Wichita State University, Wichita, Kansas
Patient Education Concepts

Karen A. Newell, PA-C
Academic Coordinator, Emory University School of Medicine, Physician Assistant Program, Atlanta, Georgia
Wound Closure

Claire Babcock O'Connell, MPH, PA-C
Associate Professor, Physician Assistant Program, University of Medicine and Dentistry of New Jersey and Rutgers University, Robert Wood Johnson Medical School, Piscataway, New Jersey
Arterial Puncture

Daniel L. O'Donoghue, PhD, PA-C
Assistant Professor, Physician Associate Program, University of Oklahoma College of Medicine, Oklahoma City, Oklahoma
Office Pulmonary Function Testing

Donald M. Pedersen, PhD, PA-C
Professor and Program Director, Physician Assistant Program, University of Utah School of Medicine, Salt Lake City, Utah
Exercise Stress Testing for the Primary Care Provider

Richard R. Rahr, MBA, EdD, PA-C
Professor and Chair, Physician Assistant Studies, School of Allied Health Sciences, University of Texas Medical Branch, Galveston, Texas
Performing an Electrocardiogram

Ted J. Ruback, MS, PA-C
Associate Professor and Head, Division of Physician Assistant Education, Director, Physician Assistant Program, Oregon Health and Science University School of Medicine; Assistant Director, Center for Ethics in Health Care, Oregon Health and Science University, Portland, Oregon
Informed Consent

Virginia Fallow Schneider, PA-C
Assistant Professor, Director, Physician Assistant Program, Baylor College of Medicine; Assistant Professor, University of Houston College of Pharmacy, Houston, Texas
Lumbar Puncture

Gary R. Sharp, MPH, PA-C
Associate Professor and Clinical Coordinator, Physician Associate Program, University of Oklahoma College of Medicine, Oklahoma City, Oklahoma
Office Pulmonary Function Testing

Shepard B. Stone, MPS, PA
Associate Clinical Professor of Anesthesiology, Yale University School of Medicine; Physician Associate–Anesthesiologist, Yale-New Haven Hospital, New Haven, Connecticut
Endotracheal Intubation

Kirsten Thomsen, PA-C
Adjunct Faculty, Department of Family and Community Medicine, University of New Mexico School of Medicine, Albuquerque, New Mexico
Standard Precautions

Dan Vetrosky, MEd, PhD Candidate, PA-C
Assistant Professor and Academic Coordinator, Department of Physician Assistant Studies, University of South Alabama, Mobile, Alabama
Nasogastric Tube Placement; Urinary Bladder Catheterization

M.F. Winegardner, MPAS, PA-C
Physician Assistant, Department of Radiation Oncology, Mercy Cancer Center, Mercy Medical Center—North Iowa, Mason City, Iowa
Joint and Bursal Aspiration

Preface

In writing this book regarding common clinical procedures for physician assistants (PAs), we hope to fill a unique need for an area of clinical practice that is vital to PA education and the practice of medicine as a PA. Our profession has prided itself on its ability to function as a part of the health care team that can fill almost any role that is needed, including the performance of clinical procedures. As the PA profession has evolved, using PAs in roles that provide greater autonomy and responsibility has served to increase the importance of a curriculum that incorporates common clinical procedures as part of the preparation of competent PAs.

In attempting to accomplish this goal we have turned to our colleagues who are involved in PA education, either as core faculty or clinical preceptors, who are very aware of the clinical procedure skills that PA practice requires. Although we recognize that this textbook does not cover every procedure that a PA may be asked to perform in practice, it does address a majority of the commonly occurring clinical procedures, and most were selected based on data that support the frequency with which PAs perform these procedures in primary care settings.

Acknowledgments

We are forever indebted to the hundreds of bright, caring, compassionate, and pioneering men and women who founded our profession. They ventured into this career with little assurance that they would have a job or a career, much less a dependable income. They have made it into one of the most rewarding professions in existence today. Their vision, dedication, endurance, ingenuity, and concern for the best interest of their patients continue to be a motivating force for us as physician assistant (PA) educators.

We would also like to recognize the hundreds of colleagues with whom we share the role and title of PA educator. These individuals often give up freely the opportunity for the greater income and greater control of their schedule that can often be found in private practice to help prepare the next generation of PAs. We find the dedication and commitment of PA educators to their profession truly inspiring.

We owe a great debt of gratitude to PA students. Without their eager thirst for information and knowledge, we would find our responsibility to teach them clinical procedures to be simply work. However, their passion and excitement about learning clinical procedures for the purpose of taking care of their patients makes this task a true pleasure.

Finally, we would like to acknowledge W.B. Saunders for its commitment to making educational materials available to PAs. Specifically, we would like to thank Shirley Kuhn for pursuing the idea of this book with us and encouraging us to take the leap of faith necessary to bring this project to fruition. We would also like to thank Helaine Tobin for her ceaseless attention to detail and for helping us navigate through the process of editing this text.

Table of Contents

Chapter 1

Informed Consent

▷ Ted J. Ruback

Procedure Goals and Objectives

Goal: To provide clinicians with the necessary knowledge and understanding of the principles of informed consent for all clinical procedures.

Objectives: The student will be able to . . .

▶ Describe the historical basis of informed consent.

▶ Describe the philosophical doctrine of informed consent.

▶ Describe the underlying principles of informed consent.

▶ List the three essential conditions that must be met to ensure effective informed consent.

▶ Describe exceptions to the requirement for informed consent.

Background and History of the Patient-Provider Relationship

Beginning in the 1970s, there has been a dramatic shift in the character of the physician-patient relationship, from one that has traditionally been paternalistic or physician-focused to one that recognizes patient autonomy and is predominantly patient-centered. This struggle between paternalism and autonomy has revolutionized the field of health care ethics and has formed the basis for the doctrine of informed consent.

Paternalism is based on the principle of beneficence, the desire to do good for the patient. The concept of informed consent asserts that the desire to do good is not a justification for overriding a competent patient's right to personal autonomy and self-determination. Although there is some question about whether consent to medical procedures can ever be truly informed, the process of obtaining informed consent from a patient has been incorporated into American society's expectation of good medical practice.

Purpose of Informed Consent

In May 2000, the House of Delegates of the American Academy of Physician Assistants adopted a policy of comprehensive "Guidelines for Ethical Conduct for the Physician Assistant Profession." The new code of ethics addresses the profession's responsibility in protecting a patient's autonomy.

"Physician assistants have a duty to protect and foster an individual patient's free and informed choices. The doctrine of informed consent means that a PA provides adequate information that is comprehendible to a competent patient or patient surrogate. At a minimum, this should include the nature of the medical condition, the objectives of the proposed treatment, treatment options, possible outcomes, and the risks involved. PAs should be committed to the concept of shared decision making, which involves assisting patients in making decisions that account for medical, situational, and personal factors."

(American Academy of Physician Assistants, 2000)

Informed consent should be obtained from a patient before all medical interventions that have the potential for harm, including diagnostic as well as therapeutic procedures. A patient, through the exercise of personal autonomy, may either agree to or refuse a proposed procedure or treatment, but it is the responsibility of the practitioner to make sure that the decision is based on complete and appropriate information. In most states, health care providers have an "affirmative duty" to disclose such information, which means that information must be volunteered and not just provided in response to questions posed by the patient. Once the information has been disclosed, the provider's obligation has been met. Weighing the risks and deciding on a course of action then becomes the responsibility of the patient or the patient's surrogate.

Legal actions against health care professionals for failure to obtain informed consent to treatment have been pursued under two separate theories of liability—one based on the concept of battery and the other on the concept of negligence (Applebaum, 1987).

Most early litigation involving informed consent argued that the provision of treatment without consent constituted battery—an intentional, nonconsensual touching of the patient. The concept of battery protects a person's physical integrity against unwanted invasion.

After 1957, most suits alleging lack of informed consent were brought under the legal theory of negligence. Under this theory, an injured patient argues that he or she was harmed by the provider's unintentional failure to satisfy a professional standard of care. When applied in an informed consent case, the alleged negligence results from a failure to disclose sufficient information about the risks or complications of a treatment.

Essential Components of Informed Consent

There are three essential conditions that must be met to ensure effective informed consent. First, the patient must have the capacity, or competence, to make an informed decision. Second, the patient must be given sufficient information about the procedure or treatment and the alternatives to allow him or her to make an informed choice. Third, the patient must give consent to treatment voluntarily, without coercion, manipulation, or duress.

Patient Capacity. There is no universally accepted test of a patient's capacity to consent to treatment. In general, an adult is presumed to be legally competent unless he or she has been formally and legally declared incompetent. Conversely, a minor is generally presumed to be legally incompetent to make medical decisions, although a number of exceptions to this rule exist and are often state-specific (e.g., emancipation). Additionally, specific legislation sometimes grants minors legal status to make some medical decisions for themselves (e.g., testing for sexually transmitted diseases as well as reproductive decisions).

Competency is usually established by assessing whether or not the patient has the capacity to understand the nature of his or her condition and the various options available and whether or not he or she is capable of making a rational decision. To make a rational choice, patients must be able to understand the treatments available as well as the likely outcomes in each case. They must also be able to deliberate and consider their options and weigh them against one another to choose the best alternative. To do so effectively, they must assess the options available in relation to a set of values and goals, without which they would have no basis for preferring one outcome to any other (Moskop, 1999). They must also be able to communicate their understanding and their decision in some intelligible way.

Adequate Information. As stated previously, the second requirement of informed consent is that the patient must be provided with adequate information with which to make a decision. The right to informed consent is embedded in the nature of fiduciary relationships, wherein one party has differential power, and thus that party has the inherent responsibility to share necessary information with the other. General categories of information that must be provided are the diagnosis, the nature of the proposed procedure, the risks and benefits of the procedure, and the available alternatives (including the alternative of not having the procedure), including the risks and benefits of each.

Disclosure of information is judged adequate by two competing standards that have emerged in the laws governing informed consent. The older standard, known as the professional standard, bases disclosure of information on the prevailing practice within the profession. The professional standard requires a health care provider to disclose the type and amount of information that another practitioner in the same specialty and "community" would disclose. The professional standard is consistent with good medical care as defined by the profession. Because the focus is not on patient understanding but rather on the accepted standard of practice defined by the profession, the professional standard is more likely to be distorted by paternalism and less likely to allow for true patient autonomy.

The second standard of disclosure, introduced in 1972, is the reasonable person standard of material risk. The reasonable person standard requires a health care provider to disclose to a patient whatever a reasonable person in the patient's position would want to know, before making a decision about an intervention. Material information is information that the practitioner recognizes that a reasonable person in the patient's position would consider to be significant to his or her decision-making about the recommended medical intervention. Risks that are not serious, or are unlikely, are not considered material. Under this standard, the critical requirement shifts from whether the disclosure met the profession's standard to whether the undisclosed information would have been material to a reasonable patient's decision-making.

The great advantage of the reasonable person standard is the focus on the preferences of the patient. A requirement for this standard is that the type and amount of information provided must be at the patient's level of understanding if he or she is truly to be autonomous as a decision maker. The disadvantages of this standard include its failure to articulate the nature of the hypothetical reasonable person. In addition, the retrospective application of this standard presents a significant problem in that any complication of a procedure is likely to seem material after it has occurred (Nora, 1998).

Although the reasonable person standard does focus more on the patient's perspective, it does not require that the disclosure be tailored to each patient's specific informational needs or desires. Instead, it bases the requirements on what a hypothetical reasonable person would want to know. There has been some movement to expand the reasonable person standard of disclosure from the needs of the hypothetical reasonable person to the needs of the specific patient. This more subjective, patient-centered approach allows greater differentiation based on patient preference, relying on the unique nature and abilities of the individual patient to determine the amount of disclosure needed to satisfy the requirements of informed consent.

In addition to providing information, the provider has the ethical obligation to make reasonable efforts to ensure comprehension. Communicating highly technical and specialized knowledge to someone who is not conversant in the subject presents a formidable challenge. Patient-centered barriers to informed consent—such as anxiety, language differences, and physical or emotional impairments—can impede the process. Lack of familiarity or sensitivity on the part of the provider to the patient's cultural and health care beliefs can act as a significant barrier to providing effective informed consent. Process-centered barriers—including readability of consent forms, timing of the consent discussion, and amount of time devoted to the process—also may reflect disrespect for the autonomy of the patient.

To optimize information sharing, explanations should be given clearly and simply, and questions should be asked frequently to assess understanding. Whenever possible, a variety of communication techniques should be used, including written forms of educational materials and videotapes. Computers represent a powerful and effective tool that may, in the future, be integrated into a clinical setting and improve patient understanding and decision-making (Jimison, 1998).

Voluntary Choice. Consent to treatment obtained using manipulation or coercion, or both, is the antithesis of informed consent. Although a health care provider's recommendation regarding treatment typically can have a strong influence on a patient's decision-making, a recommendation offered as part of the practitioner's responsibility to inform and guide a patient in his or her decision-making is not considered coercion.

Types of Informed Consent

Consent may take many forms, including implied, general, and special. Implied consent is often used when immediate action is required. In the emergency room, consent is presumed when inaction may cause greater injury or would be contrary to good medical practice. General consent is often obtained on hospital admission to provide consent for routine services and routine touching by health care staff. Special consent is required for specific high-risk procedures or treatments.

Consent obtained verbally is as binding as written consent because there is no legal requirement that consent be in written form. However, when disagreements arise, oral consent becomes difficult to prove. The health care provider should always document verbal consent explicitly in the medical record.

Written consent is the preferred form of consent. The consent form provides legal, visible proof of a patient's intentions. A well-drafted informed consent document can provide concrete evidence that some exchange of information was communicated to, and some assent obtained from, the patient. Such a document, supported by an entry in the patient's medical record, is often the key to a successful malpractice defense when the issue of consent to treatment arises.

Some states have laws that specify certain language on consent forms for certain procedures. In cases that do not require specific forms, a general consent form that identifies the patient and documents the procedure, the risks associated with it, the indications, and the alternatives can be used. Most states require a consent form to be witnessed. Because of the potential conflict of interest, usually it is not advisable to have office personnel (nursing or other staff) be the sole witness to a consent document.

A written informed consent document should be prepared with the patient's needs in mind and should be presented with the opportunity for the patient to ask questions and discuss concerns. Consent forms are often written in great detail and use medical and legal terminology that is far beyond the capacity of many patients. For true autonomy to exist in informed consent, consent forms should be understandable and should contain the patient's primary language or languages whenever possible. If necessary, an interpreter should be made available during the informed consent conference. Again, the issue of comprehension is vital to the process. Health care providers should not make the mistake of equating the written and signed document with informed consent and should take care to make sure that information-transferring communication did, in fact, occur.

Patient's Right to Refuse Treatment

Patients have the right to refuse treatment. In such circumstances, it is essential to document such refusals carefully and, most importantly, the patient's understanding of the potential consequences of refusing treatment. Again, the signature of a witness is helpful in these circumstances.

Exceptions to Informed Consent Requirements

Several types of legitimate exceptions to the right of informed consent have been described. In rare instances, courts have recognized limited privileges that potentially can protect health care providers from claims alleging a lack of informed consent. Such exceptions include emergencies, patients unable to consent, a patient waiver of consent, public health requirements, and therapeutic privilege. In all these instances, the provider has the burden of proving that the claimed exception was invoked appropriately.

According to the emergency exception, if treatment is required to prevent death or other serious harm to a patient, that treatment may be provided without informed consent. Courts have upheld that the emergent nature of the situation and the impracticality of conferring with the patient preclude the need for informed consent. This exception is based on the presumption that the patient would consent to treatment to preserve life or health if he or she were able to do so and if there were sufficient time to obtain consent. Despite this exception, a competent patient may refuse interventions even if they are life-saving. For example, courts have repeatedly recognized the rights of Jehovah's Witnesses to refuse blood products.

The care of patients who lack decision-making capacity can be provided without the patient's informed consent. This exception, however, does not imply that no consent is necessary; instead, informed consent is required from a surrogate acting on behalf of the patient. Some surrogate decision makers are clearly identifiable, for example, the legal guardians assigned to protect the best interests of persons judged to be incompetent and the parents of minor children. In other cases, surrogates are more difficult to determine.

The decision-making authority of surrogates is directed by defined standards. These standards require surrogates to rely first on any treatment preferences specifically indicated, either in writing or orally, by the patient before he or she lost decision-making capacity. Lacking such direction, surrogates are then empowered to exercise "substituted judgment," that is, to use their knowledge of the patient's preferences and values to choose the alternative that they believe the patient would choose if he or she were able to do so. In some instances, prior knowledge of a patient's preferences or values is lacking. In such situations, surrogates are directed to rely on their assessment of the patient's best interests and are encouraged to pursue the course of action they deem most likely to foster the patient's overall well-being (Buchanan, 1989).

When a surrogate's treatment choice appears clearly contrary to a patient's previously expressed wishes or best interests, the patient's provider is duty-bound to question that choice. The health care provider does not have the authority to unilaterally override the surrogate's decision but must bring the issue to the attention of an appropriate legal authority for review and adjudication.]

In the newly adopted code of ethics of the physician assistant (PA) profession, the PA's role with regard to surrogates is clearly delineated.

> When the person giving consent is a patient's surrogate, a family member, or other legally authorized representative, the PA should take reasonable care to assure that the decisions made are consistent with the patient's best interests and personal preferences, if known. If the PA believes the surrogate's choices do not reflect the patient's wishes or best interests, the PA should work to resolve the conflict. This may require the use of additional resources, such as an ethics committee.
>
> **(American Academy of Physician Assistants, 2000)**

[Informed consent, although clearly recognized as a patient's right, is not a patient's duty. Patients can choose to waive their right to receive the relevant information and give informed consent to treatment. The provider may honor the patient's right to choose someone else to make treatment decisions on his or her behalf as long as the request is made competently, voluntarily, and with some understanding that the patient recognizes that he or she is relinquishing a right. Health care providers should not feel obligated to accept the responsibility for making treatment decisions for the patient if they are asked to do so. Instead, they can request that the patient make his or her own choice or designate another person to serve as surrogate.

Sometimes medical interventions have a potential benefit not only to the patient but also to others in the community. In such rare instances, public health statutes may authorize patient detention or treatment without the patient's consent. This exception overrides individual patient autonomy in specific circumstances to protect important public health interests.

The final exception to informed consent is the concept of therapeutic privilege, which allows the health care provider to let considerations about the physical, mental, and emotional state of the patient affect what information is disclosed to the patient. The practitioner should believe that the risk of giving information would pose a serious detriment to the patient. The anticipated harm must result from the disclosure itself and not from the potential influence that the information might have on the patient's choice. The sole justification of concern that the patient might refuse needed therapy is not considered adequate to justify invoking this exception. The therapeutic privilege is extremely controversial and not universally recognized. Thus, the value of therapeutic privilege as an independent exception to informed consent is limited.]

Conclusions

The moral and legal doctrine of informed consent and its counterpart, the refusal of treatment, are products of the last half of the 20th century. During this time, judges sought to protect patient autonomy, that is, the patient's right to self-determination. Informed consent requires the health care practitioner to provide the patient with an adequate disclosure and explanation of the treatment and the various options and consequences.

Informed consent, however, is more than a legal necessity. When conducted properly, the process of communicating appropriate information to patients about treatment alternatives can help establish a reciprocal relationship between health care provider and patient that is based on good and appropriate communication, considered advice, mutual respect, and rational choices. The therapeutic objective of informed consent should be to replace some of the patient's anxiety and unease with a sense of participation as a partner in decision-making. Such a sense of participation strengthens the therapeutic alliance between provider and patient. After initial consent to treatment has occurred, a continuing dialogue between patient and practitioner, based on the patient's continuing medical needs, reinforces the original consent. In the event of an unfavorable outcome, the enhanced relationship will prove crucial to maintaining the patient's trust.

In the area of informed consent, as in every other area of risk management, the best recommendation is to practice good medicine. Informed consent is an essential part of good medical practice today and is an ethical and moral responsibility of all health care providers.

References

American Academy of Physician Assistants: Guidelines for Ethical Conduct for the Physician Assistant Profession. American Academy of Physician Assistants. Alexandria, Va, 2000.

Applebaum PS, Lidz CW, Meisel A: Informed Consent: Legal Theory and Clinical Practice. New York, Oxford University Press, 1987.

Buchanan AE, Brock DW: Deciding for Others: The Ethics of Surrogate Decision Making. Cambridge, England, Cambridge University Press, 1989.

Jimison HB, Sher PP, Appleyard R, LeVernois Y: The use of multimedia in the informed consent process, J Am Med Inform Assoc 5:245–254, 1998.

Moskop JC: Informed consent in the emergency department. Emerg Clin N Am 17:327–340, 1999.

Nora LM, Benvenuti RJ: Medicolegal aspects of informed consent. Neurol Clin N Am 16:207–215, 1998.

Bibliography

- Edge RS, Groves JR: Ethics of Health Care: A Guide for Clinical Practice. New York, Delmar Publishers, 1999.
- Gorney M, Martello J, Hart L: The Medical Record: Informing your patients before they consent. Clin Plast Surg 26:57–68, 1999.
- Jonsen AR, Siegler M, Winslade WJ: Clinical Ethics, 4th ed. New York, McGraw-Hill, 1998.
- Moy JG: Informed consent. In Pfenninger JL, Fowler GC (eds): Procedures for Primary Care Physicians. St. Louis, Mosby-Year Book, 1994.
- Taylor HA: Barriers to informed consent. Semin Oncol Nurs 15:89–95, 1999.

Chapter 2

Standard Precautions

▷ Kirsten Thomsen

Procedure Goals and Objectives

Goal: To use and understand the importance of standard precautions when interacting with a patient.

Objectives: The student will be able to . . .

▶ Describe the indications, contraindications, and rationale for adhering to standard precautions.

▶ Identify and describe common problems associated with adhering to standard precautions.

▶ Describe the essential infectious disease principles associated with standard precautions.

▶ Identify the materials necessary for adhering to standard precautions and their proper use.

Background and History

The concept of isolating patients with infectious diseases in separate facilities, which became known as infectious disease hospitals, was introduced in a published hospital handbook as early as 1877. Although infected and noninfected patients were separated, nosocomial transmission continued, largely because of the lack of or minimal aseptic procedures, coupled with the fact that infected patients were not separated from each other by disease. By 1890 to 1900, nursing textbooks discussed recommendations for practicing aseptic procedures and designating separate floors or wards for patients with similar diseases, thereby beginning to solve the problems of nosocomial transmission (Lynch, 1949).

Shortly thereafter, the cubicle system of isolation changed U.S. hospital isolation procedures as patients were placed in multiple-bed wards. "Barrier nursing" practices, consisting of the use of aseptic solutions, handwashing between patient contacts, disinfecting patient-contaminated objects, and separate gown use, were developed to decrease pathogenic organism transmission to other patients and personnel. These practices were used in U.S. infectious disease hospitals. By the 1960s, the designation of specifically designed single or multiple patient isolation rooms in general hospitals and outpatient treatment for tuberculosis caused these specialized hospitals (which since the 1950s had housed tuberculosis patients almost exclusively) to close (Garner, 1996).

The lack of consistent infectious patient isolation policies and procedures noted by the Centers for Disease Control (CDC) investigators in the 1960s led to the CDC publication in 1970 of a detailed isolation precautions manual entitled *"Isolation Techniques for Use in Hospitals,"* designed to assist large metropolitan medical centers as well as small hospitals with limited budgets.

After revision in 1983, the manual was renamed the *"CDC Guidelines for Isolation Precautions in Hospitals."* These new guidelines encouraged hospital infection control decision making with respect to developing isolation systems specific to the hospital environment and circumstances or choosing to select between category-specific or disease-specific isolation precautions. Decisions regarding individual patient precautions were to be based on factors such as patient age, mental status, or possible need to prevent sharing of contaminated articles and were to be determined by the individual who placed the patient on isolation status. Decisions regarding the need for decreasing exposure to infected material by wearing masks, gloves, or gown were to be left to the patient caregiver (Garner, 1984; Haley et al, 1985).

Issues of overisolation of some patients surfaced using the 1983 categories of isolation, which included strict isolation, contact isolation, respiratory isolation, tuberculosis (acid-fast bacilli) isolation, enteric precautions, drainage-secretion precautions, and blood and body fluid precautions. In using the disease-specific isolation precautions, the issue of mistakes in applying the precautions arose if the patient carried a disease not often seen or treated in the hospital (Garner, 1984; Haley et al, 1985), if the diagnosis was delayed, or if a misdiagnosis occurred. This happened even if additional training of personnel was encouraged. These factors, coupled with increased knowledge of epidemiologic patterns of disease, led to subsequent updates of portions of the CDC reports:

- Recommendations for the management of patients with suspected hemorrhagic fever published in 1988 (Centers for Disease Control and Prevention, 1988)
- Recommendations for respiratory isolation for human parvovirus B19 infection specific to patients who were immunodeficient and had chronic human parvovirus B19 infection or were in transient aplastic crisis (Centers for Disease Control and Prevention, 1989)
- Recommendations for the management of tuberculosis, which stemmed from increasing concern for multidrug-resistant tuberculosis, especially in human immunodeficiency virus (HIV)-infected patients in care facilities (Centers for Disease Control and Prevention, 1990)
- Recommendations for hantavirus infection risk reduction (Centers for Disease Control, 1994)
- Expansion of recommendations for the prevention and control of hepatitis C virus (HCV) infection and hepatitis C virus–related chronic disease (Centers for Disease Control and Prevention, 1998)

Body Substance Isolation

An entirely different approach to isolation, called *body substance isolation* (BSI), was developed in 1984 by Lynch and colleagues (1987, 1990) and required personnel, regardless of patient infection status, to apply clean gloves immediately before all patient contact with mucous membranes or nonintact skin, and to wear gloves if a likelihood existed of contact with any moist body substances. An apron or other barrier was also to be worn to keep the provider's own clothing and skin clean. When barriers, such as masks, could not prevent transmission by airborne routes (e.g., rubella, chickenpox), it was recommended that personnel be immunized if proof of immunity could not be documented. Additionally, when immunity was not possible, as with pulmonary tuberculosis, masks were to be worn with during all patient contact. Goggles or glasses, hair covers, and shoe covers were also used as barriers. Careful handling of all used sharps, recapping of needles without using the hands, and the disposal of used items in rigid puncture-resistant containers were stressed. Trash and soiled linen from all patients were bagged and handled in the same manner. This approach sought to protect the patient from contracting nosocomial infections and the provider from bacterial or viral pathogens that might originate with the patient.

Universal Precautions

In response to increasing concerns by health care workers and others about occupational exposure and the risk of transmission of human immunodeficiency virus, hepatitis B virus (HBV), and other blood-borne pathogens during provision of health care and first aid, the CDC, in 1987, defined a set of precautions that considered blood and certain body fluids from all patients to be potential sources of infection for human immunodeficiency virus, HBV, and other blood-borne pathogens. These recommendations became known as universal precautions (UP) and have subsequently been integrated into the *Recommendations for Isolation Precautions in Hospitals, 1996,* which includes the current Standard Precautions (SP) (Table 2–1).

Table 2–1

Recommendations for Isolation Precautions in Hospitals, Hospital Infection Control Practices Advisory Committee, 1996

Standard Precautions

Use Standard Precautions, or the equivalent, for the care of all patients.

Handwashing

Wash hands after touching blood, body fluids, secretions, excretions, and contaminated items, whether or not gloves are worn. Wash hands immediately after gloves are removed, between patient contacts, and when otherwise indicated to avoid transfer of microorganisms to other patients or environments. It may be necessary to wash hands between tasks and procedures on the same patient to prevent cross-contamination of different body sites.

Use a plain (nonantimicrobial) soap for routine handwashing.

Use an antimicrobial agent or a waterless antiseptic agent for specific circumstances (e.g., control of outbreaks or hyperendemic infections), as defined by the infection control program. (See Contact Precautions for additional recommendations on using antimicrobial and antiseptic agents.)

Gloves

Wear gloves (clean, nonsterile gloves are adequate) when touching blood, body fluids, secretions, excretions, and contaminated items. Put on clean gloves just before touching mucous membranes and nonintact skin. Change gloves between tasks and procedures on the same patient after contact with material that may contain a high concentration of microorganisms. Remove gloves promptly after use, before touching noncontaminated items and environmental surfaces, and before going to another patient, and wash hands immediately to avoid transfer of microorganisms to other patients or environments.

Mask, Eye Protection, Face Shield

Wear a mask and eye protection or a face shield to protect mucous membranes of the eyes, nose, and mouth during procedures and patient care activities that are likely to generate splashes or sprays of blood, body fluids, secretions, and excretions.

Gown

Wear a gown (a clean, nonsterile gown is adequate) to protect skin and to prevent soiling of clothing during procedures and patient care activities that are likely to generate splashes or sprays of blood, body fluids, secretions, or excretions. Select a gown that is appropriate for the activity and amount of fluid likely to be encountered. Remove a soiled gown as promptly as possible, and wash hands to avoid transfer of microorganisms to other patients or environments.

■ Table 2–1 (*Continued*)

Patient Care Equipment

Handle used patient care equipment soiled with blood, body fluids, secretions, and excretions in a manner that prevents skin and mucous membrane exposures, contamination of clothing, and transfer of microorganisms to other patients and environments. Ensure that reusable equipment is not used for the care of another patient until it has been cleaned and reprocessed appropriately. Ensure that single-use items are discarded properly.

Environmental Control

Ensure that the hospital has adequate procedures for the routine care, cleaning, and disinfection of environmental surfaces, beds, bed rails, bedside equipment, and other frequently touched surfaces and ensure that these procedures are being followed.

Linen

Handle, transport, and process used linen soiled with blood, body fluids, secretions, and excretions in a manner that prevents skin and mucous membrane exposures and contamination of clothing, and that avoids transfer of microorganisms to other patients and environments.

Occupational Health and Bloodborne Pathogens

Take care to prevent injuries when using needles, scalpels, and other sharp instruments or devices; when handling sharp instruments after procedures; when cleaning used instruments; and when disposing of used needles. Never recap used needles, or otherwise manipulate them using both hands, or use any other technique that involves directing the point of a needle toward any part of the body; rather, use either a one-handed "scoop" technique or a mechanical device designed for holding the needle sheath. Do not remove used needles from disposable syringes by hand, and do not bend, break, or otherwise manipulate used needles by hand. Place used disposable syringes and needles, scalpel blades, and other sharp items in appropriate puncture-resistant containers, which are located as close as practical to the area in which the items were used, and place reusable syringes and needles in a puncture-resistant container for transport to the reprocessing area.

Use mouthpieces, resuscitation bags, or other ventilation devices as an alternative to mouth-to-mouth resuscitation methods in areas where the need for resuscitation is predictable.

Patient Placement

Place a patient who contaminates the environment or who does not (or cannot be expected to) assist in maintaining appropriate hygiene or environmental control in a private room. If a private room is not available, consult with infection control professionals regarding patient placement or other alternatives.

Airborne Precautions

In addition to Standard Precautions, use Airborne Precautions, or the equivalent, for patients known or suspected to be infected with microorganisms transmitted by airborne droplet nuclei (small-particle residue [5 μm or smaller in size] of evaporated droplets containing microorganisms that remain suspended in the air and that can be dispersed widely by air currents within a room or over a long distance).

Patient Placement

Place the patient in a private room that has (1) monitored negative air pressure in relation to the surrounding area, (2) 6 to 12 air changes per hour, and (3) appropriate discharge of air outdoors or monitored high-efficiency filtration of room air before the air is circulated to other areas in the hospital. Keep the room door closed and the patient in the room. When a private room is not available, place the patient in a room with a patient who has active infection with the same microorganism, unless otherwise recommended, but with no other infection. When a private room is not available and cohorting is not desirable, consultation with infection control professionals is advised before patient placement.

Respiratory Protection

Wear respiratory protection when entering the room of a patient with known or suspected infectious pulmonary tuberculosis. Susceptible persons should not enter the room of patients known or suspected to have measles (rubeola) or varicella (chickenpox) if other, immune caregivers are available. If susceptible persons must enter the room of a patient known or suspected to have measles (rubeola) or varicella, they should wear respiratory protection. Persons immune to measles (rubeola) or varicella need not wear respiratory protection.

Table 2-1 (Continued)

Patient Transport

Limit the movement and transport of the patient from the room to essential purposes only. If transport or movement is necessary, minimize patient dispersal of droplet nuclei by placing a surgical mask on the patient, if possible.

Additional Precautions for Preventing Transmission of Tuberculosis

Consult CDC "*Guidelines for Preventing the Transmission of Tuberculosis in Health Care Transmission of Facilities*" for additional prevention strategies.

Droplet Precautions

In addition to Standard Precautions, use Droplet Precautions, or the equivalent, for a patient known or suspected to be infected with microorganisms transmitted by droplets (large-particle droplets [larger than 5 μm in size] that can be generated by the patient during coughing, sneezing, talking, or the performance of procedures).

Patient Placement

Place the patient in a private room. When a private room is not available, place the patient in a room with a patient(s) who has active infection with the same microorganism but with no other infection (cohorting). When a private room is not available and cohorting is not achievable, maintain spatial separation of at least 3 feet between the infected patient and other patients and visitors. Special air handling and ventilation are not necessary, and the door may remain open.

Mask

In addition to standard precautions, wear a mask when working within 3 feet of the patient. (Logistically, some hospitals may want to implement the wearing of a mask to enter the room.)

Patient Transport

Limit the movement and transport of the patient from the room to essential purposes only. If transport or movement is necessary, minimize patient dispersal of droplets by masking the patient, if possible.

Contact Precautions

In addition to Standard Precautions, use Contact Precautions, or the equivalent, for specified patients known or suspected to be infected or colonized with epidemiologically important microorganisms that can be transmitted by direct contact with the patient (hand or skin-to-skin contact that occurs when performing patient care activities that require touching the patient's dry skin) or indirect contact (touching) with environmental surfaces or patient care items in the patient's environment.

Patient Placement

Place the patient in a private room. When a private room is not available, place the patient in a room with a patient(s) who has active infection with the same microorganism but with no other infection (cohorting). When a private room is not available and cohorting is not achievable, consider the epidemiology of the microorganism and the patient population when determining patient placement. Consultation with infection control professionals is advised before patient placement.

Gloves and Handwashing

In addition to wearing gloves as outlined under Standard Precautions, wear gloves (clean, nonsterile gloves are adequate) when entering the room. During the course of providing care for a patient, change gloves after having contact with infective material that may contain high concentrations of microorganisms (fecal material and wound drainage). Remove gloves before leaving the patient's environment and wash hands immediately with an antimicrobial agent or a waterless antiseptic agent. After glove removal and handwashing, ensure that hands do not touch potentially contaminated environmental surfaces or items in the patient's room to avoid transfer of microorganisms to other patients or environments.

Table 2–1 (*Continued*)

Gown

In addition to wearing a gown as outlined under Standard Precautions, wear a gown (a clean, nonsterile gown is adequate) when entering the room if you anticipate that your clothing will have substantial contact with the patient, environmental surfaces, or items in the patient's room, or if the patient is incontinent or has diarrhea, an ileostomy, a colostomy, or wound drainage not contained by a dressing. Remove the gown before leaving the patient's environment. After gown removal, ensure that clothing does not contact potentially contaminated environmental surfaces to avoid transfer of microorganisms to other patients or environments.

Patient Transport

Limit the movement and transport of the patient from the room to essential purposes only. If the patient is transported out of the room, ensure that precautions are maintained to minimize the risk of transmission of microorganisms to other patients and contamination of environmental surfaces or equipment.

Patient Care Equipment

When possible, dedicate the use of noncritical patient care equipment to a single patient (or cohort of patients infected or colonized with the pathogen requiring precautions) to avoid sharing between patients. If use of common equipment or items is unavoidable, adequately clean and disinfect them before use for another patient.

Additional Precautions for Preventing the Spread of Vancomycin Resistance

Consult the HICPAC report on preventing the spread of vancomycin resistance for additional prevention strategies.

HICPAC, Hospital Infection Control Practices Advisory Committee.
From Centers for Disease Control and Prevention: Recommendations for Isolation Precautions in Hospitals, 1996. Available at *www.cdc.gov/ncidod/hip/isolat/isopart1.htm* and *www.cdc.gov./ncidod/hip/isolat/isopart2.htm.*

Standard Precautions

Although universal precautions were designed to address the transmission of bloodborne infections through blood and certain body fluids, they do not address other routes of disease transmission, which were addressed at the time by body substance isolation guidelines. Additionally, confusion developed as to whether one should use universal precautions and body substance isolation guidelines, since both guidelines dealt with similar circumstances but offered conflicting recommendations. The Centers for Disease Control and Prevention (CDC) guideline for isolation precautions in hospitals was revised in 1996 by the CDC and the Hospital Infection Control Practices Advisory Committee (HICPAC), which had been established in 1991 to serve in a guiding and advisory capacity to the Secretary of the Department of Health and Human Services (DHHS), the Assistant Secretary of Health of the DHHS, the Director of the CDC, and the Director of the National Center for Infectious Diseases with respect to hospital infection control practices and U.S. hospital surveillance, prevention, and control strategies for nosocomial infections. The CDC guideline revision was designed to include the following objectives:

(1) to be epidemiologically sound; (2) to recognize the importance of all body fluids, secretions, and excretions in the transmission of

nosocomial pathogens; (3) to contain adequate precautions for infections transmitted by the airborne, droplet, and contact routes of transmission; (4) to be as simple and user friendly as possible; and (5) to use new terms to avoid confusion with existing infection control and isolation systems." (Garner, 1996) The new guidelines were designed to supersede universal precautions and body substance isolation guidelines and in essence combined parts of both these previous guidelines. This synthesis of guidelines allows patients who were previously covered under disease-specific guidelines to now fall under standard precautions, a single set of recommendations. For patients who require additional precautions (defined as *transmission-based precautions,* for use when additional transmission risk exists, e.g., from airborne or droplet contamination), additional guidelines have been developed above and beyond those of standard precautions (Garner, 1996); (see Table 2–1).

Gloving, Gowning, Masking, and Other Protective Barriers as Part of Universal Precautions

All health care workers should routinely use appropriate barrier precautions to prevent skin and mucous membrane exposure during contact with any patient's blood or body fluids that require universal precautions. Gloves should be worn:

• For touching blood and body fluids requiring universal precautions, mucous membranes, or nonintact skin of all patients
• For handling items or surfaces soiled with blood or body fluids to which universal precautions apply

Gloves should be changed after contact with each patient. Hands and other skin surfaces should be washed immediately or as soon as patient safety permits if contaminated with blood or body fluids requiring universal precautions. Hands should be washed immediately after gloves are removed. Gloves should reduce the incidence of blood contamination of hands during phlebotomy, but they cannot prevent penetrating injuries caused by needles or other sharp instruments. Institutions that judge routine gloving for all phlebotomies as not necessary should periodically re-evaluate their policy. Gloves should always be available to health care workers who wish to use them for phlebotomy. In addition, the following general guidelines apply:

• Use gloves for performing phlebotomy when the health care worker has cuts, scratches, or other breaks in the skin.

- Use gloves in situations in which the health care worker judges that hand contamination with blood may occur, for example, when performing phlebotomy in an uncooperative patient.
- Use gloves for performing finger or heel sticks, or both, in infants and children.
- Use gloves when persons are receiving training in phlebotomy.

Masks and protective eyewear or face shields should be worn by health care workers to prevent exposure of mucous membranes of the mouth, nose, and eyes during procedures that are likely to generate droplets of blood or body fluids requiring universal precautions. Gowns or aprons should be worn during procedures that are likely to generate splashes of blood or body fluids requiring universal precautions.

All health care workers should take precautions to prevent injuries caused by needles, scalpels, and other sharp instruments or devices during procedures; when cleaning used instruments; during disposal of used needles; and when handling sharp instruments after procedures. To prevent needlestick injuries, needles should not be recapped by hand, purposely bent or broken by hand, removed from disposable syringes, or otherwise manipulated by hand. After they are used, disposable syringes and needles, scalpel blades, and other sharp items should be placed in puncture-resistant containers for disposal. The puncture-resistant containers should be located as close as practical to the area of use. All reusable needles should be placed in puncture-resistant containers for transport to the reprocessing area.

General infection control practices should further minimize the already minute risk for salivary transmission of human immunodeficiency virus. These infection control practices include the use of gloves for digital examination of mucous membranes and endotracheal suctioning, handwashing after exposure to saliva, and minimizing the need for emergency mouth-to-mouth resuscitation by making mouthpieces and other ventilation devices available for use in areas where the need for resuscitation is predictable.

The Application of Standard Precautions in Clinical Procedures

Standard precautions should be followed when performing any procedure in which exposure to, or transmission of, infectious agents is possible. These guidelines attempt to minimize exposure to infectious body fluids. Because it is not always possible to determine in advance whether a specific patient is infectious, these precautions should be followed routinely for all patients. The nature of performing clinical procedures often results in exposure to body fluids. Consequently, as practitioners involved in performing clinical procedures, it is imperative that we attempt to anticipate potential exposures and implement preventive guidelines to reduce exposure risks.

Additionally, it is important that the practitioner assess the health status of each patient to determine if additional precautions are warranted and, if so, apply the necessary transmission-based precautions as described in Table 2–1. Standard precautions are the current recommended behaviors designed to prevent the transmission of pathogens from patient to practitioner or practitioner to patient. It is imperative that all providers be knowledgable about standard precautions and transmission-based precautions and how to practice them competently and consistently.

References

Centers for Disease Control and Prevention: Recomendations for prevention and control of hepatitis C virus (HCV) infection and HCV-related chronic disease. MMWR Morb Mortal Wkly Rep 47:1–39, 1998.

Centers for Disease Control and Prevention: Laboratory management of agents associated with hantavirus pulmonary syndrome: Interim biosafety guidelines. MMWR Morb Mortal Wkly Rep 43:1–7, 1994.

Centers for Disease Control: Guidelines for preventing the transmission of tuberculosis in health-care settings, with special focus on HIV-related issues. MMWR Morb Mortal Wkly Rep 39:1–29, 1990.

Centers for Disease Control: Risks associated with human parvovirus B19 infection. MMWR Morb Mortal Wkly Rep 38:81–88, 93–97, 1989.

Centers for Disease Control: Management of patients with suspected viral hemorrhagic fever. MMWR Morb Mortal Wkly Rep 37:1–16, 1988.

Centers for Disease Control: Update: Universal precautions for prevention of transmission of human immunodeficiency virus, hepatitis B virus, and other blood borne pathogens in health-care settings. MMWR Morb Mortal Wkly Rep 37:377–388, 1988.

Garner JS: Guideline for isolation precautions in hospitals. Part I. Evolution of isolation practices, Hospital Infection Control Practices Advisory Committee. Am J Infect Control 24:24–31, 1996.

Garner JS: Comments on CDC guideline for isolation precautions in hospitals, 1984. Am J Infect Control 12:163–164, 1984.

Haley RW, Garner JS, Simmons BP: A new approach to the isolation of patients with infectious diseases: Alternative systems. J Hosp Infect 6:128–139, 1985.

Lynch P, Cummings MJ, Roberts PL: Implementing and evaluating a system of generic infection precautions: Body substance isolation. Am J Infect Control 18:1–12, 1990.

Lynch P, Jackson MM: Rethinking the role of isolation precautions in the prevention of nosocomial infections. Ann Intern Med 107:243–246, 1987.

Lynch T: Communicable Disease Nursing. St. Louis, CV Mosby, 1949.

Bibliography

• American College of Physicians Task Force on Adult Immunization and Infectious Diseases Society of America: Guide for Adult Immunization, 3rd ed. Philadelphia, American College of Physicians, 1994.

- Bell DM, Shapiro CN, Ciesielski CA, Chamberland ME: Preventing blood borne pathogen transmission from health care workers to patients: The CDC perspective. Surg Clin North Am 75:1189–1203, 1995.
- Cardo DM, Culver DH, Ciesielski CA, et al: A case-control study of HIV seroconversion in health care workers after percutaneous exposure: Centers for Disease Control and Prevention Needlestick Surveillance Group. N Engl J Med 337:1485–1490, 1997.
- Centers for Disease Control and Prevention: Public Health Service (PHS) guidelines for the management of health care worker exposures to HIV and recommendations for postexposure prophylaxis. MMWR Morb Mortal Wkly Rep 47:1–33, 1998.
- Centers for Disease Control and Prevention: Recommendations for follow-up of health-care workers after occupational exposure to hepatitis C virus. MMWR Morb Mortal Wkly Rep 46:603–606, 1997.
- Centers for Disease Control and Prevention: Immunization of health-care workers: Recommendations of the Advisory Committee on Immunization Practices (ACIP) and the Hospital Infection Control Practices Advisory Committee (HICPAC). MMWR Morb Mortal Wkly Rep 46:1–42, 1997.
- Centers for Disease Control and Prevention: Case-control study of HIV seroconversion in health-care workers after percutaneous exposure to HIV infected blood—France, United Kingdom, and United States, January 1988–August 1994. MMWR Morb Mortal Wkly Rep 44:929–933, 1995.
- Centers for Disease Control and Prevention: Hospital Infection Control Practices Advisory Committee: Guideline for prevention of nosocomial pneumonia. Infect Control Hosp Epidemiol 15:587–627, 1994.
- Centers for Disease Control and Prevention: Guidelines for preventing the transmission of *Mycobacterium tuberculosis* in health-care facilities, 1994. MMWR Morb Mortal Wkly Rep 43:1–132, 1994.
- Centers for Disease Control and Prevention: National Institutes for Health: Biosafety in Microbiological and Biomedical Laboratories, 3rd ed. Atlanta, U.S. Department of Health and Human Services, Public Health Service, 1993.
- Centers for Disease Control and Prevention: Update on adult immunization: Recommendations of the Immunization Practices Advisory Committee (ACIP). MMWR Morb Mortal Wkly Rep 40:1–94, 1991.
- Centers for Disease Control and Prevention: Protection against viral hepatitis: Recommendations of the Advisory Committee on Immunization Practices (ACIP). MMWR Morb Mortal Wkly Rep 39:1–27, 1990.
- Centers for Disease Control and Prevention: Update: Universal precautions for prevention of transmission of human immunodeficiency virus, hepatitis B virus, and other blood borne pathogens in health-care settings. MMWR Morb Mortal Wkly Rep 37:377–382, 387–388, 1988.
- Chin J (ed): Control of Communicable Diseases Manual, 17th ed. Washington, D.C., American Public Health Association, 1999.
- Diekema DJ, Alabanese MA, Schuldt SS, Doebbeling BN: Blood and body fluid exposures during clinical training: Relation to knowledge of universal precautions. J Gen Intern Med 11:109–111, 1996.
- Garner JS: Hospital Infection Control Practices Advisory Committee: Guidelines for Isolation Precautions in Hospitals. Infect Control Hosp Epidemiol 17: 53–80, 1996.
- Gerberding JL, Lewis FR Jr, Schecter WP: Are universal precautions realistic? Surg Clin North Am 75:1091–1104, 1995.

- Moran G: Emergency department management of blood and fluid exposures. Ann Emerg Med 35:47–62, 2000.
- National Committee for Clinical Laboratory Standards: Protection of laboratory workers from infectious disease transmitted by blood, body fluids, and tissue: Tentative guideline. NCCLS Document M29-T2, vol 11. Villanova, PA, National Committee for Clinical Laboratory Standards, 1991, pp 1–214.
- Orenstein R, Reynolds L, Karabaic M, et al: Do protective devices prevent needlestick injuries among health care workers? Am J Infect Control 23:344–351, 1995.
- Osborn EHS, Papadakis MA, Gerberding JL: Occupational exposures to body fluids among medical students: A seven-year longitudinal study. Ann Intern Med 130:45–51, 1999.
- Peter G (ed): Report of the Committee on Infectious Diseases Red Book, 25th ed. Elk Grove Village, Ill, American Academy of Pediatrics, 2000.
- U.S. Department of Labor, Occupational Health and Safety Administration: Criteria for recording on OSHA Form 200. OSHA instruction 1993, standard 1904. Washington, D.C., U.S. Department of Labor, 1993.
- U.S. Department of Labor, Occupational Safety and Health Administration: Occupational exposure to blood borne pathogens, final rule. CFR Part 1910.1030. Fed Reg 56:64004–64182, 1991.
- U.S. Department of Labor, Occupational Health and Safety Administration: Record keeping guidelines for occupational injuries and illnesses: The Occupational Safety and Health Act of 1970 and 29 CFR 1904. OMB No. 120-0029. Washington, D.C., U.S. Department of Labor, 1986.

Chapter 3

Sterile Technique

▷ Paul C. Hendrix

Procedure Goals and Objectives

Goal: To provide clinicians with the necessary knowledge and skills to perform clinical procedures using accepted sterile technique.

Objectives: The student will be able to . . .

▶ Describe the indications and rationale for practicing sterile technique.

▶ Identify and describe the history and development of the concept of sterile technique.

▶ List the principles of sterile technique.

▶ Describe the essential steps performed in the surgical hand scrub.

▶ Describe the essential steps performed in preparing and draping a sterile field.

▶ Describe the principles involved in the use of surgical caps, masks, and gowns.

▶ Describe the principles involved in the use of standard precautions.

Background and History

The teachings of Hippocrates (460 BC) were instrumental in turning the art of healing away from mystical rites to an approach that everyone could understand and practice. He stressed cleanliness to avoid infection by using boiling water and fire to clean instruments and by irrigating dirty wounds with wine or boiled water (Adams, 1929). Louis Pasteur (1822–1895) developed what would come to be known as the *germ theory of disease.* His experiments revealed that microbes could be found in the air and on the surface of every object (Dubos, 1950). He discovered that the number of microbes could be reduced on surfaces by using heat or appropriate cleansing but that they would still remain in the air. Joseph Lister (1827–1912) is considered the father of sterile technique (Godlee, 1917). When Lister learned of Pasteur's work, he began to experiment with various methods of sterile technique in surgery. He noted a significant decrease in postoperative infections after using carbolic acid to sterilize both surgical wounds and his own hands and by spraying the operative field. His antiseptic methods of performing surgery were refined over the years and eventually incorporated into hospitals worldwide.

Principles of Sterile Technique

Sterile technique is the method by which contamination with microorganisms is prevented. Adherence to protocol and strict techniques are required at all times when caring for open wounds and performing invasive procedures. To avoid infection, procedures should be performed within a sterile field from which all living microbes have been excluded. Items entering the sterile field, including instruments, sutures, and fluids, must be sterile. Although it is not possible to sterilize the skin, it is possible to reduce significantly the number of bacteria that are normally present on the skin. Before a procedure, personnel must first perform a surgical hand scrub and then don sterile gloves, sterile gown, and mask. The primary goal is to provide an environment for the patient that will promote healing, prevent infections, and minimize the length of recovery time. Using the principles of sterile technique will accomplish that goal. These principles are listed here.

- All items used within a sterile field must be sterile.
- A sterile barrier that has been permeated must be considered contaminated.
- The edges of a sterile container are considered contaminated once the package is opened.
- Gowns are considered sterile in front from shoulder to waist level, and the sleeves are considered sterile to 2 inches above the elbow.

- Tables are sterile at table level only.
- Sterile persons and items touch only sterile areas; unsterile persons and items touch only unsterile areas.
- Movement within or around a sterile field must not contaminate the field.
- All items and areas of doubtful sterility are considered contaminated.

Materials Utilized for Hand Scrub

- Chlorhexidine gluconate or povidone-iodine solutions are rapid-acting, broad-spectrum antimicrobials that are effective against gram-positive and gram-negative microorganisms. Each is prepared in combination with a detergent to give a cleansing action along with the antimicrobial effect.
- Sterile disposable scrub brushes impregnated with chlorhexidine gluconate or povidone-iodine.

Procedure for the Surgical Scrub—Timed (Anatomic) Method

Note: Two methods of surgical scrubbing are typically used: the *timed method* (Fig. 3–1), which is described here, and the *counted stroke method.* Both methods follow a prescribed anatomic pattern of scrubbing beginning with the fingernails, four surfaces of each finger, the palmar and dorsal surfaces of the hands and wrists, and extending up the arms to the elbows. The timed method requires a total of 5 minutes of scrub time. The counted stroke method requires a specific number of bristle strokes for the fingers, hands, and arms. The scrub includes 30 strokes for the fingernails and 20 strokes to each surface of the fingers, hands, wrists, and arms to the elbows.

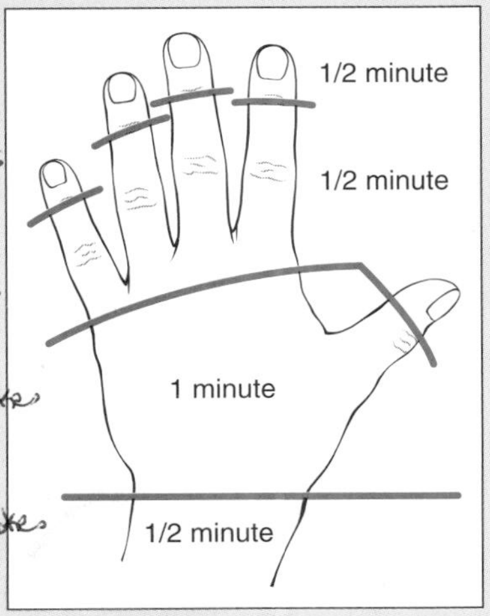

1. Organize supplies and adjust water to a comfortable temperature.
2. Wet hands and arms, prewash with soap from a dispenser, rinse.
3. Remove scrub brush from package and use nail cleaner to clean fingernails.

Figure 3–1

Procedure for the Surgical Scrub — Timed (Anatomic) Method – *(continued)*

4. Squeeze scrub brush under water to release soap from sponge.

back/forth

5. With scrub brush perpendicular to fingers, begin to scrub all four sides of each finger with a back-and-forth motion.

Circular

6. Scrub dorsal and palmar surfaces of hand and wrist with a circular motion.

7. Starting at the wrist, scrub all four sides of the arm to the elbow.

8. Transfer scrub brush to the other hand and repeat steps 5 to 7.

9. Discard scrub brush and rinse hands and arms, starting with the fingertips and working toward the elbows.

10. Allow contaminated water to drip off the elbows by keeping hands above the waist.

DO NOT DIP H₂O off finger tips

Materials Utilized to Prepare the Procedure Site

Note: Preparation trays are commercially available and typically include the listed necessary items.

- Disposable razors to remove hair from the procedure site
- Towels
- Antiseptic soap: There are multiple antiseptic skin scrubs available. The most commonly used are iodine-based soaps and solutions.
- Gauze sponges
- Large clamp or ring forceps to hold the preparation sponge or gauze

Procedure for Preparing the Operative Site

1. Scrub the skin with the antiseptic solution, beginning at the procedure site and working outward in a circular fashion toward the periphery of the field (Fig. 3–2). Make sure the area prepared is much wider than the procedure site.
Note: The scrubbing action must be vigorous, including both mechanical and chemical cleansing of the skin.

2. On reaching the outer boundary, discard the first sponge and repeat the procedure until all prepared sponges are used.
Caution: Do not return to a previously prepared area with a contaminated sponge.

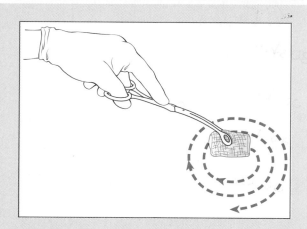

Figure 3–2

Materials Utilized for Draping a Patient and the Procedure Site

Note: Draping the procedure site and the patient follows preparing the skin.

- Drapes: typically green, blue, or gray to reduce glare and eye fatigue.
- Types of drapes: towels, sheets, split sheets, fenestrated sheets, stockinette, and plastic incision drapes.

Note: Each type of drape has a specific use, for example, fenestrated sheets have a window that exposes the procedure site, and stockinette is used to cover the extremities circumferentially. Drapes must be lint-free, antistatic, fluid-resistant, abrasive-free, and made to fit contours.

Procedure for Draping

Note: Draping is the process of maintaining a sterile field around the procedure site by covering the surrounding areas and the patient with a barrier.

1. Hold the drapes high enough to avoid touching nonsterile areas.
2. Always walk around the table to drape the opposite side.

Caution: Never reach over the patient.

3. Handle drapes as little as possible and avoid shaking out wrinkles (contaminants are present in the air).
4. When draping, make a cuff over the gloved hand to protect against touching an unsterile area, and place the folded edge toward the incision to provide a uniform outline of the surgical site and to prevent instruments or sponges from falling between layers.

Note: Any part of the drape below waist or table level is considered nonsterile. Towel clips fastened through the drapes have contaminated points and should be removed only if necessary.

5. If a hole is found in a drape after it is placed, cover it with a second drape.
6. Drapes should not be adjusted after placement. If a drape is placed improperly, either discard it or cover it with another drape.

Procedure for Maintaining a Sterile Field

Note: The sterile field includes the draped patient and any scrubbed personnel.

1. Someone outside the sterile field must hand items needed during the procedure into the sterile field. This is the reason a minimum of two individuals is required to do most procedures—one with nonsterile hands to pass instruments and supplies into the sterile field, and one with gloved hands working within the sterile field.

Procedure for Maintaining a Sterile Field – *(continued)*

Note: Sterile supplies are uniformly packaged in such a way to allow an unsterile person to open and pass them safely, without contamination, into the sterile field.

2. Contamination of supplies or personnel within the sterile field must be addressed immediately. This includes changing gowns or gloves and removing from the sterile field any instrument or supplies that have become contaminated.

3. Unsterile personnel must avoid contact with the sterile field by remaining at a safe distance (at least 12 inches away) and by always facing the field when passing to avoid accidental contact.

4. Every individual involved with the procedure must immediately call attention to any observed breaks, or suspected breaks, in sterile technique.

5. If the sterility of any item is in doubt, it must be considered contaminated, removed from the sterile field, and replaced with a sterile item.

Caution: **There is no compromise with sterility. An item is either sterile or unsterile.**

Procedure for Wearing Surgical Masks, Caps, and Gowns

Note: Because of the large numbers of potentially harmful microbes that reside in the respiratory tract, surgical masks are recommended at all times when there are open sterile items or sterile instruments present.

1. Fit the mask snugly over both the nose and the mouth and tie securely (Fig. 3–3).
2. When wearing a mask, it is advisable to keep conversation to a minimum to prevent moisture buildup.
3. Change surgical masks routinely between procedures or during a procedure if they become moist or wet.

Note: Surgical caps prevent nonsterile material from the hair entering the sterile field. The standard unisex surgical cap is adequate for women and men with short hair, but long hair requires a more voluminous cap. Both caps and masks are generally made of paper and are disposable.

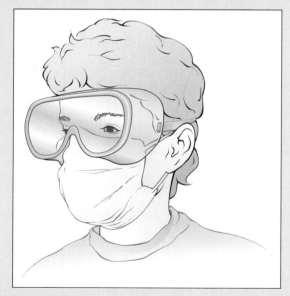

Figure 3–3

Note: For lengthy procedures, or when it is necessary to put the forearms into the sterile field, a sterile surgical gown is required (Figs. 3–4 and 3–5). Procedures for which gloves are sufficient include joint aspiration, suturing a minor laceration, and performing a lumbar puncture. A gown is required for repairing a large

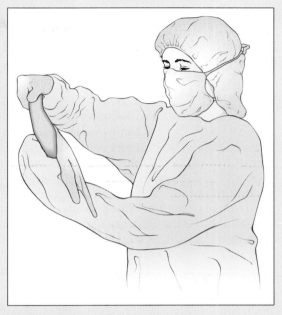

Figure 3–5

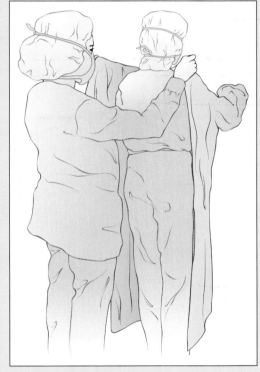

Figure 3–4

wound, for cardiac catheterization, or for any procedure that requires it by protocol. Only the front of the gown above the waist level and the lower portion of the sleeves are considered sterile. Even though the entire gown is sterile initially, it is easy to brush against a nonsterile object with the back, sides, or lower portion of the gown.

Special Considerations

Standard Precautions

In 1987, the Centers for Disease Control and Prevention (CDC) developed universal precautions, later incorporated into standard precautions, which were designed to protect health care personnel from unknown exposures from the patient and environment. The CDC stated:

Since medical history and examination cannot identify all patients who are potentially infected with bloodborne pathogens, specific precautions should be used with all patients, thereby reducing the risk of possible exposure to its minimum. (CDC, 1987)

Therefore, all procedures and patients should be considered potentially contaminated, and strict protocols should be followed to prevent exposure to blood and body fluids. The CDC advised that health care workers could reduce the risk of exposure and contamination by adhering to the following guidelines:

1. Use appropriate barrier protection to prevent skin and mucous membrane exposure when contact with blood and body fluids of any patient is anticipated. Gloves, masks, and protective eyewear or face shields should be worn during all surgical procedures and when handling soiled supplies or instruments during or after a procedure to prevent exposure of mucous membranes.
2. Wash hands and other skin surfaces immediately and thoroughly if contaminated with blood or other body fluids. Although both sterile and nonsterile personnel wear gloves during a surgical procedure, handwashing after the removal of gloves should become a routine practice for all personnel working in a procedure room.
3. Take all necessary precautions to protect against injuries caused by needles, scalpels, and other sharp instruments or devices during procedures; when cleaning used instruments; and when handling sharp instruments after a procedure. Needles should never be recapped or bent after use. Suture needles and sharps should be contained in a puncture-resistant container and sealed for proper disposal according to recommended practices and established protocols. Sharp instruments should be placed in a tray in such a way that their points are not exposed so that injury to persons working with the trays is avoided. During the procedure, care must be taken when handling suture needles to ensure that no one receives an injury by placing the needle on a needle holder and passing it with the point down.
4. Health care workers who have exudative lesions or weeping dermatis should refrain from all direct patient care and from handling patient care equipment until the condition resolves. Individuals with minor breaks in the skin should restrict scrubbing activities until the break has healed. Sterile gloves should be worn if a skin lesion is present, and the lesion covered when working in a procedure room.

The Occupational Safety and Health Administration (OSHA) has adopted these guidelines in its efforts to maintain a safe working environment. In addition, both OSHA and the CDC recommend that aspirated or drainage material never come into contact with health care providers. Thus, the use of an adequate suctioning system is important during procedures, with careful disposal protocols after the procedure is completed. For more information on standard precautions, see Chapter 2.

Disposal of Materials

1. Care should be taken to dispose of contaminated supplies and materials to avoid the transmission of infectious organisms to others.
2. Sharp objects should be disposed in appropriately marked containers.
3. Body fluids, human tissue, disposable gowns, gloves, caps, and drapes should be placed in containers marked with the appropriate biohazard warnings.
4. All receptacles containing biohazardous waste should be properly labeled and identified and processed according to institutional procedures.

References

Adams F: The Genuine Works of Hippocrates. New York, W. Wood, 1929.
Centers for Disease Control: Recommendations for prevention of HIV transmission in health-care settings. MMWR 36 (suppl. 2), 1987.
Dubos R: Louis Pasteur: Free Lance of Science. Boston, Little, Brown, 1950.
Godlee RJ: Lord Lister. London, Macmillan, 1917.

Chapter 4

Blood Pressure Measurement

▷ Randy Danielsen

Procedure Goals and Objectives

Goal: To measure accurately the systemic arterial blood pressure in any patient in any setting.

Objectives: The student will be able to . . .

▶ Describe the indications, contraindications, and rationale for performing arterial blood pressure measurement.

▶ Describe the essential anatomy and physiology associated with the performance of blood pressure measurement.

▶ Identify the necessary materials and their proper use for performing blood pressure measurement.

▶ Identify the proper steps and techniques for performing blood pressure measurement.

▶ Identify the indications for performing orthostatic blood pressure assessment.

▶ Identify the proper steps and techniques for performing orthostatic blood pressure measurement.

Background and History

Various theories about circulation and blood pressure emerged about 400 BC. Hippocrates knew about arteries and veins, but he believed veins carried air. Six hundred years later, Galen demonstrated that arteries and veins both carried blood; however, he also thought that the heart was a warming machine for two separate types of blood. He was convinced that veins and arteries were not connected and that blood flowed both backward and forward from the heart. Subsequently Galen's teachings remained unchallenged for more than 1000 years (Stevens, 1978).

It was William Harvey, in 1616, who actually disagreed with Galen by demonstrating one-way circulation of blood and theorized the existence of capillaries. Thirty years later, Marcello Malpighi was the first to view capillaries microscopically (Stevens, 1978).

The first person known to measure blood pressure was Steven Hales in 1733. A British scientist, clergyman, and amateur scientist, Hales inserted a brass pipe into the carotid artery of a mare and then attached the pipe to a windpipe taken from a goose. This flexible goose windpipe was then attached to a 12-foot glass tube. Although the experiment had little practical application at the time, it did provide valuable information about blood pressure (Wain, 1970).

Although Ritter von Basch experimented with a device that could measure the blood pressure of a human without breaking the skin, the prototype design of the sphygmomanometer was devised in 1896 by Scipione Riva-Rocci through diagnostic monitoring of the pulse (Lyons et al, 1987). He introduced a method for indirect measurement of blood pressure based on measuring the external pressure required to compress the brachial artery so that arterial pulsations could no longer be transmitted through the artery. The Riva-Rocci sphygmomanometer was described by Porter as

> an inflatable band that was wrapped around the upper arm; air was pumped in until the pulse disappeared; it then was released from the band until the pulse reappeared, and the reading was taken. (Porter, 1997)

In 1905, a Russian physician named Korotkoff first discovered the auscultatory sounds that are heard while measuring the blood pressure. While the artery is occluded during blood pressure measurement, transmitted pulse waves can no longer be heard distal to the point of occlusion. As the pressure in the bladder is reduced by opening a valve on the inflation bulb, pulsatile blood flow reappears through the generally compressed artery, producing repetitive sounds generated by the pulsatile flow. The sounds, named after Korotkoff, change in quality and intensity. The five phases of these changes are characterized in Table 4–1. Around the turn of the 20th century, blood pressure management became an accepted clinical measurement. As data increased, physicians and other clinicians were able to establish normal blood pressure ranges and identify abnormalities.

■ Table 4–1

Korotkoff Sounds*

Phase	
I	First appearance of clear, repetitive, tapping sounds; this coincides approximately with the reappearance of a palpable pulse
II	Sounds are softer and longer, with the quality of an intermittent murmur
III	Sounds again become crisper and louder
IV	Sounds are muffled, less distinct, and softer
V	Sounds disappear completely

* As the pressure is reduced during deflation of the occluding cuff, the Korotkoff sounds change in quality and intensity.
From Perloff D, Grimm C, Flack J, et al: Human blood pressure determination by sphygmomanometry. Circulation 88:2461, 1993.

Rene Laennec is credited with the invention of the stethoscope in 1816, which became a convenience for physicians who preferred not to place their ears directly on the chest wall of a patient. As already noted, in 1905, Korotkoff tried using the stethoscope to monitor the pulse while the sphygmomanometer was inflated. He discovered a more accurate blood pressure reading, plus the fact that the pulse disappeared as the cuff pressure decreased at a point in consonance with the expanding of the heart. Subsequently, the term *Korotkoff sounds* came to be used (Lyons et al, 1987).

For the accurate indirect measurement of blood pressure, the American Heart Association (AHA) recommends that the cuff size be based solely on the limb circumference (Manning, 1983). Manning, Kuchirka, and Kaminski studied prevailing cuffing habits and compared them with newly revised American Heart Association guidelines and reported their findings in *Circulation* in 1983. They found that "miscuffing" occurred in 2% of 200 blood pressure determinations in 167 unselected adult outpatients, including 72% of 85 readings taken on "nonstandard" size arms. Undercuffing large arms was the most frequent error, accounting for 84% of the miscuffings. They concluded that undercuffing elevates the blood pressure readings by an average of 8.5 mm Hg systolic and 4.6 mm Hg diastolic. It is critical, therefore, that the clinician choose the appropriate size cuff based on the circumference of a patient's bare upper arm. The bladder (inside the cuff) length should encircle 80% and the width should cover 33% to 50% of an adult's upper arm. For a child younger than age 13, the bladder should encircle 100% of the child's upper arm. A cuff that is too narrow or too large for an arm may result in an incorrect blood pressure reading. The clinician should have a full range of cuff sizes to accommodate the patient population. Cuffs that are generally available have usually been classified by the width of the bladder rather than by the length and are labeled *newborn, infant, child, small adult, adult, large adult,* and *thigh.*

More information regarding blood pressure measurements may be found in the American Heart Association's "*Recommendations for Human*

Blood Pressure Determination by Sphygmomanometers" (1994) and the American Society of Hypertension's *"Recommendations for Routine Blood Pressure Measurement by Indirect Cuff Sphygmomanometry"* (1992).

Every clinician who takes indirect blood pressure measurements should be carefully trained and should practice on a regular basis. The reading that is taken is an important tool in diagnosis, which is why it is considered one of the "vital signs."

Indications

As one of the vital signs, peripheral measurement of the blood pressure is an indirect method of determining cardiovascular function.

- Its use is indicated for evaluation of both healthy and ill patients to help assess cardiac status.
- Blood pressure measurement is a part of every complete physical or screening examination and is performed to screen for hypertension.

Contraindications

There are no absolute contraindications to measuring blood pressure. Relative contraindications include physical defects and therapeutic interventions such as indwelling intravenous catheters and renal dialysis shunts.

Potential Complications

- Complications from measurement of blood pressure may occur as a result of improper training of the individual performing the assessment.
- Overinflation or prolonged time of inflation may lead to tissue or vascular damage at the measurement site.
- Lack of proper care of or flawed equipment may give an inaccurate reading.

Review of Essential Anatomy and Physiology

In most clinical settings, blood pressure is measured by the indirect technique of using a sphygmomanometer placed over the brachial artery of the upper extremity. The brachial artery is a continuation of the axillary artery, which lies medial to the humerus proximally and

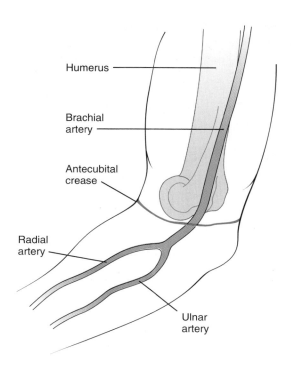

Humerus

Brachial artery

Antecubital crease

Radial artery

Ulnar artery

Figure 4–1. Location of the brachial artery.

gradually courses anterior to the humerus as it nears the antecubital fossa (Fig. 4–1). Placement of the bladder and cuff of the sphygmomanometer circumferentially over the brachial artery allows inflation of the cuff to create adequate pressure so that the artery is fully occluded when the pressure exceeds the systolic pressure within the brachial artery.

Indirect measurement of the blood pressure involves the auscultatory detection of the initial presence and disappearance of changes and the disappearance of Korotkoff sounds, which are audible with the aid of a stethoscope placed over the brachial artery distal to the blood pressure cuff near the antecubital crease. Korotkoff sounds are low-pitched sounds (best heard with the stethoscope bell) that originate from the turbulence created by the partial occlusion of the artery with the inflated blood pressure cuff.

As long as the pressure within the cuff is so little that it does not produce even partial occlusion (or intermittent occlusion), no sound is produced when auscultating over the brachial artery distal to the cuff. When the cuff pressure becomes great enough to occlude the artery during at least some portion of the arterial pressure cycle, a sound becomes audible over the brachial artery distal to the cuff. This sound is audible with a stethoscope and correlates with each arterial pulsation.

There are five phases of Korotkoff sounds used in determining the systolic and diastolic blood pressure (see Table 4–1). Phase I occurs as

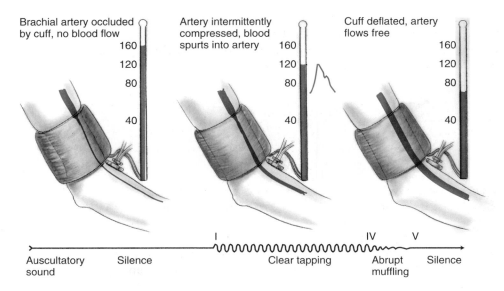

Figure 4–2. Phase 1 of Korotkoff sounds. (From Jarvis C: Physical Examination and Health Assessment, 2nd ed. Philadelphia, WB Saunders, 1996, p 196.)

the occluding pressure of the cuff falls to a point that is the same as the peak systolic pressure within the brachial artery (Fig. 4–2). The tapping sound that is produced is clear and generally increases in intensity as the occluding pressure continues to decrease. Phase II occurs at a point approximately 10 to 15 mm Hg lower than at the onset of phase I, and the sounds become softer and longer with a quality of intermittent murmur. Phase III occurs when the occluding pressure of the cuff falls to a point that allows for large amounts of blood to cross the partially occluded brachial artery. The phase III sounds are again crisper and louder than phase II sounds. Phase IV occurs when there is an abrupt muffling and decrease in the intensity of the sounds. This occurs as the pressure is close to that of the diastolic pressure of the brachial artery. Phase V occurs when the blood vessel is no longer occluded by the pressure in the cuff. At this point, the tapping sound disappears completely.

Patient Preparation

- The environment should be relaxed and peaceful. Blood pressure levels may be affected by emotions, physical activity, or the surroundings. Subsequently, the examiner should minimize any and all disturbances that may affect the reading.

- The patient is asked to be seated or to lie down, making sure that the bare arm is supported and at the level of the heart.
- Ideally, the patient should avoid smoking or ingesting caffeine for 30 minutes before the blood pressure is recorded.

Materials Utilized for Blood Pressure Measurement

- Stethoscope
- Sphygmomanometer (which includes a manometer, mercury or aneroid, with a calibrated scale for measuring pressure; inflatable rubber bladders; tubes; and valves)
- Recording instruments (Fig. 4–3)
- Appropriate size cuff. Note: A cuff that has an antimicrobial agent to help prevent bacterial growth is recommended. It has been reported that blood pressure cuffs can carry significant bacterial colonization and can actually be a source of transmission of infection (Sternlicht, 1990).

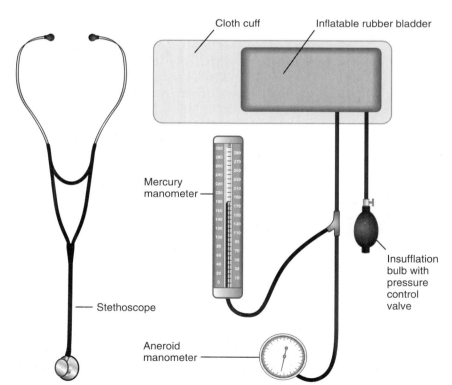

Figure 4–3. Instruments used for recording blood pressure.

Procedure for Indirect Blood Pressure Measurement

1. Check to see that the mercury level of the sphygmomanometer is at 0 or, if an aneroid device is used, that the needle rests within the calibration window.
2. Palpate the brachial artery and place the cuff so that the midline of the bladder is over the arterial pulsation.

Note: Care should be taken that the cuff is placed at approximately the horizontal level of the heart.

3. Wrap and secure the cuff snugly around the patient's bare upper arm. The lower edge of the cuff should be 1 inch (approximately 2 cm) above the antecubital crease, the point at which the bell of the stethoscope is to be placed (Fig. 4–4).

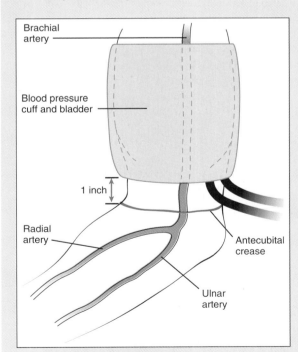

Brachial artery

Blood pressure cuff and bladder

1 inch

Radial artery

Antecubital crease

Ulnar artery

Figure 4–4

Note: Avoid rolling up the sleeve in such a manner that it may form a tight tourniquet around the upper arm.

4. Place the manometer so that the center of the mercury column or aneroid dial is at eye level and clearly visible to the examiner. Make sure that the tubing from the cuff is unobstructed.
5. Inflate the cuff rapidly to 70 mm Hg and increase by increments of 10 mm Hg while palpating the radial pulse. Note the level of pressure at which the pulse disappears and subsequently reappears during deflation.

Note: This procedure, the palpatory method, provides the necessary preliminary approximation of the systolic pressure to ensure an adequate level of inflation when the actual, auscultatory measurement is accomplished. The palpatory method is particularly useful to avoid underinflation of the cuff in patients with an auscultatory gap and overinflation in those with very low blood pressure.

Note: The auscultatory gap occurs at a point between the highest systolic reading and the diastolic reading. The Korotkoff sounds may become absent between the peak systolic measurement and diastole, resulting in underestimation of the peak systolic blood pressure if the cuff is not initially inflated to a high enough pressure.

6. Place the earpieces of the stethoscope into your ear canals, angled forward to fit snugly.
7. Switch the stethoscope head to the bell or low-frequency position.

Procedure for Indirect Blood Pressure Measurement – *(continued)*

8. Place the bell of the stethoscope over the brachial artery pulsation just above and medial to the antecubital fossa but below the lower edge of the cuff (Fig. 4–5). Hold it firmly in place, making sure the bell makes contact with the skin around the entire circumference.

Note: excessive pressure will result in stretching the underlying skin, causing the bell to function as a diaphragm. This may result in the loss of low-frequency sounds.

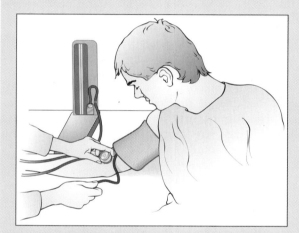

Figure 4–5

9. Inflate the bladder rapidly and steadily to a pressure 20 to 30 mm Hg above the level previously determined by palpation. Partially unscrew the valve and deflate the bladder at 2 mm per second while listening for the appearance of Korotkoff sounds.

10. As the pressure in the bladder falls, note the level of the pressure on the manometer at the first appearance of repetitive sounds, the continuation of the sounds, and when the sounds disappear.

Note: During the period of the Korotkoff sounds (see Table 4–1), the rate of deflation should be less than 2 mm per beat, thereby compensating for both rapid and slow heart rates.

11. Record the systolic and diastolic pressure immediately, rounded off upward to the nearest 2 mm Hg. The name of the patient, the date and time of measurement, the arm or site at which the measurement was taken, the cuff size, and the patient's position while taking the measurement should be noted.

Special Considerations

The Apprehensive Patient or "White Coat" Hypertension

Clinicians should obtain more than one blood pressure measurement from a patient to rule out white coat hypertension. Ambulatory monitoring is the most efficient means for accomplishing this. Unfortunately, many insurance companies do not pay for this type of monitoring. A patient's self-recorded blood pressure readings may help rule out white coat hypertension as well as assisting in monitoring a patient's therapy.

The Obese or Large Arm

If the arm circumference of the patient exceeds 41 cm, use a thigh cuff (18 cm wide) on the patient's upper arm. In patients with extremely large arms, place the cuff on the patient's forearm and listen over the radial artery. Occasionally, it may be necessary to determine the blood pressure in the leg; this may be required to rule out coarctation of the aorta or if an upper extremity blood pressure determination is contraindicated. To do this, use a wide, long thigh cuff with a bladder size of 18×42 cm and apply it to the midthigh. Center the bladder over the posterior surface, wrap it securely, and listen over the popliteal artery.

Block and Schulte discussed ankle blood pressure measurements and found that mean blood pressure readings obtained at the arm and at the ankle were statistically equivalent and concluded that ankle cuff placement provided a reliable alternative to the placement of the cuff on the arm (Block and Schulte, 1996).

Infants and Children

It is certainly true that measuring blood pressure in infants and children presents special problems because of their frequent lack of cooperation. The same measuring techniques are used as in adults. As mentioned earlier, pediatric cuff sizes are available to ensure that the bladder completely encircles the upper arm.

Elderly Patients

In elderly patients, who may have significant atherosclerosis, it is likely that the systolic pressure is overestimated by the indirect method of blood pressure measurement. Because of the tendency for the blood pressure to be more labile in elderly patients, it is important to obtain several baseline measurements before making any diagnostic or therapeutic decisions (Joint National Committee on Prevention, Detection, Evaluation, and Treatment of High Blood Pressure, 1997).

Assessment of Orthostatic Blood Pressure

The measurement of orthostatic blood pressure is an essential clinical tool for the assessment and management of patients suffering from many common medical disorders. According to Carlson (1999), orthostatic hypotension, which is a decline in blood pressure when standing erect, is the "result of an impaired hemodynamic response to an upright posture or a depletion of intravascular volume. The measurement of orthostatic blood pressure can be done at the bedside and is therefore easily applied to several clinical disorders."

Orthostatic hypotension is detected in 10% to 20% of community-dwelling older individuals (Mader et al, 1987). This condition is frequently asymptomatic, but disabling symptoms of light-headedness, weakness, unsteadiness, blurred vision, and syncope may occur.

The American Academy of Neurology's consensus statement (1996) defines orthostatic hypotension as a "reduction of systolic blood pressure of at least 20 mm Hg or diastolic blood pressure of at least 10 mm Hg within 3 minutes of standing."

Many clinicians use a combination of a drop in blood pressure combined with an increase in heart rate to determine the presence of orthostatic hypotension.

Performing these orthostatic measurements requires adequate techniques in blood pressure measurement, appropriate positioning of the patient, and proper timing of the measurements.

Materials Utilized for Measuring Orthostatic Blood Pressure

This technique requires the same equipment as previously mentioned for measuring blood pressure.

Procedure for Measuring Orthostatic Blood Pressure

1. Ask the patient about his or her ability to stand.
2. Make sure the cuffed arm is positioned so that the brachial artery is held at the level of the heart.
3. After 5 minutes of supine rest, take a baseline blood pressure and pulse.
4. Repeat the measurements immediately upon having the patient stand.
5. Repeat the measurements again 1 to 3 minutes after continued standing.

Follow-Up Care and Instructions

Obviously, the results of the blood pressure measurements will dictate the follow-up actions and instructions. Long-term observations have been made on the contributions of high blood pressure to illness and death. It is important to note that the classification of blood pressure has changed

Table 4–2

Classification of Blood Pressure

Level	Reading
Optimal level of systemic blood pressure	120 mm Hg systolic/80 mm Hg diastolic
Normal level of blood pressure	130 mm Hg systolic/85 mm Hg diastolic
High-normal blood pressure	130–139 mm Hg systolic/85–89 mm Hg diastolic
Hypertension is divided into three categories	
Stage 1	Blood pressure of 140–149 mm Hg systolic/90–99 mm Hg diastolic
Stage 2	Blood pressure of 160–169 mm Hg systolic/100–109 mm Hg diastolic
Stage 3	Blood pressure of 180 mm Hg systolic/100 mm Hg diastolic

drastically. In 1997, the sixth report of the Joint National Committee (JNC-VI) on prevention, detection, evaluation, and treatment recommended the classification found in Table 4–2.

Clinicians should explain to patients the meaning of their blood pressure readings and advise them of the appropriate need for periodic remeasurement or follow-up care. Table 4–3 is a suggested follow-up form to be given to patients after their blood pressure has been taken.

The measurement of orthostatic blood pressure is a simple technique that requires the same equipment as previously mentioned in this chapter for measuring blood pressure. Practical applications include the

Table 4–3

Blood Pressure Record and Follow-Up Recommendations

Date:		Name	Age

Blood Pressure Measurements
  Sitting
  Lying
  Standing
		Right Arm	Left Arm

Recommendations ☐ Return in ___ days ☐ Daily BP Readings ☐ Salt Restriction		Medications	Home BP Readings

BP, blood pressure.

detection of intravascular volume depletion and autonomic dysfunction and the treatment of hypertension, congestive heart failure, and other clinical disorders.

References

American Academy of Neurology: Consensus statement on the definition of orthostatic hypotension, pure autonomic failure, and multiple system atrophy. Neurology 46:1470, 1996.

American Heart Association: Human Blood Pressure Determination by Sphygmomanometry. Dallas, American Heart Association, 1994, p 24.

American Society of Hypertension: Recommendations for routine blood pressure measurement by indirect cuff sphygmomanometry. Am J Hypertens 5:207–209, 1992.

Block FE, Schulte GT: Ankle blood pressure measurement: An acceptable alternative to arm measurements. Int J Clin Monit Comput 13:167–171, 1996.

Carlson JE: Assessment of orthostatic blood pressure: Measurement, technique, and clinical applications. South Med J 92:167–173, 1999.

Joint National Committee on Prevention, Detection, Evaluation, and Treatment of High Blood Pressure: The sixth report of the Joint National Committee (JNC-VI) on Prevention, Detection, Evaluation and Treatment of High Blood Pressure. Arch Intern Med 157:2413–2416, 1997.

Lyons SA, Petrucelli RJ: Medicine: An Illustrated History. New York, Abradale Press, 1987.

Mader SL, Josephson KR, Rubenstein LZ: Low prevalence of postural hypotension among community-dwelling elderly. JAMA 258:1511–1514, 1987.

Manning DM, Kuchirka C, Kaminski J: Miscuffing: Inappropriate blood pressure cuff application. Circulation 68:763–766, 1983.

Porter R: The Greatest Benefit to Mankind: A Medical History of Humanity. New York. WW Norton, 1997.

Sternlicht AL: Significant bacterial colonization occurs on the surface of non-disposable sphygmomanometer cuffs and re-used disposable cuffs. Anesth Analg S391, 1990.

Stevens G: Famous Names in Medicine. East Sussex, England, Wayland Publishers, 1978, pp 4–6.

Wain H: A History of Medicine. Springfield, Ill, Charles C Thomas, 1970.

Bibliography

• Bates B: A Guide to Physical Examination and History Taking, 6th ed. Philadelphia, JB Lippincott, 1995, pp 276–280.

• Common problems in measuring blood pressure and recommendations for avoiding them. Available at http://www.trimlinemed.com/html/common_mistakes.html

• Gordon R: The Alarming History of Medicine/Amusing Anecdotes from Hippocrates to Heart Transplants. New York, St. Martins Press, 1994.

• Low PA, Opfer-Gehrking TL, McPhee BR: Prospective evaluation of clinical characteristics of orthostatic hypotension. Mayo Clin Proc 70:617–622, 1995.

- Perloff D, Grim C, Flack J, et al: Human blood pressure by sphygmomanometry. Circulation 88:2460–2470, 1993.
- Swartz MH: Textbook of Physical Diagnosis: History and Examination, 2nd ed. Philadelphia, WB Saunders, 1994, pp 244–245.
- Tips for taking blood pressure. Available at http://www.trimlinemed.com/html/tips_taking_blood_pressure.html

Chapter 5

Venipuncture

▷ Ken Harbert

Procedure Goals and Objectives

Goal: To obtain a venous sample of blood while observing standard precautions and with the minimal degree of risk to the patient.

Objectives: The student will be able to . . .

- ▶ Describe the indications, contraindications, and rationale for performing venipuncture.

- ▶ Identify and describe common complications associated with venipuncture.

- ▶ Describe the essential anatomy and physiology associated with the performance of venipuncture.

- ▶ Identify the necessary materials and their proper use for performing venipuncture.

- ▶ Identify the important aspects of post-procedure care following venipuncture.

Background and History

Venipuncture evolved from the practice of phlebotomy. The word *phlebotomy* is derived from two Greek words referring to "veins" and "cutting"; thus phlebotomy can be defined as the incision of a vein for bloodletting or collection. Since early times, humans have appreciated the association between blood and life itself. Many medical principles and procedures have evolved from this belief. Hippocrates (460–377 BC) stated that disease was the result of excess substances such as blood, phlegm, black bile, and yellow bile within the body. It was believed that removal of the excess of these substances would restore balance (McCall and Tankersley, 1998). From this belief arose the practice of bloodletting—the first form of phlebotomy. By the 17th and 18th centuries, phlebotomy was a major therapy for those practicing the healing arts. Lancets were among the primary instruments used by clinicians in the 18th century.

Methods and procedures associated with phlebotomy today are dramatically improved. Rarely today is phlebotomy used as a therapeutic modality (e.g., for patients with polycythemia). Instead, the primary purpose of phlebotomy is to obtain a sample of blood for diagnostic testing. The development of sophisticated laboratory equipment has reduced the need for venipuncture by requiring smaller quantities of blood for diagnostic assessments, amounts that can often be obtained by simply puncturing the skin without directly accessing the veins. There are many ways to obtain a blood sample using the venipuncture method. The procedures in this chapter describe techniques using Vacutainers, syringes, and infusion sets.

Indications

There are as many reasons to perform venipuncture as there are different disease entities. This procedure is indicated any time that a sample of venous blood is necessary in quantities larger than those readily available by finger stick methods.

Contraindications

Once the decision has been made to perform the venipuncture procedure, the next most important decision is the selection of the site from which to draw a sample. Although many suitable sites may exist, some areas should be avoided. Sites to avoid include the following:

- Obvious areas of skin infection, for example, cellulitis, skin rashes, newly tattooed areas

- Skin sites that have extensive scarring from burns, surgery, injuries, repeated venipuncture, or trauma
- Upper extremity on the ipsilateral side of a mastectomy; use of this site may affect the test results because of the presence of lymphedema, which occurs after dissection and removal of the lymphatic system
- Sites at which a hematoma is present might produce erroneous results in certain types of testing; if another site is not available for venipuncture, the sample should be drawn from the distal aspect of the hematoma
- If the patient has an intravenous (IV) line for fluids or blood transfusions, it is essential to use the opposite arm as the site of the venipuncture. If this is not possible, satisfactory samples can typically be drawn from a site distal to the IV site. When following this procedure, the IV line should be turned off for at least 2 minutes, if possible. The blood should then be drawn from a vein other than the one that the IV is placed in above the selected site. The first 5 mL of blood should be drawn and discarded before drawing the samples for testing.
- An arm with a fistula or cannula in place without specific directions from your supervising physician; if the extremity is edematous, another site should be chosen

Additionally, patients with diffuse intravascular coagulation, hyperfibrinolysis, thrombocytopenia, or qualitative platelet disorders characteristically bleed for a long time after venipunctures.

Potential Complications

Several complications may occur when performing venipuncture. These complications include the following:

- Infection of the skin (cellulitis)
- Infection of the vein (phlebitis)
- Thrombosis
- Laceration of the vein
- Hemorrhage or hematoma at the site of the puncture. The risk of complications is increased with repeated puncture at any site. The most common complication is hemorrhage or hematoma at the site of the puncture. This occurs when blood leaks into the tissues after nicking or penetrating the distal wall of the vein when inserting the needle into the vein. Using the right angle of insertion for the needle can minimize the likelihood of this complication. Also, slower insertion of the needle will reduce the likelihood of inserting it too deeply. A smaller gauge needle will also decrease the risk of hemorrhage or hematoma. If a hematoma does develop, remove the tourniquet, remove the needle, and maintain pressure on the site for at least 10 minutes.

Syncope, or fainting, can occur when performing a venipuncture. Remove the tourniquet, remove the needle, apply pressure to the site, and fix with tape. Lay the patient down and apply appropriate measures to wake the patient up. This potential complication is one of the most compelling reasons why the best position for performing a venipuncture is the supine position.

Review of Essential Anatomy and Physiology

Blood constitutes 6% to 8% of the total body weight and consists of blood cells suspended in a fluid called *plasma. Serum* refers to the substrate remaining when the fibrinogen has been removed from the plasma. The three main types of blood cells are red blood cells, called *erythrocytes;* white blood cells, called *leukocytes;* and platelets, known as *thrombocytes.* The primary function of blood is the transportation of oxygen via hemoglobin molecules within the erythrocytes. In addition, it serves to transport nutrients, waste products, components of the immune system (erythrocytes and so on), hormones, and other specialized materials throughout the body. It also plays a critical role in the constant regulation of body temperature, the regulation of fluids, and acid-base equilibrium. Finally, the platelets are responsible for preventing blood loss from hemorrhage and have their primary influence on the blood vessel walls.

Veins serve as the structures that channel the deoxygenated blood back to the heart and eventually to the lungs. The muscles within the vein walls facilitate the movement of blood within the vein; one-way valves in the vein prevent the backward flow of blood.

The cubital fossa is the triangular hollow area on the anterior aspect of the elbow. The boundaries include an imaginary line connecting the medial and lateral epicondyles superiorly, the pronator teres medially, and the brachioradialis laterally. In the cubital fossa region, the cephalic and basilic veins are often most prominent.

Because of the prominence and accessibility of these superficial veins, the cubital fossa is the site most often used for venipuncture. Considerable variations can occur in the connection of the basilic and cephalic veins. The median cubital vein crosses the bicipital aponeurosis, which separates it from the underlying brachial artery and median nerve. The median cubital vein often receives the median antebrachial vein and can bifurcate to form a median cephalic vein and a median basilic vein (Fig. 5–1). These veins may be embedded in subcutaneous tissue, making them difficult to visualize, but the use of a tourniquet occludes the veins' return and distends them, making them not only palpable but, in most instances, also visible.

Venipuncture is defined as the collection of a blood specimen or specimens from a vein for the laboratory testing of the blood sample. The tests that are performed on blood offer many important and valuable parameters

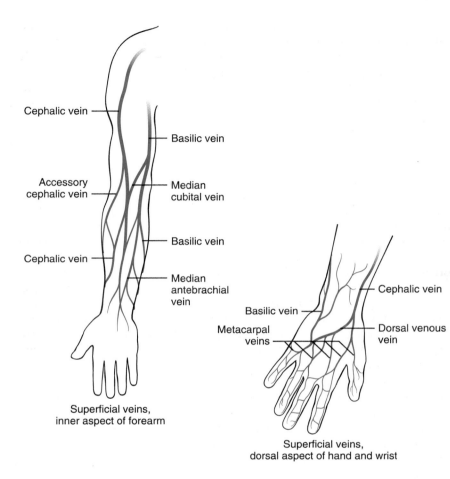

Cephalic vein

Basilic vein

Accessory
cephalic vein

Median
cubital vein

Basilic vein

Cephalic vein

Median
antebrachial
vein

Cephalic vein

Basilic vein

Dorsal venous
vein

Metacarpal
veins

Superficial veins,
inner aspect of forearm

Superficial veins,
dorsal aspect of hand and wrist

Figure 5–1. Superficial vein. *A,* Inner aspect of forearm. *B,* Dorsal aspect of hand and wrist.

for aiding in the diagnosis of a variety of different diseases. The integrity of the sample taken is dependent on using good technique, drawing from an appropriate site, and avoiding hemolysis or contamination of a sample.

Standard Precautions ▷ Practitioners should use Standard Precautions at all times when interacting with patients. Determining the level of precaution necessary requires the practitioner to exercise clinical judgment based on the patient's history and the potential for exposure to body fluids or aerosol-borne pathogens (for further discussion, see Chapter 2).

Patient Preparation

Make sure the patient has followed any preparatory instructions before drawing blood (e.g., fasting before a blood glucose or lipid profile).

- Discuss with the patient any previous experience with venipuncture to identify any potential difficulties with the procedure (e.g., fainting, vomiting).
- Discuss the need for the procedure with the patient, as well as the potential possibility of an initial stinging pain and possible bruising, while continuing to stress the importance of the patient's cooperation for a successful procedure.
- Instruct the patient to remain as still as possible while the procedure is being carried out.
- Do not say, "This will be only a little uncomfortable." The patient knows that it will hurt. Explain that you will do everything you can to minimize the discomfort, but you will need the patient's help to do so.
- Answer any and all questions that the patient may have before you begin the procedure.

Materials Utilized to Perform a Venipuncture

- Gloves: At least two pairs of nonsterile gloves (in case one set becomes contaminated; ask patient about latex allergy)
- Needles: 18 gauge to 23 gauge, single and multidraw (have a needle with a rubber sheath on the part of the needle that inserts into the Vacutainer barrel)
- Evacuated barrels: Vacutainer barrels are now available with safety release or retract features
- Evacuated tubes: serum separator tubes ethylene diaminetetraacetic acid (EDTA), sodium citrate, sodium heparin, plain, and so on (always have spare tubes so that if the vacuum is lost or there is a tube with insufficient vacuum you are prepared and do not have to repeat the venipuncture procedure)
- Labels for evacuated tubes
- Syringes: 1, 3, 5, and 10 mL, or larger (plastic or glass)
- IV butterfly infusion sets: 21, 23, or 25 gauge, or all three
- Tourniquets: ¾ inch or 1 inch for adults and ⅛ inch for children. These should be clean, wide strips of latex (check for latex allergies before beginning procedure), or an adult-child blood pressure cuff can be used. Latex-free tourniquets are available.
- Gauze pads: 2 inch × 2 inch or 4 inch × 4 inch
- Isopropyl alcohol pads, 70%
- Povidone-iodine (used for cleansing venipuncture sites for blood cultures)
- Adhesive strips (Band-Aids) (again ask patient if he or she is allergic to adhesive tape before procedure), nylon tape, and paper tape
- Sharps disposal container
- Biohazard waste container
  Note: There are many ways to obtain a blood sample using the venipuncture technique. The following procedures describe techniques using Vacutainers, syringes, and infusion sets.

Procedure for Venipuncture Using Vacutainers

Note: When performing a venipuncture, proper planning and preparation are essential to obtaining good results and ensuring a good outcome for your patient. Developing a routine, sequential plan for the venipuncture procedure helps ensure effective and efficient results with the least amount of discomfort for the patient.

1. Know which specific samples you will need to collect for the laboratory studies requested and anticipate the materials and sequence for collecting the needed samples.
2. For each laboratory study to be performed, identify the additive, additive function, volume, and specimen considerations to be followed for each using the corresponding tubes with color-coded tops. This will save the patient undue distress and will help you in obtaining the best outcome for each sample of blood and corresponding laboratory test that is to be performed.
3. Wash hands with warm water and bacteriostatic soap. Always observe standard precautions for the prevention of transmission of human immunodeficiency virus (HIV), hepatitis B and C, and other blood borne infections (Centers for Disease Control, 1989).
4. Check patient identification to ensure that the correct patient is having the procedure.
5. Check the test ordered, even if ordered by you.
6. Assemble the equipment, preparing the tubes in the right order and placing the appropriate needle on the Vacutainer barrel.

Note: In some instances, the equipment needed is dependent on the patient, the medical condition, the site to be used for the procedure, the number of samples required, and the type of setting (hospital, outpatient, pediatric ward, nursery, emergency room) where the procedure will be performed.

7. Position the patient in a manner that is both proper for the procedure and comfortable for the patient. If possible, position the patient in a supine or recumbent position. This assists the patient in relaxing and carries the least likelihood for injury to the patient if he or she experiences vasovagal syncope. If the patient is sitting up, extend his or her arm straight down from shoulder to waist.
8. Observe the patient for any of the contraindications mentioned previously.
9. Inspect the patient's surface anatomy and venous system in the chosen venipuncture site before applying the tourniquet. The cubital fossa is the most common site for sampling and IV injections. Check bilaterally, distally, and proximally to the most common site for venipuncture in the adult, which is the antecubital fossa.

Note: To augment the ability to identify the best site for venipuncture, palpation skills and the sense of touch should be refined by using the palmar aspects of gloved finger pads. Do not rely totally on vision. This can be practiced on oneself or on volunteers until the location of a vein can be identified confidently with eyes closed. Heavily pigmented skin and overlying adipose tissue can make veins difficult to visualize. In particular, difficult venipunctures can occur in patients who have had a number of venipunctures, or in patients who are using IV drugs. In these instances, selecting an adequate site may be difficult. Patients who are frequently subjected to venipuncture may be able to direct you to sites with the highest likelihood of success. A warm compress applied lightly before the procedure can facilitate vein dilatation and thus assist with the identification of an adequate vein. The selection of a good site should include a vein that is easily palpated, is large and well anchored, and does not roll when palpated.

Note: The best veins for venipuncture in the right order of choice follow:

■ Median cubital vein, which is easily palpated, well anchored, least painful, and least likely to bruise, and is usually the largest vein in the antecubital space
■ Cephalic vein, which is a large vein that is easily palpated but poorly anchored; venipuncture here can be painful to the patient
■ Basilic vein, which is easy to palpate, not well anchored, and very close to the brachial artery and the median nerve

Note: For finding difficult veins:

■ Have the patient keep the extremity below the level of the heart for a few minutes.
■ Apply a warm towel to the extremity to promote vasodilation from the heat—the towel should be less than 42°C and should be left on no longer than 2 minutes.
■ Use a blood pressure cuff inflated to a point between the systolic and diastolic pressures as a tourniquet to allow for greater control and less discomfort to the patient.
■ Carefully rub or tap the vein over the potential puncture site to increase the vein's vasodilation (should be done before the site is prepared).

10. Firmly place the tourniquet about 3 to 4 inches above the venipuncture site,

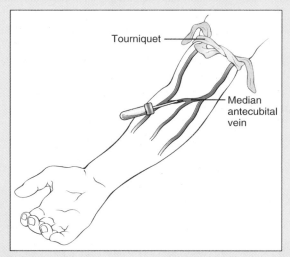

Tourniquet

Median antecubital vein

Figure 5–2

not too tight, and use a wide tube band tied with easily removable bow ties pointing up and away from the site (Fig. 5–2).

Note: Be sure the patient has no contraindications against the use of a tourniquet. Apply the tourniquet in a manner in which it can be easily removed.

Caution: Never leave the tourniquet on for more than 2 minutes. The vein may collapse if the tourniquet is too close to the puncture site.

11. After applying the tourniquet, begin palpation of the identified site to locate a desirable vein.

Note: The vein can also be tapped to cause it to dilate and become more prominent. Allow gravity to help the vein become engorged and thus enlarged. If the vein being palpated feels very tight and has no flexibility, it may be a tendon or may overlie a tendon. If it has a palpable pulse, it is an artery. Be certain of the underlying anatomy before performing the procedure.

Procedure for Venipuncture Using Vacutainers – *(continued)*

12. Put on latex gloves.
13. Before cleansing the area, secure the site by anchoring the vein distal to the venipuncture site, using a finger to apply pressure over the top of the vein and thus serving to hold the vein still.
14. Allow the area to air dry thoroughly. This is especially true when using povidone-iodine.

Note: Alcohol lyses red blood cells and can cause intense stinging. Be sure the site is dry.

15. Visualize what you are going to do and begin by stretching the skin downward below the anticipated venipuncture site with the opposite hand to anchor the vein and limit vein movement.
16. Insert the needle with the bevel facing up directly over and parallel to the vein and enter the vein or a point immediately adjacent to the vein. Insert the needle with the bevel up at about a 15- to 30-degree angle so that the needle penetrates halfway into the vessel (Fig. 5–3).

Note: Use caution when using Vacutainers because they can exert excessive vacuum, causing the vein to collapse.

17. Remove the protective covering from the threaded hub and screw the needle into the holder.

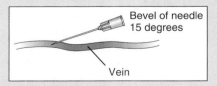

Figure 5–3

18. Place the tube inside the barrel without puncturing the top of the tube with the needle. Be sure to have extra tubes close at hand in the right order of draw.

Note: Determine the correct order of drawing the samples in the tube or slide, depending on the laboratory or the tests required, or both. This prevents interference by carryover of additives between tubes. Usually the order is as follows:

1. Blood cultures, usually performed with a syringe using *only iodine as the skin preparation*
2. Red top (chemistry, immunology, and serology panels; blood bank)
3. Gold top (chemistry, immunology, and serology panels)
4. Light blue top (requires a full draw of sample; uses include coagulation tests, such as thrombin and prothrombin times)
5. Green or lavender top (requires a full draw and inverting slowly at least eight times to prevent clotting and platelet clumping; uses include hematology, blood bank)
6. Gray top (requires a full draw to prevent hemolysis; uses include lithium, sodium heparin, and glucose levels)

This order changes when using a syringe for drawing blood (see "Procedure for Syringe Venipuncture").

Note: Inserting the needle at less than a 15- to 30-degree angle may allow the needle to puncture through the far wall of the vein.

19. Hold the needle steady and engage the Vacutainer tube. Avoid rotating the needle because this may result in excessive damage to the vessel wall.

Procedure for Venipuncture Using Vacutainers – *(continued)*

20. Move the Vacutainer tube down into the barrel so that the tube is punctured. A drop of blood will be visible at the top of the inside needle when it is in the vein. As blood flows into the last Vacutainer tube, release the tourniquet and have the patient relax his or her hand.

21. When removing the filled tube and inserting the next tube, grasp the barrel-holder securely in the nondominant hand and anchor it by holding it against the extremity to avoid inadvertently removing the needle from the lumen of the vein.

Note: The existing vacuum gently draws blood into the tubes. Most Vacutainer tubes are nonsterile and have additives. The tube will cease drawing blood when its vacuum is expired (i.e., when the tube is appropriately filled).

22. Have the next tube ready for insertion into the Vacutainer. Remove the Vacutainer tube from the holder before removing the needle.

Note: Remember that multiple tubes of blood can be drawn at this one venipuncture site without resticking the patient).

23. If multiple tubes are drawn, carefully invert tubes and mix as required for each specific tube. Do not shake the tubes vigorously because disruption of the cell membranes may result, thus altering the concentrations of intracellular and extracellular components.

24. Place tubes in easy reach in order of desired draw.

25. Carefully remove the needle from the skin.

26. Once the needle is removed completely, apply firm pressure for hemostasis by holding a sterile 2 inch × 2 inch covering over the site while the arm is outstretched or raised. Avoid bending the arm. Apply firm pressure to the site until the bleeding stops, for at least 3 to 4 minutes.

27. Dress the site with gauze and tape or adhesive strip (ask about allergies before applying dressing).

Note: If the procedure was unsuccessful, do not attempt to repeat it at the same site until healing has occurred.

28. Discard the needle in a puncture-resistant sharps container.

29. Be sure to agitate all tubes gently by tilting them back and forth to ensure adequate mixing of blood with the additive agent.

30. Clean any blood spillage with appropriate cleaning agent.

31. Label all Vacutainer tubes according to facility procedure (Fig. 5–4).

32. Properly dispose of all contaminated materials in the appropriate biohazardous waste container.

33. Recheck the patient and the venipuncture site and apply a dressing.

34. Make sure the patient is feeling fine and shows no signs of vertigo, light-headedness, or discomfort before leaving.

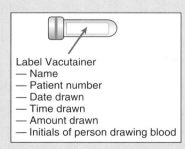

Label Vacutainer
— Name
— Patient number
— Date drawn
— Time drawn
— Amount drawn
— Initials of person drawing blood

Figure 5–4

Procedure for Syringe Venipuncture

Note: Syringes may be used for venipuncture when the patient's veins are small or fragile and Vacutainer tubes may cause the veins to collapse. Use of a syringe allows for greater control. The procedure for using a syringe follows the same steps as for using the Vacutainer tubes except it differs in the order of samples drawn, the aspiration of blood into the syringe, and the transfer of blood into the vacuum tubes.

The order of draw is as follows:

- Blood cultures, using only iodine as a skin preparation
- Light blue top (requires a full draw of sample; uses include coagulation tests such as thrombin and prothrombin times)
- Lavender top (requires a full draw and inverting at least eight times slowly to prevent clotting and platelet clumping; uses include hematology, blood bank)
- Green top
- Gray top (requires a full draw to prevent hemolysis; uses include lithium, sodium heparin, and glucose levels).
- Red top (chemistry, immunology, and serology panels; blood bank)

1. Cleanse the site, select the venipuncture site, and palpate the vein in the same manner as when using a Vacutainer system. The steps associated with the entry into the vein are the same as well.
2. Once the needle is in the vein, pull back gently on the syringe plunger while holding the syringe securely to keep the needle in the vein.
3. Using the syringe to brace against you, pull back on the plunger and fill the syringe with the desired amount of blood needed for the tubes to be filled.
4. Release the tourniquet and complete the dressing procedure using the same technique as described for the Vacutainer system.
5. When transferring from the syringe to the tubes, remove the needle from the syringe and replace it with an 18- or 19-gauge needle.
6. Take extreme care to puncture the tubes in the right order and allow the tubes to fill by using the pressure of the vacuum tube.
7. Do not use the plunger to fill the tubes.

Note: Use caution with a syringe, because the temptation will be to push the blood sample into the vacuum tube using the syringe plunger, which will affect the sample. Vacuum tubes draw blood into the tubes using their own vacuum. The Vacutainer system consists of vacuum tubes, a needle holder (Vacutainer barrel), and a disposable multisample or single-sample needle (Fig. 5–5). New multisample needles have guard sheaths.

8. Continue with the same labeling procedure and ensure the status of the patient before allowing him or her to leave.

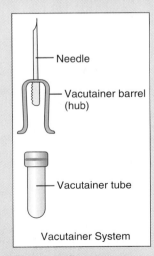

Needle

Vacutainer barrel (hub)

Vacutainer tube

Vacutainer System

Figure 5–5

Procedure for a Butterfly Set Venipuncture

Note: An IV infusion set or butterfly can be used for venipuncture when you are drawing from a hand or a foot or from a very small or difficult vein. The procedure for cleansing the site and site selection are the same as for the syringe and Vacutainer procedures; however, new sites could include the hand and the foot with the infusion set.

1. Insert the needle at a lesser angle than for either of the other methods.

Caution: It is important to take great care with the needle so as not to miss the vein.

Note: Infusion sets come in different sizes of needles, and the appropriate one for the adult, child, or difficult vein should be selected carefully.

2. Attach a syringe to the set and be careful not to use excessive suction from the syringe as the blood is drawn slowly and carefully.

Note: The infusion set has plastic "wings" that are attached to a short length of flexible plastic tubing, which is then attached to either a syringe or IV tubing.

Note: As soon as the needle is in the vein, blood will be visible in the tubing, and this will allow for easy access by the syringe.

3. Fill the tube with the appropriate amount of blood, release the tourniquet, and attach a needle. Transfer to the appropriate tubes using the same order as for a syringe.

4. When using a safety infusion set, slide the safety cover over the needle and discard the set.

5. In order to prevent an accidental restick with the infusion set needle, hold the base of the needle or the wings as you remove the needle, and do not let go of the needle base until it is being placed in the biohazard sharps container.

Special Considerations

- If no blood is obtained, change the position of the needle carefully. Move it forward or backward. Watch for formation of a hematoma. If this occurs, stop the procedure. Also consider adjusting the angle of the needle.
- If blood stops flowing into the vacuum tube, the vein may have collapsed. Resecure the tourniquet to increase venous filling. If this is not successful, remove the needle, take care of the puncture site, and redraw.
- Never draw from a thrombosed or scarred vein. Thrombosed veins lack resilience, feel cordlike, and roll easily.
- Never attempt venipuncture in an artery. Arteries pulsate, are very elastic, and have a thick wall. If you see bright red blood, be cautious: Remove the tourniquet, carefully remove the needle, and apply a firm steady pressure for at least 10 minutes.

- Never draw above an IV site. The fluid may dilute the specimen; collect from the opposite arm. Do not use alcohol when drawing a blood alcohol sample.
- Never draw over scars or new tattoo sites. It is difficult to puncture the scar tissue, and the needle and the tourniquet should not come in contact with the inflamed tattoo site. Edematous extremities with swollen tissue alter the test results.
- Avoid leaving a tourniquet on for more than 2 minutes. This can cause hemoconcentration of nonfilterable elements. The hydrostatic pressure causes some water and filterable elements to leave the extracellular space.
- Make sure the venipuncture site is dry.
- When using a syringe, avoid drawing the plunger back too forcefully.

Follow-up Care and Instruction

- Advise the patient that he or she may experience some minor discomfort and discoloration at the site of the venipuncture for the following 48 to 72 hours.
- Instruct the patient to keep the site clean and dry to reduce the likelihood of infection.
- Educate the patient about signs of infection and phlebitis and advise him or her to call or return to the office if such signs are seen.

References

Centers for Disease Control and Prevention: Guidelines for the prevention of transmission of human immunodeficiency virus and hepatitis B virus to health care and public safety workers. MMWR 38:1–36, 1989.
McCall RE, Tankersley CM: Phlebotomy Essentials. Philadelphia, JB Lippincott, 1998, pp 2–4.

Bibliography

- Bardes CL: Essential Skills in Clinical Medicine. Philadelphia, FA Davis, 1996, pp 104–106.
- Chesnutt MS, Dewar TN, Locksley RM, Turee JH: Office and Bedside Procedures. Norwalk, Connecticut, Lange, 1992, pp 27–29.
- Fischbach F: A Manual of Laboratory and Diagnostic Tests, 5th ed. Philadelphia, JB Lippincott, 1996, pp 25–27.
- Greene HL, Fincher RM, Johnson WP, et al: Clinical Medicine, 2nd ed. St. Louis, CV Mosby, 1996, pp 874–878.
- Jacobs DS, DeMott WR, Grady HJ, Horvat RT: Laboratory Test Handbook. Lexicomp, 1996, pp 197–200.

- Jandl JH: Blood: Texbook of Hematology. Boston, Little, Brown, 1997, pp 53–55.
- McClatchey KD: Clinical Laboratory Medicine. Baltimore, Williams & Wilkins, 1996, pp 84–90.
- Sacher RA, McPherson RA: Wildmann's Clinical Interpretation of Laboratory Tests, 11th ed. Philadelphia, FA Davis, 2000, p 31.
- Wallach J: Interpretation of Diagnostic Tests, 7th ed. Philadelphia, Lippincott Williams & Wilkins, 2000, pp 3–17.

Chapter 6

Obtaining Blood Cultures

▷ Darwin Brown

Procedure Goals and Objectives

Goal: To obtain a blood culture sample successfully while observing standard precautions and with the minimal degree of risk to the patient.

Objectives: The student will be able to . . .

► Describe the indications, contraindications, and rationale for obtaining a blood culture sample.

► Identify and describe common complications associated with obtaining a blood culture sample.

► Describe the essential anatomy and physiology associated with obtaining a blood culture sample.

► Identify the materials necessary for obtaining a blood culture sample and their proper use.

► Identify the important aspects of patient care after a blood culture sample is obtained.

Background and History

A blood culture is performed when an infection of the blood (bacteremia or septicemia) is suspected in the presence of fever, chills, low blood pressure, or other symptoms. The blood culture helps identify the infection's origin and provides a basis for determining appropriate antimicrobial therapy.

Bacteremia is a microbial infection of the bloodstream. Identification of pathogens within the bloodstream is accomplished primarily by blood culture. Culturing blood is one of the most important procedures that can be performed in individuals who are severely ill and febrile as well as those in whom an intravascular infection is suspected. Isolation and identification of an infectious agent from the blood have obvious diagnostic significance and also provide an invaluable guide for selecting the most appropriate antimicrobial agent for therapy (Hoeprich and Rinaldi, 1994).

The sources of bacteremia include focal sites of infection most often associated with the respiratory tract, the genitourinary tract, the abdomen, and the skin and soft tissues. The infecting organism typically reflects the organisms indigenous to the site.

Until approximately 1985, broth culture was the most conventional blood culture method. Conventional broth culture methods call for inoculating blood to liquid media contained in bottles or tubes. Today there is a wide variety of different media to choose from. The obtained cultures are incubated either aerobically or anaerobically for 7 to 14 days at 35°C. They are then examined visually every day for evidence of growth; in addition, blind subcultures and smears are prepared at scheduled intervals.

Indications

Blood cultures are a useful diagnostic tool for the evaluation of patients with history and clinical physical examination findings that are indicative of bacteremia or septicemia.

- Blood cultures should be obtained only if there is reasonable suspicion of a bloodstream infection (bacteremia). A thorough history and physical examination can provide important information for determining the potential of an infectious state.
- Documentation should be made of the specific infecting organism in bacteremia or focal infection sites.
- Blood cultures are useful for monitoring the efficacy of pharmacologic treatments of blood borne infections.
- Other specific indications for obtaining blood cultures include severely ill and febrile patients, suspected infective endocarditis, intravascular catheter site infection, meningitis, osteomyelitis, septic arthritis, bacterial pneumonia, and fever of unknown origin.

Contraindications

There are few true contraindications to obtaining blood cultures.

- Patients currently being treated with warfarin (Coumadin) should be carefully assessed to determine if the benefit of performing the procedure outweighs the potential risk.
- Obtaining blood cultures should be avoided at the site of an active skin infection because of the probability of introducing bacteria into the blood circulation and the increased possibility of contamination of the culture by organisms originating from the infected structures.
- If multiple previous blood cultures have failed to identify an infecting agent, the likelihood of obtaining a useful result diminishes and must be considered in view of all the available clinical evidence.

Potential Complications

Complications resulting from the collection of a blood culture are limited.

- The development of a hematoma at the site of the venipuncture is not uncommon.
- Continued bleeding from the puncture site may also occur.
- Other possible complications include the development of a localized skin infection or phlebitis.
- Contaminated blood samples may result in the inappropriate use of antibiotics, which, in turn, may enhance selection for multidrug-resistant organisms. This may increase the rate of nosocomial infections and antibiotic-related complications, possibly raising health care costs (Chien, 1998).

In general, contamination should be suspected if:

- A common component of the skin flora is recovered and the patient's history does not warrant consideration of a "nonpathogen" as being significant.
- A mixture of several kinds of bacteria is recovered.
- Growth is found in only one of several specimens from separate venipunctures (Hoeprich, 1994).

Review of Essential Anatomy and Physiology

It is important to be aware of the specific anatomy of each area at which blood cultures will be obtained. It is generally accepted that

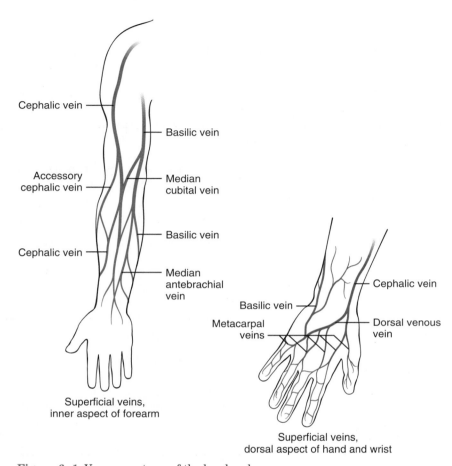

Figure 6–1. Venous anatomy of the hand and arm.

for each septic episode, at least two sets of blood culture specimens should be collected. This results in two separate venipunctures at different sites. The median cubital vein is usually the easiest to locate. Other acceptable locations include the cephalic and basilic veins and veins in the back of the hand (Fig. 6–1). For more information regarding the anatomy and physiology of veins see Chapter 5.

Standard Precautions ▷ Practitioners should use Standard Precautions at all times when interacting with patients. Determining the level of precaution necessary requires the practitioner to exercise clinical judgment based on the patient's history and the potential for exposure to body fluids or aerosol-borne pathogens (for further discussion, see Chapter 2).

Patient Preparation

Instruct the patient about the need for the procedure and the potential benefits and risks associated with having the procedure performed.

- Explain that the procedure includes skin preparation and the potential need to use two separate venipuncture sites.
- If the patient notes an allergy to iodine, use chlorhexidine or 70% isopropyl alcohol for site cleansing.

Materials Utilized for Obtaining Blood Cultures

- 20-mL syringe with 21-gauge needle or vacuum tube adapter and needle
- 70% isopropyl alcohol swabs or wipes
- 1% to 2% tincture of iodine, povidone-iodine, or chlorhexidine gluconate swabs or wipes
- Alcohol swabs for cleaning blood culture bottle tops
- Aerobic and anaerobic vacuum blood culture bottles with properly identified patient labels
- Tourniquet
- Gloves
- 2-inch × 2-inch gauze pads
- Bandages

Procedure for Obtaining a Blood Culture

1. Identify the patient. Ask the patient to state his or her name and then check and confirm other identification information.
2. Initial setup: Assemble and lay out equipment for collecting the blood culture specimen. Wash your hands before putting on gloves.
3. Position the patient. Make sure patient is in a comfortable position and that the arm is supported appropriately.
4. Apply tourniquet 3 inches above intended site. Locate an appropriate vein and then release tourniquet.
5. Clean the site using sterile 70% isopropyl alcohol wipes; starting at the intended site, move outward in concentric circles (Fig. 6–2). Repeat this two to three times, being sure to use a new, clean wipe each time.
6. Next apply povidone-iodine in the same manner two to three times and allow site to air dry. Once dry, the site should not be touched again. Sterile gloves must be worn if the site is to be repalpated.
7. Replace the tourniquet and remove the iodine with 70% isopropyl alcohol just before venipuncture.
8. Perform the venipuncture using a syringe or vacuum tube system.

Procedure for Obtaining a Blood Culture – *(continued)*

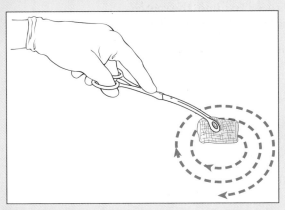

Figure 6–2

9. Draw blood in the correct order. If specimens for multiple laboratory tests are to be obtained, always collect the blood culture specimens first, and then fill the other tubes as needed. Swab the top of the blood culture bottle with an alcohol wipe before blood insertion. Inoculate anaerobic bottle, followed by aerobic bottle.

10. Release the tourniquet after the first tube has been filled. The tourniquet should not be left on for more than 1 minute.

11. After the specimen has been collected, remove the needle and apply pressure until bleeding has stopped.

12. Immediately dispose of the needle in the proper container. Do not attempt to recap needles.

13. After the specimen has been collected, label all cultures with appropriate patient information, which should include patient's full name, identification number, culture site location, time, date, and your initials.

14. Clean the patient's arm of iodine before placing an adhesive bandage. Check to make sure the site is not bleeding before covering with bandage.

15. Pick up and account for all materials before leaving the patient's room. Remove your gloves and wash your hands. Thank the patient for his or her cooperation.

Special Considerations

The issue of using indwelling central catheters for obtaining blood cultures is somewhat controversial, and studies are conflicting (DesJardin et al, 1999). If a blood sample for culture is to be obtained during the placement of a central venous catheter, the catheter must be one that is placed in a completely sterile manner above the chest. If an indwelling central venous or arterial catheter is already in place, samples must be taken from both the catheter port and peripheral venipuncture sites to rule out line sepsis (Chein, 1998).

For infants, collect 1 to 5 mL of blood per 100-mL blood culture bottle (Hall, 1995).

Follow-Up Care and Instructions

• Advise the patient that he or she may experience some minor discomfort and discoloration at the site of the venipuncture for the following 48 to 72 hours.

- Instruct the patient to keep the site clean and dry to reduce the likelihood of infection.
- Explain to the patient the signs of hematoma, infection, and phlebitis and instruct him or her to call or return to the office or clinic if any of these occur.
- Advise the patient to report any adverse events associated with the venipuncture. These may include development of a hematoma or continued bleeding from the venipuncture site.

References

Chien JW: Making the most of blood cultures. Postgrad Med 104:120, 1998.

DesJardin JA, Falagas ME, Ruthazer R, et al: Clinical utility of blood cultures drawn from indwelling central venous catheters in hospitalized patients with cancer. Ann Intern Med 131:641–647, 1999.

Hall G: Microbiology. In Tietz NW (ed): Clinical Guide to Laboratory Tests, 3rd ed. Philadelphia, WB Saunders, 1995, p 904.

Hoeprich PD, Rinaldi MG: Diagnostic methods for bacterial, rickettsial, mycoplasmal, and fungal infections. In Hoeprich PD, Jordan MC, Ronald AR (eds): Infectious Diseases: A Treatise of Infectious Processes, 5th ed. Philadelphia, JB Lippincott, 1994, pp 169–171.

Bibliography

- Flynn JC: Procedures in Phlebotomy, 2nd ed. Philadelphia, WB Saunders, 1999.
- Lehmann CA (ed): Saunders Manual of Clinical Laboratory Science. Philadelphia, WB Saunders, 1998.

Chapter 7

Inserting Intravenous Catheters

▷ Ellen Davis-Hall

Procedure Goals and Objectives

Goal: To insert an intravenous (IV) line successfully while observing standard precautions and with the minimal degree of risk to the patient.

Objectives: The student will be able to . . .

▶ Describe the indications, contraindications, and rationale for insertion of an IV line.

▶ Identify and describe common complications associated with IV line insertion.

▶ Describe the essential anatomy and physiology associated with the insertion of an IV line.

▶ Identify the necessary materials for insertion of an IV line and their proper use.

▶ Identify the important aspects of patient care after insertion of an IV line.

Background and History

Once William Harvey described the circulation of blood in 1628, experimentation with this system was inevitable. It was in 1656, however, that Sir Christopher Wren used a quill and bladder to inject opium intravenously into a dog, and IV therapy was begun (Gardner, 1982). Because of the sepsis accompanying such endeavors, IV therapy did not come into general use until the 1920s (Weinstein, 1997).

Little controversy exists over the value of IV therapy, and its use is widespread. Performance of this activity is highly technical and demands careful instruction and supervised experience. Various professionals and technicians can initiate IV therapy. This is regulated by state law and may vary.

Indications

Indications for IV therapy include:

- The administration of fluids (e.g., in clinical situations such as volume depletion, burn injury, blood loss, heat illness, shock, electrolyte imbalance)
- The provision of rapid and efficient delivery of medications (e.g., in various medical and surgical states and emergencies)
- The administration of blood or blood products

Contraindications

There are few contraindications to IV therapy.

- Venipuncture should be avoided at the site of an active skin infection, because of the probability of introducing bacteria into the blood circulation.
- IV lines should not be inserted distal to any area of preexisting thrombophlebitis.
- Lower extremity venipunctures should be avoided in the elderly and in patients with peripheral vascular disease and venous insufficiency. These compromised veins will not be effective vessels for fluid or medication administration, and the veins may suffer further injury.

Potential Complications

Local

- Thrombosis or thrombophlebitis is the result of mechanical trauma to the vein at the time of insertion and the subsequent indwelling nature of the IV cannula. To prevent or minimize these complications, it is important to avoid trauma at time of insertion, tape the cannula securely to prevent movement, and avoid inserting IV lines in close proximity to joints. Infiltration of an IV line may cause the patient discomfort and increase the risk of infection and local tissue damage. Close observation and early detection will prevent or minimize this complication.

- Local infection may also develop but can usually be avoided by adherence to sterile technique and regular dressing changes at the puncture site.

Systemic

- Catheter embolization is a rare occurrence that results from shearing off of a distal portion of the catheter end by the beveled needle tip. This may occur when either an over-the-needle or a through-the-needle catheter is advanced into the vein and is then pulled back over or through the needle. This serious complication is avoidable by strict adherence to proper technique.
- Septicemia can usually be avoided by adherence to sterile technique and established institutional IV line care protocols.
- Pulmonary embolism may occur when a small blood clot that may form near the IV site dislodges and travels through the circulation until it lodges in the small capillary bed of the lungs. Avoidance of lower extremity veins helps prevent this occurrence.
- Air embolism occurs when air, inadvertently left in or allowed into the IV tubing, travels into the bloodstream. This can be avoided by careful attention to flushing all lines before connection.

Review of Essential Anatomy and Physiology

The anatomy of the veins that are most commonly considered for IV line placement is presented in Figure 7–1. Use of veins in the arm is recommended because they are most accessible, most comfortable for the patient, and the easiest to secure for long-term therapy. Often the easiest access is available on the dorsal aspect of the hand and the lower aspects of the arm; the metacarpal and cephalic veins are used most frequently. Valves may be palpable as knotlike lumps in a vein. These valves, as well as bifurcations, should be evaluated to ascertain adequate length and straightness for threading of the IV needle and catheter.

The choice of a vein for IV line insertion is based on the prescribed therapy, the duration of therapy, the condition of the extremity and the patient in general, and the condition, size, and location of the veins.

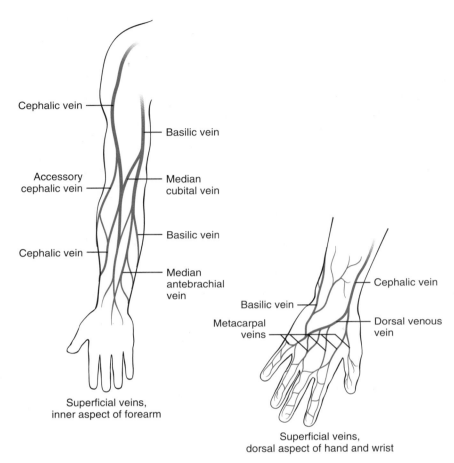

Figure 7–1. Anatomy of the veins most commonly considered for intravenous (IV) line placement.

Standard Precautions ▷ Practitioners should use Standard Precautions at all times when interacting with patients. Determining the level of precaution necessary requires the practitioner to exercise clinical judgment based on the patient's history and the potential for exposure to body fluids or aerosol-borne pathogens (for further discussion, see Chapter 2).

Patient Preparation

- The patient should be informed of the indications for the IV line, the benefits and risks associated with the procedure, and the steps involved in the procedure. The patient may be anxious or afraid of the IV line itself or the anticipated pain, and explaining the procedure may help alleviate some of the anxiety.

- Inquire about iodine, latex, and tape allergies.
- The patient should also be advised of the need to limit movement of the extremity once the IV line is in place.
- Occasionally, in pain-sensitive individuals, an injection of lidocaine (Xylocaine) 0.5% to 1.0%, to raise a wheal at the puncture site, may help minimize discomfort. This can be accomplished with a needle as small as 27 gauge. This may be especially helpful when a larger gauge butterfly or catheter is required. The patient should be warned, however, of the "bee sting and burn" nature of the lidocaine injection. The patient must be carefully screened for the possibility of previous allergic reactions to lidocaine before using this technique.

Materials Utilized for Inserting Intravenous Lines

■ Intravenous catheter or butterfly
  Note: There are a large number of catheters available for IV cannulation. The most common choice is the *over-the-needle catheter*. An alternative to this is the *butterfly* or winged small vein needle. The use of these two types of infusion devices is the focus of this section. They are presented in Figure 7–2. The gauge of the catheter or butterfly needle is chosen based on the vein used and the purpose of the infusion. A plan to administer blood, for example, demands a larger gauge, such as 16 gauge, whereas IV fluids alone can be administered with a needle having a gauge as small as 23.
■ Gloves and eye protection
■ Povidone-iodine or alcohol swabs, or both
■ Intravenous fluid
■ Administration set (tubing with a drip chamber, a roller clamp flow regulator, and a standard connector that fits into the hub of the cannula or butterfly needle)

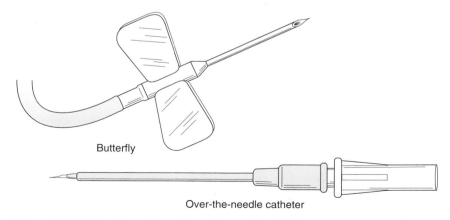

Butterfly

Over-the-needle catheter

Figure 7–2. Butterfly needle and over-the-needle catheter.

- Tourniquet
- 1/2 inch tape
- Arm board (if necessary to prevent flexion of a joint near the IV insertion point)
- Scissors to trim hair (if necessary)
- 2 inch × 2 inch or 4 inch × 4 inch gauze bandages or other occlusive dressing
- IV catheter pole
- Biohazardous waste and needle containers
- Antibiotic ointment (optional)

Procedure for Inserting an Intravenous Catheter

1. Apply the tourniquet above the elbow to ensure adequate filling of the veins, first to one arm and then to the other to identify the best vein for IV catheter insertion.

Note: The most distal vein that is large enough to accommodate the size of the required butterfly needle or catheter should be chosen.

2. Palpate the veins for firmness and stability.

Note: Selection of the vein should be determined more by how the vein feels than by how it looks. Choose a vein that is straight and void of palpable valves for at least 1 inch proximal to your intended insertion site.

3. Release the tourniquet and recheck all supplies. Make certain that all necessary materials are within easy reach, the fluids are hung, and the tubing is flushed with the IV solution.

4. Reapply the tourniquet above the elbow.

5. If tourniquet pressure does not distend the vein adequately, ask the patient to open and close the hand several times, tap or pat the vein lightly, apply a warm moist towel, or have the patient place the extremity lower than the heart to facilitate vein dilatation.

6. Apply gloves and eye protection.

7. Cleanse the puncture site with a povidone-iodine swab followed by an alcohol swab. If an alcohol swab alone is used, the cleansing should be a 30-second preparation.

8. With the nondominant hand, hold the patient's hand or arm and retract the skin distal to the insertion site toward the fingers.

Note: This serves to make the skin taut and anchor the vein to help prevent it from "rolling" (Fig. 7–3).

9. Puncture the vein using direct or indirect entry:

Note: Direct entry (one step) is useful for larger veins.

- Warn the patient of the "stick."
- With the dominant hand, insert the butterfly or catheter needle (bevel up) through the skin at a 15- to 30-degree angle at the site of anticipated vein entry.

Procedure for Inserting an Intravenous Catheter – *(continued)*

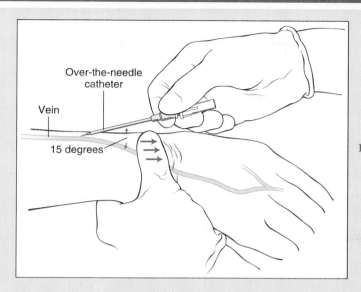

Figure 7–3

■ As soon as the skin is punctured, and with one continuous motion, drop the hub down close to the skin, if needed, and enter the vein from the top (see Fig. 7–3).

Note: Indirect entry (two steps) is useful for smaller veins.

■ Warn the patient of the "stick."
■ With the dominant hand, insert the butterfly or catheter needle (bevel up) through the skin and tissue at a 15- to 30-degree angle slightly distal to the anticipated point of vein entry.
■ Relocate the vein and while maintaining the distal anchor, enter the vein either from the top or the side. A "pop" may be felt with vein puncture.

Note: If the vein is successfully entered, there will be a flashback of blood into the butterfly or catheter hub tubing.

10. After the initial appearance of the flash, advance the catheter 2 to 3 mm further to help ensure that the catheter is not inadvertently removed from the vein when the stylette is removed.
11. If the IV line insertion attempt is unsuccessful (no flashback), pull the butterfly and intact catheter back slightly, but not out of the skin.
12. Reassess the location and anchoring of the vein and advance the butterfly or catheter again in the direction of the vein. If the attempt is unsuccessful, the tourniquet should be released and the butterfly or catheter removed (Heckman, 1993).
13. Apply pressure for 1 minute and then attempt insertion at a more proximal site or in the other extremity.
14. Once removed from the skin puncture, properly discard the butterfly or catheter.

Caution: Never reuse a catheter.

15. Once the flashback is achieved, the vein can be cannulated with the butterfly needle or catheter.

Procedure for Inserting an Intravenous Catheter – *(continued)*

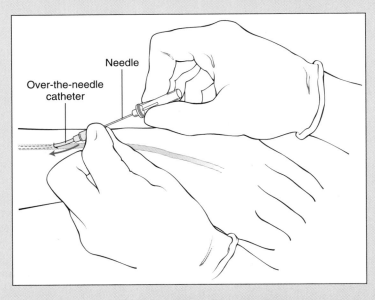

Figure 7–4

Over-the-Needle Catheter Cannulation

- Hold the needle base firmly in place with the nondominant hand while advancing the catheter with the dominant hand over the needle and threading into the vein all the way to the catheter hub (Fig. 7–4).
- Hold the catheter flange in place with the nondominant hand.

- Apply light pressure to the vein proximal to the indwelling catheter tip with the little finger of the nondominant hand, release the tourniquet, and remove the needle portion with the dominant hand (Fig. 7–5).
- Attach the administration set and release proximal pressure on the vein (Fig. 7–6). The infusion may begin.

Caution: Once the stylette has been withdrawn from the catheter (even partially), it

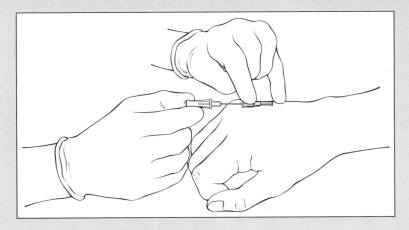

Figure 7–5

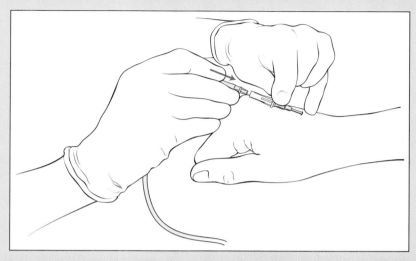

Figure 7–6

should never be reinserted. Attempting to do so can result in the shearing off of a small portion of the distal catheter, which then floats free in the circulatory system. This small piece of catheter floats until it lodges in a smaller vessel and potentially creates a site for embolism and infarction.

Butterfly Needle Cannulation

■ Once the flashback is noted, thread the needle in gently up the distended vein

to its hub with the dominant hand (Fig. 7–7). Be careful not to puncture the vein's posterior wall.
■ Hold the plastic butterfly portion of the IV line in place against the skin with the nondominant hand and apply light pressure to the vein proximal to the indwelling needle tip with the little finger of this hand.
■ Release the tourniquet and attach the administration set.
■ Last, release the proximal pressure on the vein and begin the infusion.

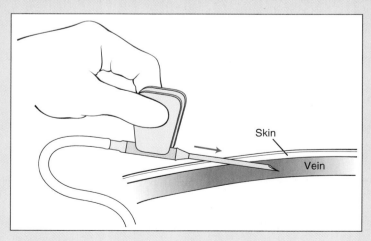

Figure 7–7

Procedure for Inserting an Intravenous Catheter – *(continued)*

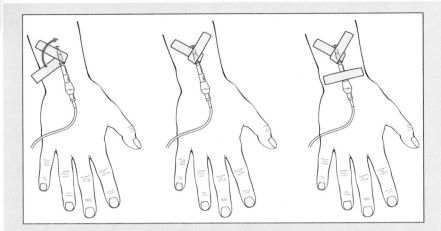

Figure 7–8

16. Inspect the site for any signs of swelling. If swelling is observed, turn off the infusion of fluids and remove the IV line. Apply pressure to the site for at least 3 to 5 minutes. Insertion of the IV line should next be attempted at a more proximal site or in the other extremity.

17. Secure the butterfly or catheter with chevron taping. Slip a 4- to 5-inch-long piece of 1/2-inch tape under the base of the IV line, adhesive side up, and then cross over the hub to adhere it to the skin proximal to the insertion site.

18. Tape the distal end of the administration set tubing to the skin. Avoid taping over the insertion site (Fig. 7–8).

Note: Some institutions recommend the use of an antibiotic ointment at the IV insertion site.

19. Apply either a gauze bandage or an occlusive dressing over the site.

20. Loop and secure the tubing separate from the butterfly or catheter (Fig. 7–9).

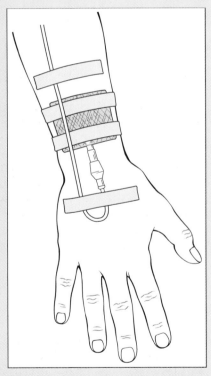

Figure 7–9

Special Considerations

- Butterfly IV line equipment is especially useful in the pediatric population. It has also been termed a *scalp vein IV line* because of this historically useful site for infants (Weinstein, 1997). However, scalp veins are no longer the first choice for IV access in babies. With small IV catheters available, the sites currently recommended are the hand, forearm, upper arm, foot, and antecubital fossa. Proper securing of the IV line in children is paramount.
- In the geriatric population, the smallest catheter possible (based on infusion indication) should be used. Skin care is an important consideration, with careful securing of the catheter onto the often fragile skin. A tourniquet may not be necessary. Although the site selection process is the same as the one for adults presented earlier, in geriatric patients, the smaller vessels may be fragile and rupture easily. At the other extreme, the larger, hardened, distended veins may represent sclerotic vessel walls, which may make puncture and threading difficult. It is important to avoid lower extremity IV lines in this population.

Follow-Up Care and Instructions

- Instruct the patient receiving IV therapy or the caregiver to notify the IV therapist if there is burning, stinging, redness, bleeding, or swelling at the insertion site. These may be initial signs of infection. The IV solution should be discontinued immediately if these symptoms occur.
- The rare patient on home IV therapy will require additional education in regard to fluid management, dressings, and possible complications. The most common complication of any IV therapy is phlebitis, which is often a result of movement of the needle or catheter within the vein. This vein may appear indurated, tender, erythematous, hardened, and very warm to the touch. The IV line should be removed immediately (Way, 1994). If the patient experiences significant discomfort, oral analgesics and warm, moist soaks to the area may be administered (Sager and Bomar, 1980).

References

Gardner C: United States House of Representatives honors the National Intravenous Therapy Association, Inc. J Natl Intravenous Ther Assoc 5:14, 1982.

Heckman J: Emergency Care and Transportation of the Sick and Injured. Rosemont, Ill, American Academy of Orthopaedic Surgeons, 1993.

Sager D, Bomar S: Intravenous Medications. Philadelphia, JB Lippincott, 1980.

Way L: Current Surgical Diagnosis and Treatment. Norwalk, Conn, Appleton & Lange, 1994 .

Weinstein S: Plummer's Principles and Practices of Intravenous Therapy. New York, Lippincott-Raven, 1997.

Chapter 8

Arterial Puncture

▷ Claire Babcock O'Connell

Procedure Goals and Objectives

Goal: To obtain a high-quality sample of arterial blood while observing standard precautions and with a minimal degree of risk to the patient.

Objectives: The student will be able to . . .

▶ Describe the indications, contraindications, and rationale for performing an arterial puncture.

▶ Identify and describe common complications associated with arterial punctures.

▶ Describe how to perform an Allen test.

▶ Describe the essential anatomy and physiology associated with the performance of an arterial puncture.

▶ Identify the materials necessary for performing an arterial puncture and their proper use.

▶ Properly perform the actions necessary to collect an arterial sample of blood.

▶ Identify the important aspects of post-care after an arterial puncture.

Background and History

Gaining intentional access to the circulatory system has been practiced for centuries. As discussed in Chapter 5, at approximately 400 years BC, Hippocrates exposed the view that disease was a result of excess substances such as blood, phlegm, black bile, and yellow bile within the body. Resulting from this view, it was believed that the removal of the excess could restore balance. Bloodletting, which involved cutting into a vein with a sharp instrument to release blood from the circulatory system, was commonplace.

Accessing the arterial system specifically is a relatively recent procedure. The first recorded arterial puncture was performed in 1912, and the first arterial sample used for blood gas analysis was obtained in 1919. However, routine blood gas analysis was not practiced until after 1953 with the introduction of technology designed to measure oxygen pressure (McCall and Tankersley, 1998).

Indications

Arterial puncture is indicated whenever a sample of arterial blood is required. Unlike venous blood, the level of dissolved gases in an arterial sample is constant throughout the arterial system. Therefore, a sample obtained from any arterial site represents the true level of gases dissolved in the blood within the arterial system. Arterial blood is preferred whenever an assessment of the level of dissolved gases is needed for diagnostic or therapeutic purposes. The following is a list of conditions that may necessitate arterial sampling:

- Diagnosis of an acute dysfunction in CO_2/O_2 exchange or acid-base balance: Conditions include severe exacerbations of asthma, suspected pulmonary thromboembolism, coma of unknown cause, suspected drug overdose, and cardiac arrhythmias that are refractory to medical intervention.
- Monitoring the severity and progression of a documented disease process in patients with a chronic condition that affects CO_2/O_2 exchange or acid-base balance: Progressive chronic obstructive pulmonary disease (COPD) may be monitored through changes from baseline arterial blood gas values. Patients receiving long-term oxygen therapy should be monitored when changes in status occur and periodically to document status.
- After therapeutic hyperventilation therapy or cardiopulmonary resuscitation, arterial blood gas determinations assist with the need to quantify the patient's response to therapeutic interventions, thus monitoring a return to baseline or the need for further intervention.

Procurement of an arterial sample may be preferred for a specific laboratory test that offers the most accurate assessment when performed on arterial blood. An arterial blood sample is preferable to venous blood samples when assessing ammonia levels, carbon monoxide levels, and lactate levels. Other laboratory tests can be performed using an arterial sample when venous access cannot be readily obtained, such as emergency situations of severe hypovolemia.

Contraindications

- Arterial puncture for blood sampling is absolutely contraindicated whenever the arterial pulse is not palpable.
- For the radial artery, negative results of a modified Allen test (collateral circulation test) suggest an inadequate collateral blood supply to the hand, and an alternate arterial site should be selected. To perform the Allen test, have the patient make a tight fist and elevate the hand; occlude both the radial and ulnar arteries using firm pressure for approximately 1 minute until the hand appears blanched. Lower the hand while maintaining pressure and instruct the patient to open the fist. Release only the ulnar compression while maintaining the radial artery pressure. Color should return to the entire hand within 15 seconds (positive test). Failure of color to return to normal indicates occlusion of the collateral circulation (negative test); radial artery puncture in this setting may result in ischemia and gangrene distal to the site and should not be attempted (Fig. 8–1).
- Attempting an arterial puncture when surface landmarks are not visible is not recommended.
- Arterial puncture is inadvisable in the presence of arterial disease, including atherosclerosis, arterial inflammatory conditions, or known or suspected aneurysm.
- The higher pressure inherent to the arterial system makes arterial puncture a considerably higher risk in a patient with a coagulopathy or in one undergoing anticoagulant therapy; a possible future need for such therapy should also be considered.

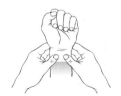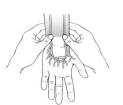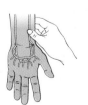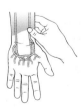

Figure 8–1. Modified Allen test. (Redrawn from Pfenninger JL, Fowler GC: Procedures for Primary Care Physicians. St. Louis, Mosby-Year Book, 1994, p 343.)

- Arterial puncture should also be avoided in a patient undergoing therapy for end-stage renal disease who may need arteriovenous shunt placement in the future.
- Local skin irritations, including infections (such as cellulitis), chronic skin rashes, and burned areas should be avoided. If these conditions are present in the site desired for arterial puncture, an alternative site should be selected.

Potential Complications

Arterial puncture is an invasive procedure with the potential for significant complications and must be performed with priority given to the safety of the patient. Any break from the proper safe technique can cause injury to the patient, which may result in loss of form and function to the body distal to the arterial puncture site. The risk of complications is increased any time repeated punctures are attempted at the same site.

- The most common complication is hemorrhage or hematoma formation at the puncture site. This occurs more often in brachial and femoral punctures than in radial punctures. Using the smallest gauge needle acceptable for the task will help to decrease the risk of hemorrhage or hematoma formation. Hematoma development can best be minimized by prompt pressure placed on the puncture site continuously for 10 minutes after the procedure is complete.
- Thrombosis is more common at the radial artery than at the brachial or femoral artery. It is more likely if the arterial puncture is performed on a vessel with occlusive disease. Thrombosis may lead to ischemia and gangrene distal to the puncture. Thrombosis may also cause distal embolization of a clot or plaque with resultant arterial occlusion. The potential for loss of function of the hand or fingers is considerable if arterial embolism occurs and is not quickly recognized and treated. The likelihood of thrombosis can be reduced by varying the site of repeated puncture and by using the smallest gauge needle possible. It is imperative to check for collateral circulation (Allen test) before a radial puncture.
- A transient arterial spasm may occur during or after arterial puncture. If this occurs, continue to monitor and assess the collateral circulation. If the circulation remains impaired, vascular consultation should be obtained. If the collateral circulation is compromised, immediate surgical intervention is warranted.
- Nerve damage may result from the inadvertent direct needle insertion into the nerve bundle or by excessive nerve compression secondary to a large hematoma in the adjacent area. If the patient has a coagulopathy that delays clotting, the risk is increased.

• Infection is rare when proper technique is followed. Proper sterile technique and avoidance of broken or damaged skin when choosing the site for arterial puncture will minimize this risk.

Review of Essential Anatomy and Physiology

Radial Artery

The radial artery is the site most frequently used for arterial puncture. It is close to the skin surface and readily accessible. It also carries the lowest risk of complications. The radial artery runs along the lateral aspect of the anterior forearm and can be easily palpated between the styloid process of the radius and the flexor carpi radialis tendon. The point of maximal pulsation is just proximal (1 to 2 cm) to the transverse wrist crease.

Before attempting radial artery puncture, check for collateral circulation by performing the Allen test. The distal forearm and wrist should be slightly hyperextended and placed on a firm surface. A small, rolled towel placed under the wrist helps achieve hyperextension. The forearm, wrist, and towel can be secured to an armboard with tape for greater stability if necessary.

Brachial Artery

The brachial artery can be accessed if the radial artery has recently been punctured or is otherwise not available (Fig. 8–2). It carries a greater risk of complication, including trauma to the basilic vein or median nerve. If occlusive complications occur, there is greater potential for tissue loss distal to the artery because the collateral circulation is less extensive. The brachial artery courses along the medial surface of the

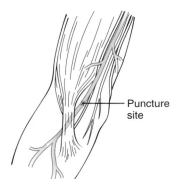

Puncture site

Figure 8–2. The right brachial artery, its branches, and the anatomic site for brachial artery puncture. (Redrawn from Pfenninger JL, Fowler GC: Procedures for Primary Care Physicians. St. Louis, Mosby-Year Book, 1994, p 345.)

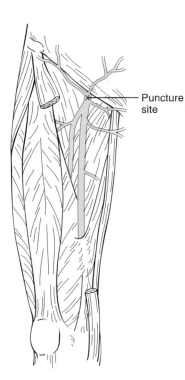

Puncture site

Figure 8–3. The right femoral artery and branches. (Redrawn from Pfenninger JL, Fowler GC: Procedures for Primary Care Physicians. St. Louis, Mosby-Year Book, 1994, p 345.)

antecubital fossa and should be accessed above the antecubital crease. The arm should be fully extended and secured to a firm surface, ulnar side up.

Femoral Artery

The femoral artery should be punctured only if radial or brachial artery access is not possible or advisable (Fig. 8–3). If the patient is severely volume depleted or is in shock, the femoral artery may be the only pulse with enough pressure to obtain arterial blood. The femoral artery can be located using the mnemonic NAVEL (*n*erve, *a*rtery, *v*ein, *e*mpty space, *l*ymphatics) from lateral to medial in the inguinal crease. The patient should be supine on a firm surface with hip extended and rotated externally.

Standard Precautions ▷ Practitioners should use Standard Precautions at all times when interacting with patients. Determining the level of precaution necessary requires the practitioner to exercise clinical judgment based on the patient's history and the potential for exposure to body fluids or aerosol-borne pathogens (for further discussion, see Chapter 2).

Patient Preparation

- The patient should be educated concerning the purpose of the test and advised of the potential level of discomfort and complications associated with performing the procedure.
- If consent forms are available, consent should be obtained.
- It is important that the patient remain as still as possible during the procedure.

Materials Utilized for Arterial Puncture

- 3- to 5-mL glass or special heparinized syringe made for arterial blood gas collection.
  Note: If not available, use plastic syringe and heparinize (see further on).
- 21- to 25-gauge, ½- to ⅝-inch needle
- Bag or cup of ice for transport
- Iodine-containing skin preparation pads
- Cork board or rubber for needle safety
- Rubber stopper or plug for syringe
- Sterile gloves, two pair
- Sterile gauze, 2 inch × 2 inch or 4 inch × 4 inch
- Arm board
- Tape—½ to 1 inch
- Goggles
- 1:1000 lidocaine *without* epinephrine, 1 to 2 mL
- Syringe and needle for local anesthesia

Procedure for Arterial Puncture

1. Secure and stabilize the site by placing the patient's arm on the arm board and securing with tape.
2. Put on sterile gloves
3. Cleanse skin with an iodine solution (e.g., povidone-iodine [Betadine], iodophor).

Note: Some practitioners prefer to follow this with an alcohol cleansing. Allow the area to air dry.

4. Coat the syringe and needle with heparin; use a plain plastic syringe if a preheparinized syringe is not available. Heparinize by aspirating 0.5 mL heparin, 10,000 U/mL, and pulling the plunger to the end of the syringe while holding the syringe and needle vertically. Slowly push back on the plunger to evacuate the heparin. The syringe and needle are now adequately coated with heparin.

Note: Heparinization of the syringe is necessary to prevent coagulation of the sample.

Procedure for Arterial Puncture – *(continued)*

Local Anesthesia

Note: Traditionally, arterial puncture has been performed without the use of local anesthesia. Several studies have proved that there is a significant decrease in pain when local anesthesia is administered before arterial puncture. Concerns that local anesthesia would inhibit proper placement by obliterating landmarks have been unfounded. The use of local anesthesia does make arterial puncture a "two-stick" procedure rather than a "one-stick" procedure. However, the intensity of the pain associated with arterial puncture may support the use of the less painful stick required with local anesthesia.

Note: Use a small amount (1 to 2 mL) of lidocaine *without* epinephrine to anesthetize the local area. Overzealous anesthesia may obscure landmarks or dull the pulse.

5. Put on sterile gloves. Advance the needle to just above the periosteum on each side of the artery without entering or making direct contact with the artery. Aspiration should be attempted before injecting the anesthetic to ensure that the anesthetic is injected into the surrounding tissues and not a blood vessel.

Note: Allow several minutes for the anesthetic to take effect before performing the arterial puncture. (For more information regarding local anesthesia techniques, refer to Chapter 22.)

6. Palpate the artery with the nondominant hand and locate the point of maximal pulsation.
7. Face the patient. Hold the syringe like a dart or a pencil with the bevel facing proximally.
8. Insert the needle at a 45- to 60-degree angle (60- to 90-degree angle for femoral puncture) (Fig. 8–4).

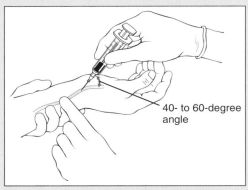

40- to 60-degree angle

Figure 8–4. Redrawn from Pfenninger JL, Fowler GC: Procedures for Primary Care Physicians. St. Louis, Mosby-Year Book, 1994, p 345.

9. Advance the needle until blood is seen entering the hub.
10. If no blood is seen, pull back until the needle is just below the skin and redirect the point 1 mm to either side. Do not exit completely.
11. Once blood enters the hub of the needle, the arterial pressure should cause blood to fill the syringe spontaneously.
12. In severely hypotensive patients, slight aspiration may be required, but this is rarely necessary.
13. Collect 3 mL of blood and then remove the needle with a swift, smooth motion.
14. Immediately apply firm, continuous pressure to the area for a minimum of 10 minutes, longer if the patient is hypertensive or is receiving anticoagulant therapy. Pressure should be applied even if no sample is obtained (Fig. 8–5).

Note: It is not advisable to have the patient apply the pressure; an assistant is recommended.

15. Hold the syringe and needle upright and allow any air bubbles to rise; tapping gently on the side of the syringe may help. Expel any air from the syringe.

Procedure for Arterial Puncture – *(continued)*

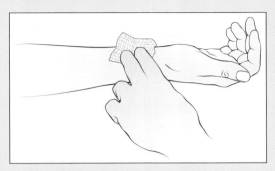

Figure 8–5. Redrawn from Potter P: Fundamentals of Nursing, 4th ed. St. Louis, Mosby-Year Book, 1997.

16. Insert the needle into a cork or rubber piece for safety; remove the needle from the syringe and close the syringe with a rubber stopper.

17. Gently roll the syringe between your palms to ensure uniform mixing of the sample with the heparin.
18. Label the syringe and place it on ice for immediate transport to the laboratory.
19. Check the arterial puncture site for hematoma formation and adequate distal perfusion.
20. Return to the patient for a repeat check in 5 minutes and again in 15 minutes. Monitor for any changes in color, temperature, or function. Inquire if the patient has experienced any numbness, increased pain, or coldness.

Special Considerations

- Prompt analysis of the sample is imperative. Delay in analysis or improper chilling will cause the blood to dissociate from the hemoglobin, thus affecting oxygen levels.
- If air is trapped in the syringe, an open system exists, which may cause O_2 to be dissolved into the sample, causing a relative decrease in PCO_2 and an increase in PO_2. The use of a Vacutainer system will also allow O_2 to enter the sample. A plain plastic syringe may lose O_2 through diffusion.
- In the presence of leukocytosis ($>100,000/mm^3$) or thrombocytosis ($>10^6/mm^3$), consumption of O_2 may be great because of the breakdown of the excess cells. This will be accompanied by a release of CO_2, causing a pseudoacidosis. A delay in analysis or improper chilling will enhance this effect. The PCO_2 rises approximately 3 to 10 mm Hg/hour in an uniced specimen, but it is stable for approximately 1 to 2 hours in a properly iced specimen.
- Excess heparin in the syringe will cause a decrease in pH. This is due to the low pH of heparin as well as the dilutional effects on the bicarbonate present in the sample.

Follow-Up Care and Instructions

- Patients who have undergone this procedure must be monitored to ensure that hemostasis has been achieved.

- Advise the patient that a small amount of tenderness and ecchymosis may result from the procedure.
- Advise the patient to seek evaluation if he or she experiences increasing pain, redness, or coolness of the extremity distal to the arterial puncture site.

Reference

McCall RT, Tankersley CM: Phlebotomy Essentials, 2nd ed. Philadelphia, JB Lippincott, 1998.

Bibliography

- Bhardwaj D, Norris A, Won DT: Is skin puncture beneficial prior to arterial catheter insertion? Can J Anaesth 46:129–132, 1999.
- Chestnutt MS, Dewar TN, Locksley RM, Chestnutt M: Office and Bedside Procedures. New York, McGraw-Hill, 1996, pp 116–127.
- Fowler GC: Arterial puncture. In Pfenninger JL, Fowler GC (eds): Procedures for Primary Care Physicians. St. Louis, Mosby-Year Book, 1994, pp 340–347.
- Giner J, Casan P, Belda J, et al: Pain during arterial puncture. Chest 110: 1443–1445, 1996.
- Gomella LG: Clinician's Pocket Reference, 8th ed. New York, McGraw-Hill, 1997, pp 225–227.
- Lightowler JV, Elliot MW: Local anesthetic infiltration prior to arterial puncture for blood gas analysis: A survey of current practice and a randomised double blind placebo controlled trial. J R Coll Phys Lond 31:645–646, 1997.
- Macklis RM, Mendelsohn ME, Mudge GH: Introduction to Clinical Medicine, 3rd ed. Philadelphia, Lippincott-Raven, 1994, pp 123–129.
- Marini JJ, Wheeler AP: Critical Care Medicine: The Essentials. Philadelphia, Lippincott Williams & Wilkins, 1197, pp 105–107.
- Okeson, GC, Wulbrecht PH: The safety of brachial artery puncture for arterial blood sampling. Chest 114:748–751, 1998.

Chapter 9

Injections

▷ Robert J. McNellis

Procedure Goals and Objectives

Goal: To perform an injection successfully while observing universal precautions and with the minimal degree of risk to the patient.

Objectives: The student will be able to . . .

▶ Describe the indications, contraindications, and rationale for administering an injection.

▶ Identify and describe common complications associated with administering injections.

▶ Describe the essential anatomy and physiology associated with performing an injection.

▶ Identify the materials necessary for performing an injection and their proper use.

▶ Identify the important aspects of patient care after an injection.

Background and History

This chapter covers the most common procedures for parenteral administration of medications. Although *parenteral* means any route other than enteral (gastrointestinal), it ordinarily refers to methods of giving drugs by injection. The most common routes of parenteral medication administration are intradermal, subcutaneous, intramuscular (IM), and intravenous. Intravenous procedures are covered in Chapter 7.

Injections are part of the armamentarium of most medical disciplines. In addition to this common ground, each specialty has its own particular applications (Brokensha, 1999).

The first experiments with intravenous injections were carried out in 1642 by a gentleman's hunting servant in eastern Germany. Similar experiments were performed in 1656 by Christopher Wren (an astronomer, mathematician, and architect in Oxford, England) and by a group of scientists associated with the physicist Robert Boyle. These experiments were prompted by new knowledge about blood circulation provided by William Harvey in 1628. The first books on the applications of intravenous infusions in humans were published in 1664 and 1667. Bladders of animals or enema syringes were used as instruments. Because of lethal accidents, the infusions soon fell out of favor (Feldman, 2000).

Reinier de Graaf has been attributed with the invention of the injection syringe in the late 1660s. De Graaf studied under anatomist Johannes van Horne at the newly established University of Leyden in Holland. As a young student, De Graaf helped Van Horne prepare anatomic specimens, and he used the injection syringe to introduce liquids and wax into the prepared blood vessels as a coloring and preservation medium.

In 1853, Charles Pravaz, a French surgeon in Lyon, invented a small syringe, the piston of which could be driven by a screw, thus allowing exact doses. A sharp needle with a pointed trocar could be introduced into a vessel, making dissection unnecessary. Pravaz used his syringe for obliteration of arterial aneurysms by injection of ferric sesquichlorate. Pravaz's syringe initiated the invention of a great number of various calibrated syringes made of glass or metal combined with glass. The calibrated syringes were commonly used in the treatment of syphilis by mercurialization.

Also in 1853, in a paper entitled "A New Method of Treating Neuralgia by Direct Application of Opioids to the Painful Point," Alexander Wood introduced his hollow needle in London, England. Within 5 years, injections of morphine had become enormously popular; thriving practices developed in response to what was seen as a potent, benign, and beneficial treatment. Patients were treated with hundreds of injections. Their doctors seemed blissfully unaware of the systemic effects of the drug they were injecting and the nature of the demand for the new treatment.

Charles Hunter, another English physician, was discouraged from using the new technique when his first two patients developed local abscesses. In 1858, he discovered that patients gained just as much benefit from injections distant from the painful site. Hunter coined the term *hypodermic* and claimed that his treatment was superior. Physicians debated the merits of the two physicians' claims and decided in Hunter's favor. During the debate, physicians continued with both treatments, apparently blind to the addiction underlying the huge and increasingly lucrative demand (Howard-Jones, 1971).

Since the 19th century, there have been great advances in understanding the mechanisms of action of parenteral medications and improvements in the technology of injections. However, the basic principles remain the same. Today, injections can be given in any space or potential space; they can be administered hypodermically under direct vision or guided by ultrasonography or radiography, as well as through the use of endoscopic techniques. The widespread use of needleless (jet) injection systems is just on the horizon. Delivery systems that are less invasive, such as nasal sprays, transdermal patches, and continuous infusion devices, may make injections less and less common.

Indications

Indications include an illness or injury that requires parenteral medication to improve, treat, or maintain the patient's condition, as well as administration of vaccines for disease prevention.

Contraindications

Potential contraindications to injections include the following conditions:

- Allergy to the intended medication
- Lack of a suitable site for injection
- Coagulopathy
- Occlusive peripheral vascular disease
- Shock
- Impairment of peripheral absorption

Potential Complications

- Anaphylactic or toxic reaction to the medication: Treatment is supportive for anaphylaxis and may vary depending on the severity of the reaction. Medication to reverse the toxic effect of the drug should be readily available. Risk of anaphylaxis can be minimized by always asking the patient about allergies or checking medical alert bracelets before injection.

- Medication error: Errors can often be avoided by using the "five rights" as guidelines for the administration of medication. These guidelines ensure that the right drug is given to the right patient in the right dose by the right route at the right time.
  - Right drug: The medication label should be checked three times: when the drug is taken from storage, when the amount of drug is removed, and when the container is returned to storage.
  - Right patient: Always check the patient's identification bracelet or ask the patient to state his or her name.
  - Right dose: Errors in dose are minimized when the unit system is used and a pharmacist prepares drugs. If a drug dose for an infant or child must be calculated, it is important to have a second person check the arithmetic, because even a small error could lead to a serious overdose. It is good practice to have a second person always double check doses of heparin, insulin, and epinephrine.
  - Right route: Only give injections of substances prepared for parenteral use; it should say "injectable" on the label. Avoid giving an inadvertent intravenous injection by drawing back before pushing the drug.
  - Right time: It is important to know why a drug is ordered for a certain time. Be sure to document when drugs were given.
- The practitioner is responsible for the medications that are administered. Administer only those drugs prepared personally or those that were prepared by the pharmacist, unless there is an emergency situation.
- Infection or abscess at the site: Infection typically occurs as the result of improper aseptic technique. Sterile abscesses can occur after injecting concentrated or irritating solutions. Rotating injection sites can minimize this complication. Injections should be avoided at sites that are inflamed, edematous, or irritated or at sites with moles, birthmarks, scar tissue, or other lesions.
- Lipodystrophy or atrophy of subcutaneous fat, which is caused from repeated injections at the same site: Rotating injection sites can minimize this complication.
- Injection pain: Minimize the use of irritating solutions given subcutaneously to reduce pain. Techniques to reduce the pain of intramuscular injections include having the patient relax the muscle, avoiding extrasensitive areas, waiting until the antiseptic is dry before injecting the medication, using a new needle for injection, inserting and withdrawing the needle rapidly, massaging the muscle after injection to distribute the medication better and increase its absorption, and using ice or topical spray to numb the area before injection.

Review of Essential Anatomy and Physiology

Intradermal injections are given in the outer layers of the skin. There is little systemic absorption of intradermally injected agents, so this type of injection is given primarily to produce a local effect. The ventral forearm is the most commonly used site because of its easy accessibility and lack of hair. In extensive allergy testing, the outer aspect of the upper arms and the area of the back between the scapulae are used.

Subcutaneous injections are given into the adipose tissue beneath the skin. The most common sites are the outer aspects of the upper arm, anterior thigh, loose tissue of the lower abdomen, upper buttocks, and upper back (see Fig. 9–1).

Intramuscular injections deposit medication deep into muscle, tissue, where it can be readily absorbed. The rate of drug absorption is faster than with the subcutaneous route but slower than with the intravenous route.

Intramuscular sites (Fig. 9–2) include the following:

- Deltoid muscle: The deltoid muscle is located on the lateral side of the humerus. Place four fingers across the deltoid muscle, with the top finger along the acromion process. The injection site is two to three fingerbreadths below the acromion process (Fig. 9–3). Injecting lower or more posterior in the muscle can result in injury to the radial and ulnar nerves or brachial artery.
- Dorsogluteal (gluteus medius): Locate the posterior superior iliac spine and the greater trochanter of the femur. Draw an imaginary line between the two landmarks. The injection site is above and lateral to the line. A less accurate method is dividing the buttocks into quadrants. The vertical dividing line extends from the gluteal fold up to the iliac crest. The injecting horizontal line extends from the medial fold to the lateral aspect of the buttock. The injection site is the upper outer quadrant, about 2 to 3 inches below the iliac crest. The risk of injury to the sciatic nerve can be great at this site; injury can cause paralysis of the affected leg (Fig. 9–4).
- Ventrogluteal (gluteus medius and gluteus minimus): Place the heel of your hand over the greater trochanter. Point the thumb toward the groin and fingers toward the head. Place the index finger over the

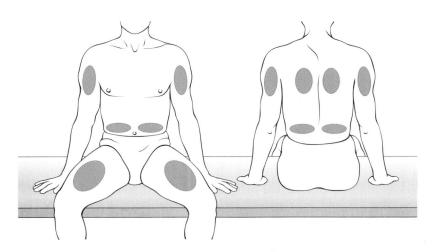

Figure 9–1. Sites for subcutaneous injection.

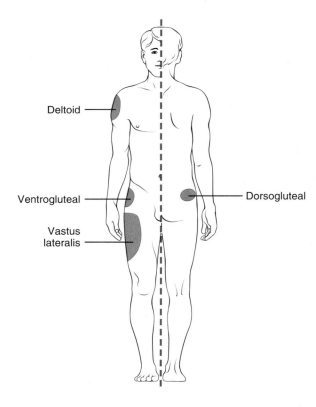

Figure 9-2. Sites for intramuscular injection.

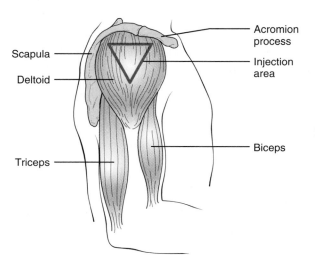

Figure 9-3. Deltoid muscle.

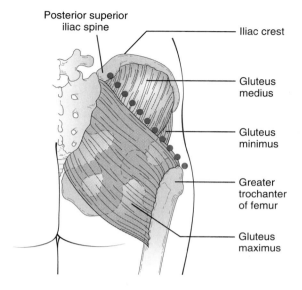

Figure 9–4 labels:
Posterior superior iliac spine
Iliac crest
Gluteus medius
Gluteus minimus
Greater trochanter of femur
Gluteus maximus

Figure 9–4. Inject above and lateral to dotted line.

anterosuperior iliac spine and extend the middle finger along the iliac crest. The index finger and middle finger form a V. Inject into the center of the V. The muscles of this site are deep and away from major nerves and blood vessels (Fig. 9–5).

- Vastus lateralis muscle: This muscle is located at the anterolateral aspect of the thigh and extends from a handbreadth above the knee to a handbreadth below the greater trochanter of the femur. The middle third of the muscle is the best site for injection. This site is a well-developed muscle that lacks major nerves and blood vessels. The branches of the lateral femoral cutaneous nerve are located superficially, and a few cases of damage to these branches have been reported. It is the preferred site for infants, children, and adults (Fig. 9–6.)

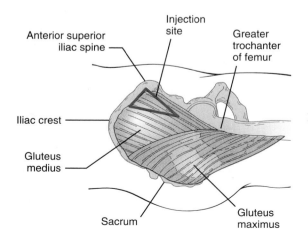

Figure 9–5 labels:
Injection site
Anterior superior iliac spine
Greater trochanter of femur
Iliac crest
Gluteus medius
Sacrum
Gluteus maximus

Figure 9–5. Ventrogluteal site.

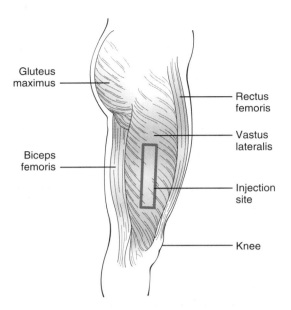

Gluteus maximus

Biceps femoris

Rectus femoris

Vastus lateralis

Injection site

Knee

Figure 9–6. Vastus lateralis site.

Parenteral medication administration provides longer action and avoids the first-pass metabolic effects of the liver. Each route of administration has advantages and disadvantages.

- Intradermal injections (ID) are advantageous for their slow absorption, which is an advantage when testing for allergies.
- Its disadvantages are that only small amounts of drug may be administered and it requires an aseptic technique.
- Subcutaneous (SC) injections have the advantage of faster onset of drug action than exists with the oral route.
- Disadvantages include the need for aseptic technique, their greater expense over oral medication, and only a small volume can be administered, some drugs can irritate tissues and cause pain, and they can produce anxiety.
- Intramuscular injections have the advantage of minimizing pain from irritating drugs, larger volumes of drug can be administered than with the subcutaneous route, and the drug is rapidly absorbed.
- Disadvantages include the requirement for aseptic technique, and that blood vessels and nerves can be damaged, and it can produce anxiety.

Standard Precautions ▷ Every practitioner should use Standard Precautions at all times when interacting with patients, especially when performing procedures. Determining the level of precaution necessary requires the practitioner to exercise clinical judgment based on the patient's history and the potential for exposure to body fluids or aerosol-borne pathogens (for further discussion, see Chapter 2).

Patient Preparation

- Ask the patient if he or she is allergic to any medications and the type of reaction that occurs.
- Explain to the patient why it is necessary to administer the injection.
- Inform the patient of the benefits and risks in understandable language.
- Inform the patient which site will be used for administering the injection.
- Tell the patient that there will be a sting or pricking sensation felt when the needle is inserted.
- Warn the patient of potential side effects, and advise the patient of signs and symptoms to watch for.
- Ask again about allergies.

Materials Utilized for Administering an Injection

- Appropriate medication
- Syringe and needle
- Materials for cleansing the skin: alcohol pad, most commonly saturated with 70% isopropyl alcohol
- Sterile or nonsterile gloves
- Needle disposal box
- Bandage strips and gauze pads
  Note: Medication comes in many forms:
  - Ampule containing a single dose of drug
  - Vial containing single or multiple drug doses
  - Vial containing powder to which a sterile diluent or solvent must be added with some drugs
  - Prefilled cartridge package
  - Syringe
  Note: Syringes range in size from a capacity of 1 mL to 50 mL, but syringes larger than 5 mL are rarely used for injections. A 2- or 3-mL syringe is adequate for most subcutaneous and intramuscular injections. Most institutions use plastic syringes, although some medications in prefilled cartridges require cartridge syringes (e.g., Tubex).
  Note: Insulin syringes have a capacity of 1 mL and are calibrated in units. There is a syringe designed for use with each strength of insulin. For example, a syringe marked U100 is coded to match the label of a vial of insulin that contains 100 units/mL. Tuberculin syringes also have a capacity of 1 mL, but they are long, slender, and calibrated in 0.01-mL

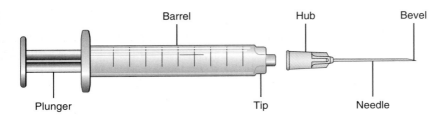

Figure 9–7. Parts of a syringe and needle.

units. This fine calibration makes it possible to administer very small amounts of potent drugs, such as those used for intradermal skin testing.

■ Barrel of the syringe, handle of the plunger, and hub of the needle

Note: These parts must, of necessity, be handled during the preparation and administration of an injection, but the inside and tip of the barrel and the shaft of the plunger must be kept sterile, as must the entire length of the needle (Fig. 9–7).

■ Needle

Note: Needles that are commonly used for injections vary in length from ½ to 1½ inches; they vary in diameter from 14 to 26 gauge (the larger the gauge, the smaller the diameter). A common size for a subcutaneous injection is 25 gauge, ⅝ inch; the needle for an intramuscular injection is larger and longer: 18 to 22 gauge, 1½ inches. Typically, needles for intradermal injections are 26 or 27 gauge and ½ to ⅝ inch long. Needles are packaged individually to permit greater flexibility in selecting the right needle for a specific patient. A syringe and needle may be packaged together if the size of the needle is relatively standard, such as an insulin or tuberculin syringe and needle.

Note: The length of the needle is determined by the size and weight of the patient and whether the drug will be injected subcutaneously or intramuscularly. The gauge depends on the viscosity of the fluid to be injected. A thin, watery, nonsticky solution can be injected easily through a fine-gauge needle (25 or 26), but a thicker, sticky solution requires a larger gauge needle (20 to 22).

Note: Many institutions are beginning to move toward needleless or safety needle systems for injections. In these systems, medication can often be drawn through vials without needles and after the injection, needles retract into the plunger, or a sheath covers the needles. Follow the manufacturer's instructions for proper use of these systems.

Procedure for Aspirating from an Ampule

1. Identify the patient.
2. Wash your hands and put on gloves.
3. Select and assemble the appropriately sized needle and syringe (use filter needle with glass ampule if the medication requires it).
4. Remove the liquid from the neck of the ampule by flicking it or swinging it quickly in a downward, spiraling motion while holding it by the top (Fig. 9–8A).
5. Tap around the neck of the ampule.
6. Protect your fingers with gauze if the ampule is made of glass.
7. Carefully break off the top of the ampule (for a plastic ampule twist the top) (see Fig. 9–8B).
8. Aspirate fluid from the ampule (see Fig. 9–8C).
9. Remove any air from the syringe as needed.
10. Clean up and dispose of working needle and ampule in accordance with your institution's policy for disposing of contaminated materials and sharp objects (see Chapter 2).

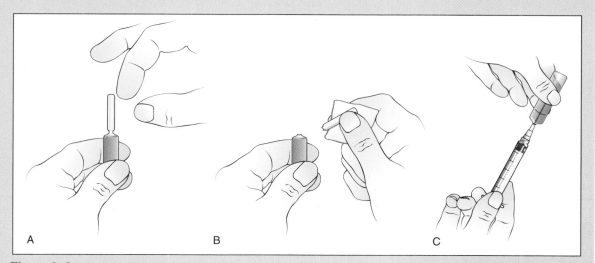

A   B   C

Figure 9–8

Procedure for Aspirating from a Vial

1. Identify the patient.
2. Wash hands and put on gloves.
3. Disinfect the top of the vial with an alcohol pad.
4. Select a syringe with a volume twice the required amount of drug or solution and add the needle.

Procedure for Aspirating from a Vial – *(continued)*

5. Draw up as much air as the amount of solution that will be aspirated.
6. Insert the needle into the top of the vial and turn upside down (Fig. 9–9*A*).
7. Push air out of the syringe into the vial (see Fig. 9–9*B*).
8. Aspirate the required amount of solution.

Note: Make sure the tip of the needle is below the fluid surface.

9. Pull the needle out of the vial.
10. Remove air from the syringe as needed (see Fig. 9–9*C*).
11. Clean up and dispose of materials in accordance with your institution's policy for disposing of contaminated materials and sharp objects (see Chapter 2).

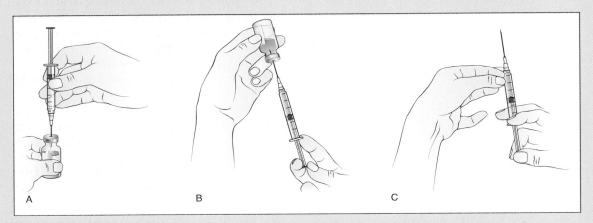

A   B   C

Figure 9–9

Procedure for Administering an Intradermal Injection

1. Identify the patient.
2. Wash hands and put on gloves.
3. Select a tuberculin syringe with a 26- or 27-gauge needle: ½- to ⅝-inch long is generally used.
4. Using aseptic technique, withdraw the appropriate amount of medication from the vial or ampule.
5. With the patient sitting up, have him or her extend the forearm and lay on a flat surface with the ventral side exposed.
6. Cleanse the surface of the ventral forearm about two to three fingerbreadths distal to the antecubital space using an alcohol pad.

Note: Be sure the test site is free of hair and lesions. Allow the skin to dry completely before administering the injection.

Procedure for Administering an Intradermal Injection – *(continued)*

7. While holding the patient's forearm in your hand, stretch the skin taut with your thumb.

8. With your free hand, hold the needle at a 15-degree angle to the patient's arm, with its bevel facing up.

9. Insert the needle about ⅛ inch below the epidermis (Fig. 9–10). Stop when the needle bevel is under the skin, and inject the antigen slowly. You should feel some resistance as you do this, and a wheal or bleb should form as you inject the antigen. If no wheal forms, you have injected the antigen too deeply; withdraw the needle and administer another test dose at least 2 inches from the first site.

10. Withdraw the needle at the same angle at which it was inserted.

11. Do not rub the site. This could cause irritation of the underlying tissue and may affect the test results.

12. Dispose of the syringe and needle according to your institution's policy regarding disposal of contaminated items (see Chapter 2).

13. Document which agents were given, including the lot number and expiration date; where, how (which specific injection method), and when they were given; and by whom.

14. Assess the patient's response in 24 to 48 hours.

Note: In patients hypersensitive to the test antigen, a severe anaphylactic response can result. This requires immediate epinephrine injection and other emergency resuscitation procedures. Be especially alert after giving a test dose of penicillin or tetanus antitoxin.

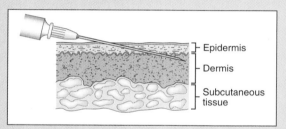

Epidermis

Dermis

Subcutaneous tissue

Figure 9–10

Procedure for Administering a Subcutaneous Injection

1. Identify the patient.

2. Wash hands and put on gloves.

3. Select a 2- to 3-mL syringe with a 24- to 26-gauge needle that is ⅜ to 1 inch long, depending on the amount of subcutaneous fat.

Note: A longer needle is needed for an obese adult, a shorter needle for a thin child.

4. Using aseptic technique, withdraw the appropriate amount of medication from the vial or ampule.

5. Select an appropriate site.

6. Rotate sites according to a planned schedule for patients who require repeated injections. Use different areas of the body unless contraindicated by the specific drug.

7. Position and drape the patient.

8. Cleanse the injection site with a sterile alcohol pad, beginning at the center of the site and moving outward in a circular motion.

Procedure for Administering a Subcutaneous Injection – *(continued)*

Note: Allow the skin to dry so that alcohol is not introduced into subcutaneous tissues as the needle is inserted.

9. With the nondominant hand, pinch the skin around the injection site.
10. Inject the needle with the bevel up at a 45-degree angle (Fig. 9–11). If a fat fold is more than 1 inch, the needle may be injected at a 90-degree angle.

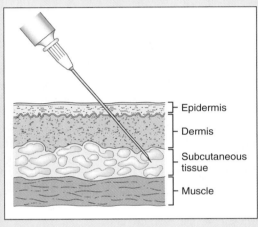

Figure 9–11

Epidermis

Dermis

Subcutaneous tissue

Muscle

11. Release the patient's skin to avoid injecting into compressed tissue and irritating nerve fibers.
12. Pull back on the plunger slightly. If no blood is aspirated, begin injecting the drug slowly. If blood appears on aspiration, withdraw the needle, prepare another syringe, and repeat the procedure.
13. After injection, remove the needle gently but quickly at the same angle used for insertion.
14. Cover the site with an alcohol sponge or sterile gauze pad and massage the site gently (unless contraindicated, e.g., heparin) to distribute the drug and facilitate absorption.
15. Remove the sponge and check the injection site for bleeding.
16. Dispose of the syringe and needle according to your institution's policy regarding disposal of contaminated items (see Chapter 2).
17. Document the medication given, including the lot number and expiration date; where, how (specific injection method), and when it was given; and by whom.

Special Considerations

Administering Insulin

Note: To establish more consistent blood levels, rotate insulin injection sites within anatomic regions. Absorption varies from one region to another. Preferred insulin injection sites are the arms, abdomen, thighs, and buttocks.

1. Make sure the type of insulin, dose, and syringe are correct.
2. When combining different types of insulin in a syringe, make sure they are compatible. Regular insulin can be mixed with all types.
3. Before drawing up insulin suspension, gently roll and invert the bottle to ensure even particle distribution. Do not shake the bottle, because this can cause foam or bubbles to develop, changing the potency and altering the dose.

Administering Heparin

Note: The preferred site for heparin injections is the lower abdominal fat pad, 2 inches beneath the umbilicus, between the iliac crests. Injecting heparin into this area, which is not involved in muscular activity, reduces the risk of local capillary bleeding. Always rotate the sites from one side to the other.

Note: Do not administer any injections within 2 inches of a scar, bruise, or the umbilicus.

Note: Do not aspirate to check for blood return because this may cause bleeding into the tissues at the site.

Note: Do not rub or massage the site after the injection. Rubbing can cause localized minute hemorrhages or bruises.

Note: If the patient bruises easily, apply ice to the site for the first 5 minutes after the injection to minimize local hemorrhage.

Procedure for Administering an Intramuscular Injection

1. Identify the patient.
2. Wash hands and put on gloves.
3. Select a 2- to 5-mL syringe with an 18- to 22-gauge needle 1 to 2 inches in length, depending on the injection site and the amount of muscle mass of the patient.
4. Using aseptic technique, withdraw the appropriate amount of medication from the vial or ampule and then draw about 0.2 cc of air into the syringe.
5. Select an appropriate intramuscular site.
6. Position and drape the patient.
7. Cleanse the injection site with a sterile alcohol sponge, beginning at the center of the site and moving outward in a circular motion. Allow the skin to dry so that alcohol is not introduced into subcutaneous tissues as the needle is inserted.
8. With the thumb and index finger of your nondominant hand, press down and stretch the skin of the injection site.

Note: This reduces the thickness of subcutaneous tissue that must be pierced to reach the muscle. This is required in an obese patient. If the patient is emaciated, raise the underlying muscle mass by pinching the tissue between the thumb and index finger.

9. Position the syringe at a 90-degree angle to the skin surface, with the needle a couple of inches from the skin. Quickly and firmly thrust the needle through the skin and subcutaneous tissue deep into the muscle (Fig. 9–12).
10. Hold the syringe with your nondominant hand, if desired. Pull back slightly on the plunger with your dominant hand. If no blood is aspirated, place your thumb on the plunger rod and slowly inject the medication into the muscle.

Note: A slow, steady injection rate allows the muscle to distend gradually and accept the medication under minimal pressure. There should be little or no resistance

Procedure for Administering an Intramuscular Injection – *(continued)*

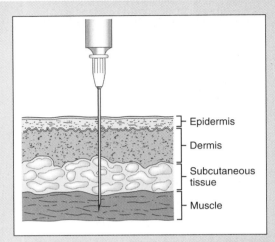

Figure 9–12

against the force of injection. The air bubble added to the syringe when it was prepared should follow the medication into the injection site to create an air block and prevent tracking of the medication back into the subcutaneous tissue (Fig. 9–13*A and B*).

11. If blood appears in the syringe on aspiration, the needle is in a blood vessel. If this occurs, withdraw the needle, prepare another injection with new equipment, and inject another site. Do not inject the bloody solution. (Follow your institution's policy for disposal of contaminated items.)

12. After the injection, gently but rapidly remove the needle at a 90-degree angle.

13. Cover the injection site immediately with an alcohol sponge or sterile gauze pad, apply gentle pressure and, unless contraindicated, massage the muscle to help distribute the drug and promote absorption.

14. Remove the alcohol sponge and inspect the injection site for signs of active bleeding. If bleeding continues, apply pressure to the site.

15. Dispose of the syringe and needle according to your institution's policy regarding disposal of contaminated items (see Chapter 2).

16. Document the medication given, including the lot number and expiration date; where, how (specific injection method), and when it was given; and by whom.

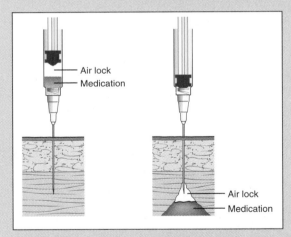

Figure 9–13

Procedure for Administering a Z-Track Intramuscular Injection

Note: The Z-track method of intramuscular injection prevents leakage of medication back into subcutaneous tissue after the injection is given. It is used with certain drugs—primarily iron preparations—that irritate or discolor subcutaneous tissue. Lateral displacement of the skin before injection helps seal the drug in the muscle after the skin is released. This procedure requires careful attention to technique, because leakage into subcutaneous tissue can cause patient discomfort or may permanently stain tissue if an iron preparation is being given. This type of injection is given only in the outer upper quadrant of the buttocks.

1. Identify the patient.
2. Wash hands and put on gloves.
3. Select a 3- to 5-mL syringe with two 20-gauge needles at least 2 inches long.
4. Using aseptic technique, withdraw the appropriate amount of medication from the vial or ampule and then draw about 0.2 to 0.5 cc of air into the syringe. Remove the first needle and attach the second needle to prevent introduction of medication from the outside of the first needle into the subcutaneous tissue.

Note: For this type of injection, be sure to provide privacy for the patient.

5. Select an appropriate site in an upper outer buttock.
6. Position and drape the patient in the prone or lateral position.
7. Cleanse the area with a sterile alcohol pad.
8. Displace the skin laterally by pulling it about ½ inch away from the injection site (Fig. 9–14A and B).

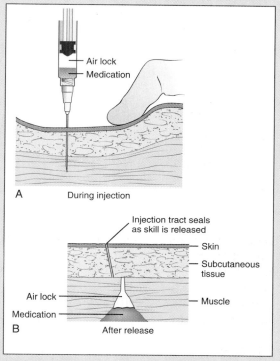

Figure 9–14

9. Insert the needle into the muscle at a 90-degree angle.
10. Pull back on the plunger slightly. If no blood is aspirated, inject the drug slowly, followed by the air, which helps clear the needle and prevents tracking of the medication through the subcutaneous tissue.
11. Encourage the patient to walk or move around in bed to facilitate absorption from the injection site.
12. Dispose of the syringe and needle according to your institution's policy regarding disposal of contaminated items (see Chapter 2).

13. Document the medication given, including the lot number and expiration date; where, how (specific injection method), and when it was given; and by whom.

Caution: Never inject more than 5 mL into a single site using the Z-track method.

Note: Alternate gluteal sites to avoid repeated injections in the same site. If the patient is on bed rest, encourage active range of motion exercises or perform passive range of motion exercises to facilitate absorption from the injection site.

Note: If you must inject more than 5 mL of solution, divide the solution and inject it at two separate sites unless the gluteal muscles and vastus lateralis are well developed. Intramuscular injections can traumatize local muscle cells, causing elevated serum levels of enzymes (creatine phosphokinase [CPK]) that can be confused with the elevated enzyme levels resulting from damage to cardiac muscle, as in myocardial infarction. Oral or intravenous routes are preferred for administration of drugs that are poorly absorbed by muscle tissue, such as phenytoin, digoxin, chlordiazepoxide, diazepam, and haloperidol.

Special Considerations

Pediatric Patients

- Subcutaneous injections are usually administered into the thigh of infants and into the deltoid area of older children.
- The preferred sites for intramuscular injections are the anterolateral aspect of the upper thigh and the deltoid muscle of the upper arm.
- Among most infants, the anterolateral thigh provides the largest muscle mass and is therefore the recommended site.
- The deltoid can also be used with the thigh when multiple injections (such as vaccinations) are needed.
- In toddlers and older children, the deltoid may be used if the muscle mass is adequate.
- Never use the gluteal muscles, which develop from walking, as the injection site for children younger than age 3 or for those who have been walking less than a year.
- The buttock should not be used routinely in children because of the risk of sciatic nerve injury (Bergeson et al, 1982).

Follow-Up Care and Instructions

- Immediately dispose of needle and syringe properly in an appropriate needle disposal ("sharps") container.

Caution: Never recap needles. It is important to follow this advice diligently to help minimize the 800,000 to 1 million needle stick injuries reported in the United States each year (see Chapter 2) (Jagger, 1988).

- Monitor the patient's response, especially after injections of large doses of antibiotic. Patient should be monitored for approximately 30 minutes for signs of anaphylaxis.
- Instruct the patient to report a new onset of fever, joint pain, shortness of breath, or rash. Also, tenderness, erythema, or ecchymosis at the injection site should be reported to the health care provider.

References

Bergeson PS, Singer SA, Kaplan AM: Intramuscular injections in children. Pediatrics 70:944–948, 1982.

Brokensha G: The hollow needle: Inappropriate injection in practice. Aust Prescr 22:145–147, 1999.

Feldman H: History of injections. Laryngorhinootologie 79:239–246, 2000.

Howard-Jones N: The origins of the hypodermic medications. Sci Am 224: 96–102, 1971.

Jagger J: Rates of needlestick injury caused by various devices in a university hospital. N Engl J Med 319:284–288, 1988.

Bibliography

- Centers for Disease Control: General recommendations on immunization recommendations of the Advisory Committee on Immunization Practices (ACIP). MMWR 43(RR01); 1–38, 1994.
- American Diabetes Association: Insulin administration. Diabetes Care 23(Suppl 1):S86, 2000.
- D'Angelo HH, Welsh NP (eds): Medication Administration and IV Therapy Manual, 2nd ed. Springhouse, PA, Springhouse, 1993.
- De Vries PGM, Henning RH, Hogerzeil HV: WHO Guide to Good Prescribing: The Use of Injections. World Health Organization, 1995. Available at http://www.med.rug.nl/pharma/ggp.htm
- Elkin MK, Perry AG, Potter PA: Nursing Interventions and Clinical Skills, 2nd ed. St. Louis, CV Mosby, 1999.
- Gilles FH, French JH: Postinjection sciatic nerve palsies in infants and children. J Pediatr 58:195–204, 1961.
- Newton M, Newton D, Fudin J: Reviewing the "big three" injection routes. Nursing 22:34–42, 1992.
- Smith SF, Duell DJ, Martin BC: Clinical Nursing Skills: Basic to Advanced Skills. Upper Saddle River, NJ, Prentice Hall Health, 2000.

Chapter 10

Performing an Electrocardiogram

▷ Richard R. Rahr

Procedure Goals and Objectives

Goal: To perform an electrocardiogram (ECG) safely and accurately.

Objectives: The student will be able to . . .

▶ Describe the indications, contraindications, and rationale for performing an ECG.

▶ Identify and describe common complications associated with performing an ECG.

▶ Describe the essential anatomy and physiology associated with the performance of an ECG.

▶ Identify the materials necessary for performing an ECG and their proper use.

▶ Accurately describe the steps in completing an ECG.

Background and History

In early experiments, Luigi Salvori demonstrated that stimulation of a charged glass rod attached to a frog's leg muscle would cause contraction of the muscle as if the frog willed it to do so (1790). Later, Kollickes and Mueller hooked a dissected frog's heart to the leg muscle; the frog's leg twitched with contraction each time the heart beat (1855). This was followed in 1880 by a crude capillary electrometer developed by Ludig and Waller that recorded the electrical activity of the heartbeat from the skin surface. However, it was not until 1901 that Einthoven invented a useful electrocardiography machine that passed light over a moving wire to produce the PQRSTU waveform that is used today (Fig. 10–1).

Einthoven was the scientist who developed the first three leads that bear his name as an axis triangle. The equilateral triangle at which leads I, II, and III come together is known as Einthoven's triangle. Einthoven's law states that the height of the R waves in leads I and III is equal to the height of the R waves in lead II.

Indications

The 12-lead electrocardiography procedure has revolutionized the standard of care in cardiology. Numerous advances in the study and function of the heart have led to sophisticated technology since the 12-lead ECG

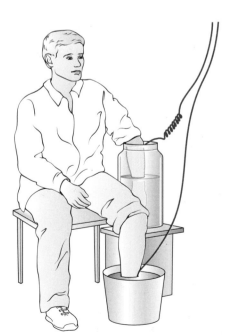

Figure 10–1. Electrocardiographic methodology in 1911. (Redrawn from Rawlings RR: Electrocardiography. Redmond, Wash, SpaceLab, 1991, p 26.)

was invented. The use of cardiac catheterization, echocardiography, nuclear medicine imaging, and magnetic resonance imaging (MRI) has dramatically changed the way cardiology is practiced. The 12-lead electrocardiography procedure, however, remains an effective and efficient method to screen for cardiovascular disease and monitor patients with acute and chronic coronary artery disease.

The ECG remains a useful and relatively inexpensive method used to detect the following:

- Ischemic heart disease, including myocardial infarction
- Heart block
- Dysrhythmia (including wide ventricular tachycardia)
- Electrolyte disturbances
- Abnormality in chamber size or myocardial hypertrophy

The use of the 12-lead ECG is essential in the following scenarios:

- At accidents or emergency calls; it increases the paramedic's capability to find true heart disease, with chest pain specificity of 62% to 90% (Taylor et al, 1998)
- Raises the sensitivity for finding true heart disease from 71% to 90% (Taylor et al, 1998)
- Gives hospital personnel early warning signs of a patient's condition when being transported for thrombolytic treatment or advanced arrhythmias; in some medical centers, thrombolytic drugs are started by the paramedic at the emergency site before the patient even reaches the hospital

The 12-lead ECG is critical and instrumental in reducing morbidity and mortality in coronary artery disease patients and also provides the practitioner with the tool needed to detect early warning signs and administer necessary treatment and reperfusion.

Contraindications

The only relative contraindications to performing the procedure follow:

- Concern that the recording equipment may be malfunctioning
- Allergy to the electrode adhesive

Potential Complications

- The most common complication of the 12-lead ECG is misinterpretation. A false-negative (normal) reading and interpretation could lead to death if practitioners ignore the possibility of a wrong interpretation.

In addition, a normal ECG does not necessarily mean a patient may not have underlying cardiac pathology.

- Other potential complications with the test are erroneous results that occur from errors in lead placement. It is always reasonable to repeat the ECG if the expected waveform pattern for a set of leads seems uncharacteristic or different from that expected.
- Since the procedure uses electrodes that are attached to the patient's skin either by adhesives or suction, the skin may tear easily in elderly or diabetic patients, creating the potential for infection.
- Although extremely unlikely, it is remotely possible that a patient could receive an electrical shock from the attachment of wires that have a short in the electrical circuit of the apparatus. Today, machines are protected by a third ground wire to prevent this complication from occurring.

Review of Essential Anatomy and Physiology

A general review of the anatomy and physiology of the heart is necessary to understand the relevance of the 12-lead ECG. The heart is a complex organ with the primary function of pumping blood through the pulmonic and systemic circulation. It is composed of four muscular chambers: right atrium and left atrium (collecting chambers) and right ventricle and left ventricle (pumping chambers) (Fig. 10–2). In addition, an

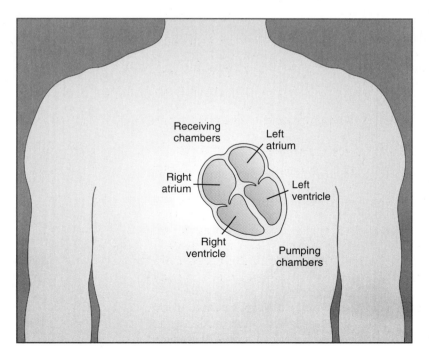

Figure 10–2. Anatomy of the heart.

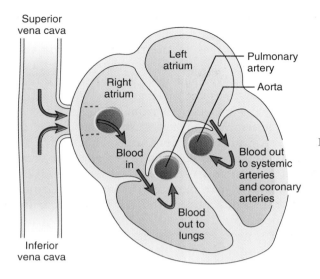

Figure 10–3. The heart box.

intricate network of specialized nerve cells coordinate the sequential contractions of the chambers to make it an effective pump. Two large vessels arise from the heart: the pulmonary artery from the right ventricle and the aorta from the left ventricle. These large vessels each have a valve (pulmonic and aortic valves, respectively) that opens to accommodate forward flow during systole and close to prevent retrograde flow during diastole. The atria and ventricles are also separated by a valve. The right atrium and ventricle are separated by the tricuspid valve, and the left atrium and ventricle are separated by the mitral valve. Similar to the pulmonic and aortic valves, these valves open to accommodate forward flow and close to prevent retrograde flow. In contrast to the pulmonic and aortic valves, the tricuspid and mitral valves open during diastole and close during systole. The left main and right coronary arteries arise from the root of the aorta. The coronary sinus drains into the right atrium.

Poorly oxygenated blood enters the right atrium of the heart from the superior and inferior vena cava, where it typically fills and empties 60 to 100 times per minute in correlation with the cardiac cycle. The atria are under low pressure and thus are thin-walled. The majority of the blood flows passively from the right atrium into the right ventricle (70%), and the forceful atrial contractions during late diastole cause the remaining portion of the atria to fill (30%). Blood is then propelled by the right ventricle into the pulmonary circulation (pulmonary artery). Blood is returned to the left atrium by four pulmonary veins that contain oxygenated blood. The left ventricle pumps the blood into the aorta, coronary arteries and, eventually, the systemic arteries to oxygenate the body tissues (Fig. 10–3). The function of the larger and thicker walled left ventricle is essential and is most important for maintaining the blood pressure necessary to effect forward flow to the systemic circulation. The coronary arteries fill with oxygenated blood during diastole to bring oxygenated blood to the myocardium. The coronary arteries fill passively during systole to supply oxygenated blood to the myocardium. Deoxygenated blood from the myocardium returns to the right atrium via the coronary sinus.

In order to understand the normal physiologic electrical depolarization of the heart, it is important to understand the electrical pathways in the heart (Fig. 10–4). Contraction of the heart is coordinated by a few regions of the heart that possess specialized myocytes with the ability to generate cyclic depolarizations of the myocardium. The sinoatrial (SA) node is located in the right atrium near the junction of the superior vena cava and the right atrium and has an intrinsic electrical depolarization rate of approximately 60 to 100 beats per minute. The atrioventricular (AV) node is located between the right atrium and the right ventricle and has an intrinsic electrical depolarization rate of 45 to 60 beats per minute. Arising adjacent to the AV node and traveling through the myocardium of the ventricular septum and the left and right ventricles are the specialized His bundle and Purkinje fibers, which possess the ability to conduct electrical impulses at a high rate of speed.

The sinoatrial node fires 60 to 100 times a minute; because this is the highest rate of automaticity in the heart, it is the site that usually initiates the cardiac electrical impulse during the normal cardiac cycle. This impulse then rapidly depolarizes the left and right atria (by spreading the impulse through intranodal tracks) until the electrical impulse reaches the AV node. The velocity with which the electrical impulse is conducted then slows considerably in the AV node, causing a delay between the atrial contraction and the ventricular contraction. After the delay in the AV node, the impulse again moves very rapidly through the His bundle, the right and left bundle branches (the left further divides into the anterior and posterior fascicles), and the Purkinje fibers, resulting in the nearly simultaneous depolarization of the right and left ventricles (Fig. 10–5).

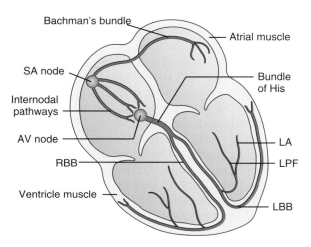

Figure 10–4. Electrical pattern of the heart. SA, sinoatrial node; AV, atrioventricular; RBB, right bundle branch; LBB, left bundle branch; LPF, left posterior fascicle; LA, left atrium.

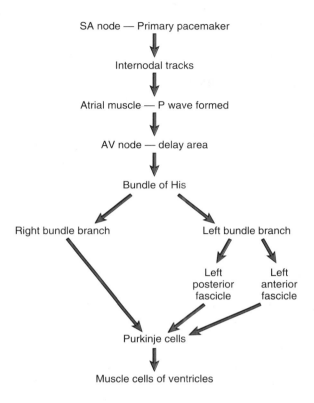

SA node — Primary pacemaker

Internodal tracks

Atrial muscle — P wave formed

AV node — delay area

Bundle of His

Right bundle branch

Left bundle branch

Left posterior fascicle

Left anterior fascicle

Purkinje cells

Muscle cells of ventricles

Figure 10–5. Electrical sequence of the normal heart. SA, sinoatrial.

The atria and ventricles are separated by a fibrous connective tissue that acts much like an insulator. This fibrous insulator prevents the spread of the electrical impulse from the atria to the ventricles through any area except the AV node. This insulating mechanism allows the atria and ventricles to beat in a synchronized and orchestrated fashion that results in effective and efficient forward flow of blood through the heart.

The electrical activity of the heart can be measured on the surface of the body by electrocardiography. The action potentials of the cardiac cells are related to the conventional system of labeling the electrocardiographic waveform with PQRST. The resulting waveform (ECG) has a P wave, which represents the depolarization of atrial tissue; a QRS interval, which represents the depolarization of the ventricles; and a T wave, which represents the repolarization of the ventricles. No waveform is noted on surface ECGs for the repolarization of the atrium (Fig. 10–6).

Patient Preparation

Preparing the patient for the ECG is important. Time should be spent explaining the activities associated with the procedure and answering the patient's questions. The steps described for preparing the patient's

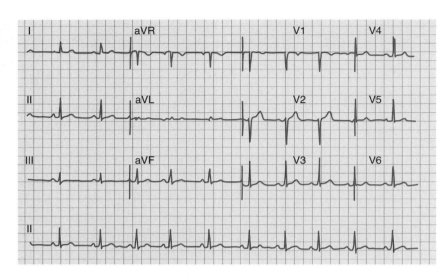

Figure 10–6. Electrocardiographic 12-lead tracing.

skin help ensure the optimal conditions for recording the ECG. The following steps should be performed in preparing the patient.

- Introduce yourself to the patient.
- Explain about the 12-lead electrocardiography procedure, and then proceed by carefully draping the patient's chest area.
- Identify the six precordia (some practitioners choose to mark them with a felt-tipped pen).
- If necessary, shave any hair in the area.
- Cleanse the skin surface with alcohol and rub with a mild abrasive pad.
- Wipe skin again with alcohol to rid surface of any residue.
- Apply the six adhesive electrodes.

Materials Utilized for Electrocardiography

- ■ The main unit or material needed to do a routine 12-lead ECG is a standard electrocardiography machine on a cart. Most modern systems today have a resting electrocardiographic analysis system with quick reference readout.
- ■ Electrodes for the six precordial sites
- ■ Razor to shave hair from a male patient's chest
- ■ Alcohol to clean skin surface of oil
- ■ Felt pen to mark site (optional)
- ■ Abrasive pad to remove epidermal skin layer at each electrode site; pad is used gently to remove the epidermal layer of skin at the six precordial sites until the felt-pen mark is gone

Procedure for Performing the Electrocardiogram

Note: Following are the steps for performing a routine 12-lead ECG at the patient's bedside.

1. Assemble supplies (leads, alcohol, abrasive pads, and so on).
2. Verify the order on the patient's chart.
3. Verify the patient's identity.
4. Wash your hands.
5. Plug in power cord and then turn on electrocardiography machine.
6. Position the patient in a comfortable supine position and provide a drape or gown that maintains the patient's modesty, yet affords adequate access to the patient's chest for the necessary lead placement.
7. Cleanse skin area at the six precordial skin placement areas on the chest.
8. Attach limb and precordial leads (refer to Figs. 10–7 and 10–8 for the correct placement of the leads).

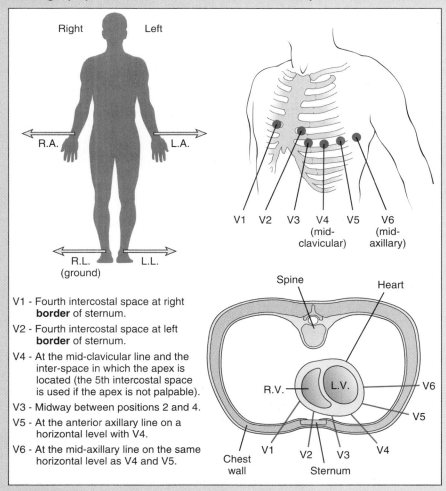

V1 - Fourth intercostal space at right **border** of sternum.

V2 - Fourth intercostal space at left **border** of sternum.

V4 - At the mid-clavicular line and the inter-space in which the apex is located (the 5th intercostal space is used if the apex is not palpable).

V3 - Midway between positions 2 and 4.

V5 - At the anterior axillary line on a horizontal level with V4.

V6 - At the mid-axillary line on the same horizontal level as V4 and V5.

Figure 10–7

Procedure for Performing the Electrocardiogram – *(continued)*

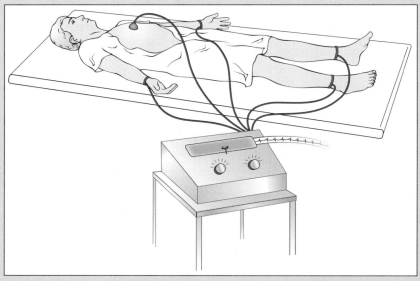

Figure 10–8

9. Check to see that all leads are connected.
10. Enter patient's information.
11. Ask the patient to lie quietly for 30 seconds.
12. Press the 12-lead button or the record ECG button to record the tracing.
13. "Acquired data" message will appear, but wait until the "ECG acquisitions complete" message appears.
14. Enter number of extra copies desired.
15. Print report for chart and heart reading station.
16. Press "store" and "data in store" to compare at time of next tracing.
17. Enter your name, date, and identification number.
18. Remove adhesive electrodes.
19. Assist patient with cleaning up and redressing as necessary.
20. Clean patient's room of used supplies.

Special Considerations

When there is a patient who has difficulty keeping in one position for 30 seconds because of pain, shortness of breath, or confusion, it may take more than one person to complete the procedure. Small children who are fearful of the procedure can present an increased challenge to the practitioner-technician.

Follow-Up Care and Instructions

- No follow-up care is necessary other than carefully removing the adhesive electrodes from the skin.
- Patients should be advised about when they can anticipate receiving the results and interpretation of the ECG.

Bibliography

- Constant J: Essentials of Learning Electrocardiography: A Complete Course for the Non-Cardiologist. New York, Parthenon, 1997.
- Dubin D: Rapid Interpretation of EKGs. Tampa, Fla, Cover, 1996.
- Goldschlager N, Goldman MJ: Electrocardiography: Essentials of Interpretation. Los Altos, Calif, Lange Medical, 1984.
- Lewis KM, Handal KA: Sensible ECG analysis. Albany, NY, Delman, 2000.
- Lipman BC: ECG Pocket Guide. Chicago, Ill, Year Book Medical, 1987.
- Murphy KR, Pelton JJ: ECG Essentials. Chicago, Ill, Quintessence, 1991.
- Rawlings CA: Electrocardiography. Redmond, Wash, Spacelabs, 1991.
- Schamroth L: An Introduction to Electrocardiography. Oxford, England, Blackwell Scientific, 1976.

Chapter 11

Exercise Stress Testing for the Primary Care Provider

▷ Donald M. Pedersen

▷ Charles S. King

Procedure Goals and Objectives

Goal: To identify appropriate candidates for exercise stress testing and to administer the test safely.

Objectives: The student will be able to . . .

► Describe the indications, contraindications, and rationale for performing exercise stress testing.

► Identify and describe common complications associated with exercise stress testing.

► Describe the essential anatomy and physiology associated with the performance of an exercise stress test.

► Identify the necessary materials and their proper use for performing an exercise stress test.

► Identify the important aspects of patient care after an exercise stress test.

Background and History

Coronary artery disease (CAD) remains a major cause of death and disability in the United States despite advances in disease prevention. There are considerable costs associated with treating this disease, which are compounded by expenses related to time lost from work and lost wages. Since the 1950s, electrocardiographic analysis during exercise has remained the most reproducible objective sign in the evaluation of the patient with possible ischemic heart disease. The physiologic stress of exercise can elicit cardiovascular abnormalities not present at rest. Although exercise testing was initially used as a diagnostic tool, it is also a powerful predictor of subsequent cardiac events. Exercise stress testing provides a controlled environment for observing the effects of increased oxygen demand on the myocardium, and it can be used to determine the adequacy of perfusion to the working myocardium.

The exercise stress test is a valuable tool for detecting CAD and for evaluating medical therapy and cardiac rehabilitation after myocardial infarction.

Electrocardiographic changes during exercise can provide evidence of ischemia if significant stenosis from CAD is present. Healthy persons who are asymptomatic may be considered candidates for exercise testing if they engage in strenuous or high-risk occupations. The American College of Sports Medicine (ACSM) recommends an exercise test for all women age 50 and older and all men age 40 and older who plan to engage in vigorous exercise. The American College of Sports Medicine does not recommend exercise testing for asymptomatic, healthy persons who are not planning vigorous exercise, regardless of the person's age (Pate et al, 1991).

In addition to the standard exercise stress test, other methods of cardiovascular stress testing include scintigraphy and echocardiography. Exercise stress scintigraphy uses a radioactive tracer to enhance abnormal areas of myocardial blood flow and can be performed with pharmacologic agents instead of exercise if a patient's condition warrants. Echocardiography has been used in combination with exercise or pharmacologic stress testing as another form of noninvasive cardiac evaluation.

Indications

By exposing the cardiopulmonary system to increased metabolic demands using standardized methods and protocols of stress, the clinician is provided a useful tool in detecting the initial presence of cardiopulmonary pathology and for assessing the efficacy of various therapies and rehabilitation programs. Alone, or in concert with established and developing imaging modalities, stress testing adds a valuable adjunct to the well-thought-out history and physical examination. It is indicated for the following:

- To establish the initial diagnosis of obstructive CAD
- To stratify risk and monitor treatment of patients with previously diagnosed or treated CAD
- To screen asymptomatic individuals (CAD risks or occupations that place the public at risk)
- To assess exercise capacity in patients with valvular, congenital abnormalities or congestive heart failure (CHF)
- To document and monitor therapy in those with exercise-related heart dysrhythmia

As with all laboratory testing, exercise stress testing should be used to augment an already high clinical suspicion of disease that is based on a quality history and physical examination. Accordingly, the rationale for using exercise stress testing in the primary care setting should be based on the "predictive value" of the given test. Attention should be paid to the prevalence of the disease in the patient population under consideration (i.e., the pretest probability of detecting pathology in a given patient).

The sensitivity and specificity of exercise stress testing with electrocardiographic monitoring alone have been validated for its use in detecting CAD by comparison of ST segment changes (depression or elevation) with the "gold standard" of coronary angiography (Gianrossi et al, 1989). "True positives" (i.e., the percentage of patients with disease, who have electrocardiographic changes indicative of ischemia) are the measures of sensitivity in exercise stress testing, which in the general patient population varies from 40% to 90% (Fletcher et al, 1992). The sensitivity of exercise stress testing in detecting cardiac pathology other than CAD is less clear.

The occurrence of "false negatives" (i.e., those tests in which there is an absence of diagnostic electrocardiographic changes in the presence of true CAD) can be minimized by sound test candidate selection and practicing good testing technique (i.e., achieving target heart rate, getting quality data, and so on). The specificity of exercise stress testing with electrocardiographic monitoring alone, described as the percentage of normal patients (i.e., those without CAD) who manifest no electrocardiographic changes indicative of CAD, is reported to be 84% (Fletcher et al, 1992). False-positive results (i.e., tests in which ECG changes suggest CAD that cannot be substantiated by subsequent coronary angiography) are often associated with patient selection (gender), electrocardiographic abnormality (left ventricular hypertrophy), Q waves at baseline, and associated drug therapy (digoxin).

Both sensitivity and specificity are improved when the pretest probability of detecting the target pathology in a group of patients is high at the onset. Prevalence tables for a variety of illnesses are published and usually broken down by gender, age, and clinical presentation (Gibbons et

Table 11–1

Pretest Probability of Coronary Artery Disease by Age, Gender, and Symptoms

Age (yr)	Gender	Typical—Definite Angina Pectoris	Atypical—Probable Angina Pectoris	Nonanginal Chest Pain	Asymptomatic
30–39	Men	Intermediate	Intermediate	Low	Very low
	Women	Intermediate	Very low	Very low	Very low
40–49	Men	High	Intermediate	Intermediate	Low
	Women	Intermediate	Low	Very low	Very low
50–59	Men	High	Intermediate	Intermediate	Very low
	Women	Intermediate	Intermediate	Low	Very low
60–69	Men	High	Intermediate	Intermediate	Low
	Women	High	Intermediate	Intermediate	Low

High, greater than 90%; intermediate, 10% to 90%; low, less than 10%; very low, less than 5%.

Adapted from Pate RR, Blair SN, Durstine JL, et al: Guidelines for Exercise Testing and Prescription. American College of Sports Medicine, 4th ed. Philadelphia, Lea & Febiger, 1991, p 87.

al, 1997). An example of the prevalence of CAD in Western society is detailed in Table 11–1.

Designing a strategy for determining the appropriateness of testing in a given population is often as much an art as a science. An incremental testing strategy for detecting CAD in individuals with a normal resting electrocardiogram, as well as those with abnormal resting electrocardiograms, is detailed in Figure 11–1.

When considering the predictive value of exercise treadmill testing with electrocardiographic monitoring, it may be the clinical history alone that provides the best guidance. It has been reported that the highest predictor of positive stress testing in either gender is the presentation of "typical" angina pectoris as opposed to atypical or nonanginal symptoms (Weiner et al, 1979). Enhancement of predicted value may be appreciated with the use of newer, more sophisticated computer analysis of exercise electrocardiographic ST-segment changes, although many of these methods require further validation. The appropriate addition of imaging by radionuclide or, most recently, echocardiography can improve both specificity and sensitivity of exercise stress testing.

Stress testing with electrocardiographic monitoring (with or without an imaging modality) is most commonly used in patients in whom the suspicion for cardiac ischemia is high based on clinical history and physical examination.

The American College of Cardiology guidelines for exercise stress testing consider symptomatic adult patients with at least an intermediate pretest probability of CAD (including those with right bundle branch block or <1 mm resting ST depression, or both) candidates for exercise treadmill testing with electrocardiographic monitoring alone (Gibbons et al, 1997). Patients with suspected CAD (i.e., high pretest probability as dictated by age, symptoms, and gender, <1 mm of ST depression) who have abnormal electrocardiograms (ECGs) that are at least in part

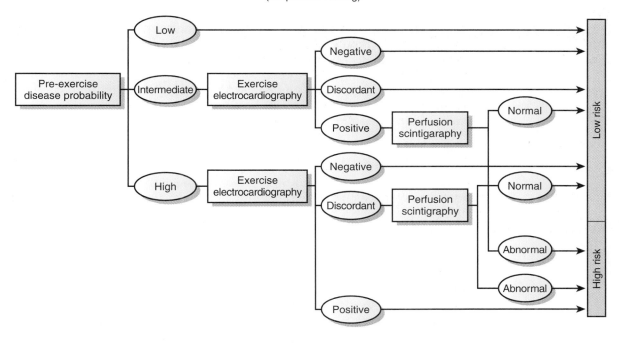

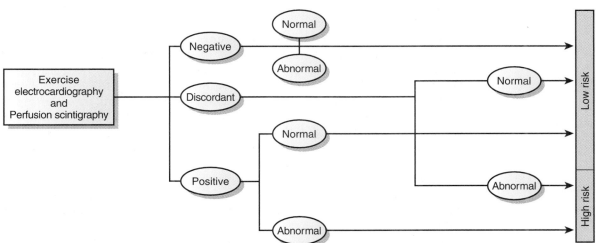

Figure 11–1. Incremental testing strategy for coronary artery disease (CAD) risk using serial results of pretest clinical risk (high, intermediate, low), exercise electrocardiography, and radionuclide perfusion scintigraphy. Top panel shows sequential testing in patients with a normal baseline electrocardiogram (ECG). Bottom panel uses combined electrocardiographic and perfusion scintigraphy (uniform) testing in patients with an abnormal baseline ECG. Results of these tests define low- and high-risk groups. (Negative exercise test (ET), <1 mm ST[1], >85% maximal heart rate; discordant ET, <1 mm ST[1], >85% maximal heart rate; positive ET, ≥1 mm ST[1], <85% maximal heart rate). (Adapted from Ladenheim ML, Kotler TS, Pollack BH, et al: Incremental prognostic power of clinical history, exercise electrocardiography and myocardial perfusion scintigraphy in suspected coronary artery disease. Am J Cardiol 59:270–277, 1987.)

attributed to glycoside therapy (digitalis), left ventricular hypertrophy, left bundle branch block, or other baseline electrocardiographic abnormalities are candidates for exercise stress testing; however, an imaging modality should also be used to improve test sensitivity-specificity.

In addition to its purely "diagnostic" applications, exercise stress testing may be used to assess previous therapy. After infarction, patients are often "risk-stratified" before hospital discharge through the use of exercise stress testing in a "submaximal" protocol. Typically, patients without recurrence of angina symptoms are stressed to 70% of their age-predicted maximal heart rate while symptoms and the ECG are assessed. This testing alerts the provider to those patients who are likely to have recurrent symptoms with activities of daily living and also provides reassurance to the patient and family about the safety of leaving the hospital.

Patients receiving antianginal agents or those who have undergone or are being considered for revascularization procedures (percutaneous transluminal coronary angioplasty [PTCA], coronary artery bypass graft [CABG]), or both, may benefit from a functional assessment of areas of myocardium treated. After initiation of antiarrhythmic therapy (pharmacologic or a device), especially in patients with a history of exercise-related abnormalities, exercise stress in a "controlled" environment can evaluate management as well as provide reassurance to the patient. Functional testing using exercise is often directed toward assessing cardiovascular capacity or response in healthy individuals as well as a variety of those with known pathology.

Functional testing can often be offered to those who have undergone congenital heart defect repair, valvular replacement or repair, or cardiac transplantation in an effort to provide a baseline or document improvement in those who were previously physically restricted. Patients who suffer from stable but chronic heart failure, diabetes, chronic renal insufficiency, or pulmonary pathology fall into the group that benefits from functional exercise testing. With the exception of asymptomatic patients with multiple cardiac risk factors and patients with occupations that place the public at risk, exercise treadmill testing with electrocardiographic monitoring should not be considered a "screening tool." The indiscriminate use of exercise stress testing in an effort to expose "silent ischemia" leads to misleading false-positive results that are financially burdensome and lead to undue patient worry (Sox et al, 1989).

Contraindications

As in any testing modality, the anticipated benefits of information provided the clinician by a test should outweigh the potential risks associated with obtaining this information. There are few absolute contraindications to performing exercise treadmill testing, but the test administrator must always weigh the anticipated benefits carefully against the perceived risks of the test.

- Generally, exercise stress testing is likely to "worsen" myocardial ischemia in patients already suffering from myocardial infarction or unstable angina. Testing should be delayed until rest pain is absent and the infarction has stabilized and been appropriately treated.
- Patients with symptoms of congestive heart failure should be stabilized to the point at which they are likely to be able to perform the planned test protocol and are not having pulmonary edema.
- Patients with symptomatic conduction abnormalities, such as high-degree atrioventricular block and symptomatic supraventricular tachycardia, and most ventricular tachycardia, and patients with demonstrated "chronotropic incompetence" should not be stressed until an adequate ventricular rate in response to increased metabolic demand can be anticipated or controlled.
- Pacemaker therapy is not a contraindication to exercise stress testing, but reprogramming the rate and response settings may be necessary and an imaging modality used if evidence of ischemia is being sought. Persistent ventricular or supraventricular tachycardia should be corrected before testing. Some antiarrhythmic agents may prevent patients from reaching "target" heart rate during testing, and the addition of an imaging modality may improve the value of the test.
- Severe systemic arterial hypertension defined as a pretest systolic pressure greater than or equal to 200 mm Hg or pretest diastolic pressure greater than or equal to 110 mm Hg is generally considered an absolute contraindication. Excessive myocardial wall stress imparted by this degree of hypertension exerts a significant increase in myocardial oxygen demand at baseline. These patients are better candidates for testing when their hypertension is controlled.
- Exercise stress testing in patients with severe aortic stenosis is prohibited because the myocardial oxygen demand at baseline is already significantly elevated. Although testing is used in determining the timing of surgery, it is reserved for patients who have not yet manifested associated angina, syncope, or congestive heart failure.

Other clinical conditions that should be controlled before exercise stress testing follow:

- Recent pulmonary embolism or infarct and severe peripheral vascular disease (deep venous thrombosis, phlebitis, claudication)
- Limitations to ambulation (cerebrovascular accident, orthopedic disability, severe vertigo-dizziness)
- Inability of the patient to follow instructions (mental disability, catatonia, psychosis)

Relative Contraindications

In some patients, the anticipated benefits of exercise testing outweigh the higher than average risks or impediments. These "relative contraindications" are usually more minor versions of the previously mentioned "absolute contraindications" and as such, are not prohibitive. Common examples follow:

- Presence of preexisting electrocardiographic abnormalities when the examiner is focusing on nonelectrocardiographic criteria: Examples are data such as new left ventricular segmental wall motion abnormality seen on echocardiography or perfusion defects and redistribution abnormalities in the setting of radionuclide studies.
- The patient who cannot mount an adequate heart rate response to exercise stress testing (beta-blocker pharmacologic therapy), has an inability to exercise because of ambulation difficulties, or is not otherwise willing to work physically
- Patients using agents such as dobutamine, dipyridamole, or adenosine, which cause pharmacologic stress and may increase myocardial oxygen demand or myocardial perfusion during which the ECG, blood pressure, heart rate, and imaging can be observed for changes suggesting ischemia

Potential Complications

- The risks of cardiac stress testing via a treadmill, cycle ergometer (use of a stationary bike with varying degrees of resistance), or arm exercise testing (use of an exercise wheel analogous to the pedals of a bicycle with varying degrees of resistance) are small when attention is paid to appropriate patient selection. Pooled data suggest that approximately 0.5 death per 10,000 tests in large heterogeneous populations can be expected (Gordon and Kohl, 1993).
- Most sudden death episodes during stress testing occur in middle-aged and older individuals with advanced atherosclerotic CAD. A detailed medical history and physical examination will often identify individuals at higher risk for complication associated with stress testing. Ironically, these individuals are the very group for which stress testing is most often indicated. Specifically, they are individuals with diabetes mellitus, multiple organ system failure, ambulatory impairment associated with orthopedic disorders, and electrolyte imbalance. Proper patient monitoring provided by well-trained individuals who can administer emergent care is essential to reduce known complications.
- Complications related to the mechanics of walking on an exercise treadmill include, but are not limited to, injury sustained from a fall; prolonged episodes of myocardial oxygen demand in excess of supply, resulting in prolonged myocardial ischemia or infarct, or both; hemodynamically significant tachycardia or bradycardia; and sudden cardiac death.

- Aggressive efforts at screening patients for contraindications before performing stress testing may significantly reduce the incidence of complications. Continuous patient monitoring for rhythm disturbances, ST-segment changes, and other electrocardiographic manifestations of myocardial ischemia, as well as disruptions in the patient's cognitive and psychomotor function, can minimize the incidence of complications associated with exercise stress testing.

Review of Essential Anatomy and Physiology

Dynamic or isotonic exercise (muscular contraction resulting in movement) is preferred for testing because it puts a volume stress rather than a pressure load on the heart. It can also be performed in increments. According to the American Heart Association statement on exercise standards, when dynamic exercise is begun or enhanced, oxygen uptake by the lungs quickly increases. After the second minute, oxygen uptake usually remains relatively stable (steady state) at each level of intensity of exercise. During steady state, heart rate, cardiac output, blood pressure, and pulmonary ventilation are maintained at reasonably constant levels.

Maximal oxygen consumption ($\dot{O}_2max$) is the highest level of oxygen consumption a subject can achieve during maximal exercise. During exercise, a physically fit subject will progressively increase his or her oxygen consumption, cardiac output, and pulmonary ventilation as the circulatory system provides blood and oxygen to the exercising tissues. The definition of a unit of metabolic equivalent (1 MET) is the total oxygen consumption measured in milliliters of oxygen per kilogram of body weight per minute for an adult sitting quietly at rest. 1 MET has been measured at approximately 3.5 mL/kg per minute. MET can be used as a work equivalent when comparing the level of physical work during different activities or different exercise protocols (Cintron, 1996).

Heart rate is one of the determinants of myocardial oxygen consumption, and thus peak heart rate is used as an indirect index of the workload imposed on the heart during exercise. Tables and formulas are available to provide the expected peak heart rate that should be attained during an exercise test carried out to maximal effort. The maximal achieved heart rate is usually expressed as a percentage of maximal predicted heart rate. A test that is limited by noncardiac factors at an attained heart rate less than 85% of maximal heart rate (MHR) may not have challenged the circulatory cardiac reserve enough to attain predictive validity. The percent of maximal heart rate at which symptoms or electrocardiographic evidence of myocardial ischemia occurs is an indicator of severity of the cardiac impairment, the individual's disability, and a rough index of prognosis.

During graduated exercise performed by normal subjects, heart rate and systolic blood pressure increase progressively. The product of the maximal achieved heart rate and blood pressure is called the *double product* or *rate-pressure product* and serves as an index of myocardial oxygen consumption. At rest, for example, the heart rate may be 70 and the systolic blood pressure 120, giving a double product of 8400. During exercise, the double product may exceed 30,000. When subjects cannot achieve a double product of 18,000 without signs or symptoms of cardiac disease, cardiac reserve is severely impaired, indicating a poor prognosis (Cintron, 1996; Fletcher et al, 1992).

A normal or negative test is one in which the end points are achieved without the appearance of symptoms, signs, or electrocardiographic findings that suggest the presence of cardiac disease. A negative test usually indicates a low statistical probability for the presence of clinically important cardiac disease.

The normal physiologic response to exercise may be altered by a number of cardiac diseases. Coronary atherosclerosis is the most common and limits the dilatory capacity of the coronary arteries. This restricts the amount of blood available to the myocardial tissues. Heart rate, blood pressure, myocardial contractility, and left ventricular chamber diameter and wall thickness all determine myocardial oxygen demand. The increase in heart rate, systolic blood pressure, and myocardial contractility induced by exercise is balanced by an increase in myocardial blood flow. Since myocardial oxygen extraction is almost maximal, even at rest, an imbalance between oxygen demand and blood supply quickly leads to myocardial ischemia and its clinical counterparts—angina, electrocardiographic changes, transient myocardial mechanical dysfunction, and occasionally cardiac rhythm disorders. The most common objective finding in patients with physiologically limiting coronary atherosclerosis who are subjected to exercise testing is electrocardiographic ST-segment depression, with or without anginal symptoms (Fig. 11–2).

Patient Preparation

- Explain the reason for the test to the patient and make sure he or she understands.
- The patient should have been given a physical examination and had a medical history taken that focused on cardiopulmonary and orthopedic systems before scheduling the test. Attention to the use of beta-blocker therapy, cardiac glycosides, and medicines altering the patient's state of consciousness should be considered before testing. With the use of an imaging modality, it is not always necessary for the patient to discontinue beta-blocker or digitalis therapy, although these medicines can alter the quality of the study by modifying the patient's maximal heart rate response or cause an abnormal baseline ECG. The physical examination should be directed toward eliciting signs or symptoms of orthopedic disease, peripheral vascular disease (claudication), or neurologic abnormalities that would limit the patient's ability to perform ergometry.

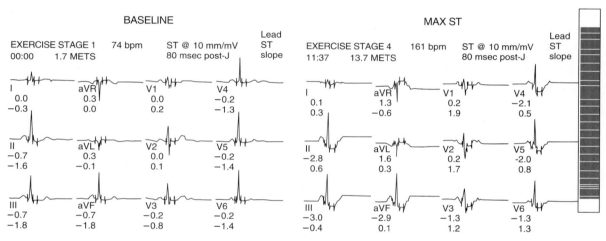

Phase name	Stage name	Time in	Speed	Grade	Workload	Heart rate	BP	RPP	VE count
		Stage	*mph*	*%*	*METS*	*bpm*	*mm Hg*	*bpm*mm Hg*	*ves/min*
PRETEST	SUPINE	0:00	1.0	0.0	1.7	74	142/78	14500	0
EXERCISE	STAGE 1	3:00	1.7	10.0	4.6	102	158/74	17100	0
	STAGE 2	3:00	2.5	12.0	7.0	106	166/72	22700	0
	STAGE 3	3:00	3.4	14.0	10.1	137			0
	STAGE 4	3:00	4.2	16.0	13.4	162			0
RECOVERY		6:06	0.0	0.0	1.0	103			0

40 yr   White   Male   BRUCE   Total exercise time: 12:00

Wt: Ht: Max HR: 162 bpm 90% of Max Predicted 180 bpm   25 mm/sec

Med: Max BP: 166/72   Maximum workload: 13.7 METS   10 mm/mV

100 Hz

Reason for termination: Max HR attained

Comments:

BASELINE   MAX ST

EXERCISE STAGE 1   74 bpm   ST @ 10 mm/mV   Lead   EXERCISE STAGE 4   161 bpm   ST @ 10 mm/mV   Lead
00:00   1.7 METS   80 msec post-J   ST slope   11:37   13.7 METS   80 msec post-J   ST slope

I	aVR	V1	V4		I	aVR	V1	V4
0.0	0.3	0.0	−0.2		0.1	1.3	0.2	−2.1
−0.3	0.0	0.2	−1.3		0.3	−0.6	1.9	0.5
II	aVL	V2	V5		II	aVL	V2	V5
−0.7	0.3	0.0	−0.2		−2.8	1.6	0.2	−2.0
−1.6	−0.1	0.1	−1.4		0.6	0.3	1.7	0.8
III	aVF	V3	V6		III	aVF	V3	V6
−0.7	−0.7	−0.2	−0.2		−3.0	−2.9	−1.3	−1.3
−1.8	−1.8	−0.8	−1.4		−0.4	0.1	1.2	1.3

Figure 11–2. Examples of electrocardiographic changes indicative of a positive exercise stress test. Compare baseline ST segments (Bruce protocol—stage 1—1.7 METs) with exercise ST segments at 11:37 (Bruce protocol—stage 4—13.7 METs) in this 40-year-old man with a positive exercise stress test. ST segments are measured 0.08 second after the J point. Note significant ST-segment depression of 0.2 mm in leads II, III, aVF, and V$_2$–V$_6$. BP, blood pressure; bpm, beats per minute; HR, heart rate; MAX ST, maximal ST; METS, metabolic equivalent; RPP, rate-pressure product.

- In an attempt to minimize patient anxiety and hopefully maximize performance in this patient-dependent test, written instructions that outline patient responsibilities and address common concerns and questions should be offered. A detailed description of the test procedure should occur before patient preparation, and questions should be solicited and addressed.
- In preparation for the test, the patient should be told to abstain from smoking and to wear comfortable clothing and sturdy footwear.
- Much information is gained when the examiner "walks the patient" back to the testing area. Information regarding gait, balance, respiratory reserve, and overall physical ability identifies individuals for whom treadmill testing is prohibitive and in whom pharmacologic stress might be considered.

Materials Utilized for Performing Exercise Stress Testing

General Environment

Note: Treadmill testing is usually conducted in a laboratory environment; however, family practitioners and internists often use any extra available space for this type of procedure. The space should be adequate for the testing team who must attend the patient during the testing. This typically involves the test proctor and one or more technicians.

■ Temperature control and adequate ventilation essential to maximize patient performance

Note: Generally, temperatures between 22° and 26°C are comfortable for exercise, especially if adequate air movement is present. In geographic locations where environmental humidity is greater than 50%, the testing environment temperature must be adjusted down to accommodate for this. Often, a portable fan improves exercise performance.

■ Adequate lighting for patient assessment and patient comfort and safety

Note: In the setting of diagnostic imaging modalities, adjustable lighting, usually in the form of a dimmer switch, can be a useful feature.

■ Room for readily available emergency equipment
■ Crash cart
■ Portable defibrillator
■ Supplemental oxygen supply
■ Curtains to ensure patient privacy as well as provide enough separation between patients to allow for normal conversation promotes patient comfort and performance
■ A sink, supply of towels, and wash cloths for the patient to use after exercise

Testing Equipment

■ Treadmill

Note: Treadmill weight capacity should equal or exceed a patient weight of 350 pounds, the system should have a variable range of speeds and degree of incline (1 to 8 miles per hour and 0 to 20 degrees) and should optimally be electronically controlled by and in synchrony with the testing clock. A dedicated electrical source should be used for the treadmill and electrocardiograph system to avoid interruption during studies. A standard treadmill platform should be equal to or exceed 50 inches in length and 16 inches in width (Pina et al, 1995). Padded handrails and emergency stop switches, which are readily visible and accessible to both patient and staff, afford added safety. The area directly behind the treadmill (often referred to as the run-out area) should be kept clear of obstruction and afford the patient safe egress from the treadmill at any time. Typically, a reclining chair or bed should be stationed proximal to the treadmill to afford the patient recumbence in the recovery period.

- Imaging equipment
- Echocardiogram
- Radionuclide camera
- Continuous oscilloscopic monitoring of a minimum of three leads, and preferably 12 leads, in the Mason-Likar configuration
- ST-segment templates, baseline correction software, and automatic dysrhythmia alerts are helpful but not essential to the safe conduct of testing.
- Machine-patient interface, specifically the electrocardiographic electrode placement

   Note: Commercially available silver–silver chloride electrodes with adhesive attachment offer excellent electrocardiographic signal transmission.

- The addition of a "tube shirt," using elasticized medical mesh material, adds stability to electrodes.
- The cable array should arise from a central module, which should be attached by a belt worn about the patient's waist.

   Note: Attention paid to confirming quality signals before testing will serve the examiner in ensuring good data for interpretation.

- Blood pressure monitoring equipment consists of a variety of available devices, ranging from automated systems that use oscillatory signaling to a standard manual mercurial sphygmomanometer and stethoscope.

   Note: In high-volume, experienced laboratories, manual cuff measurement is still the standard, offering reliable blood pressure monitoring but requiring specially trained personnel. Attention should be paid to using appropriately sized blood pressure cuffs in the variety of patients seen in a laboratory, as well as routine maintenance and calibration of manometers. Attention to basic details, such as placing the manometer at the level of the patient's heart, as well as routine cleaning and calibration, will ensure accurate and reliable blood pressure monitoring.

   Note: Laboratories using stationary bicycle ergometers for individuals with specific orthopedic, peripheral vascular or neurologic limitations to weight-bearing on a treadmill test should have similar automated resistance control features. Commercially available stationary bicycles use either mechanically braked or electronically braked flywheels for this purpose. Often, software, that interfaces with the ECG and bicycle ergometer will "ramp" the degree of stress on a preprogrammed basis. As with treadmill testing, the cycle ergometer area must be free of other equipment and afford rapid egress from the bicycle for the recovery period. Attention to seat height and handlebar adjustments can improve the chances of maximal exercise performance and data quality. Numerous tables have been computed to project METs for cycle ergometry, but generally speaking, maximal oxygen uptake is lower on cycle ergometry than on treadmill testing.

An arm ergometer uses not only dynamic arm exercise but also the musculature of the chest, back, buttocks, and legs for body stabilization. Individuals with lower extremity impairment, such as orthopedic or vascular disease, can often be stressed safely with this equipment; however, difficulty often arises with electrocardiographic signal quality because of electrical mechanical interference with upper body musculature activity. Close attention to detail in skin preparation for electrode placement can often overcome this technical limitation.

Imaging Equipment

In an effort to increase the sensitivity and specificity of exercise stress testing, an imaging modality is useful. Its typical application is in the patient with an abnormal baseline ECG for whom stress-related changes might not be quantifiable. Examples of this are left bundle branch block; prior myocardial infarction with Q waves; ST-T abnormalities of any cause, including digitalis effect; or individuals taking beta-blockers in whom failure to achieve target heart rate may occur. Pacemaker-dependent patients may benefit from adjunctive cardiac imaging. Equipment ranges from scintigraphy cameras for radionuclide imaging to two-dimensional cardiac ultrasonography. Although beyond the scope of this discussion, cardiac ultrasonography or radionuclide imaging can be applied in patients undergoing ergometry or those who are stressed with pharmacologic agents such as dobutamine, dipyridamole, or adenosine. In the application of stress echocardiography, an echocardiographic bed with a "cutaway" in the mattress—affording the sonographer apical access with the patient in the left lateral decubitus position (before and after exercise or during pharmacologic stress)—markedly improves image quality. A variety of commercially available systems afford continuous loop (rest and stress) imaging, as well as comparative (before and after) formatting.

Emergency Equipment

Exercise testing is a common and safe procedure, even in the outpatient setting, but still presents some risk. Accordingly, basic emergency equipment should be readily available to the testing team. The majority of diagnostic exercise stress tests are performed on a population with at least a moderate pretest probability of CAD. Thus, the testing facility must have appropriate emergency equipment, pharmaceuticals, and personnel trained in their use.

Table 11–2

Emergency Preparedness for Exercise Stress Testing

Emergency Equipment for Exercise Stress Testing

Nasal cannula, nonrebreathing oxygen mask, airways (oral), oxygen tank (portable for transport)
Defibrillator (portable)
Bag-valve-mask hand respirator (Ambu bag)
Syringes and needles
Intravenous tubing, solutions, and stand
Suction apparatus and supplies (gloves, tubing, and so on)
Adhesive tape

A written protocol that clearly outlines the responsibilities of each testing team member should be composed and periodically reviewed. Mock emergency drills should be carefully planned, executed, and critiqued using a variety of scenarios on a regular basis in an effort to remain prepared for the inevitable medical emergency that affects all laboratories. At a minimum, the emergency equipment listed in Table 11–2 should be close to the testing area and should be considered "ready" on a regular basis.

When generating emergency protocols, the testing team must decide the limits of its response. In the outpatient setting, basic cardiac life support and early Emergency Medical Service (EMS) activation are the mainstays of the emergency response, whereas stress testing facilities within the confines of hospitals or medical centers may offer advanced cardiac life support procedures (endotracheal intubation), highly specialized personnel, and equipment. Emergency medications and solutions should also be available in these settings (Table 11–3).

Table 11–3

Emergency Medications and Solutions

Medications	Intravenous Fluids
Atropine	Normal saline (0.9%)
Epinephrine	D5W
Isoproterenol	
Procainamide	
Verapamil	
Bretylium	
Lidocaine	
Dobutamine	
Adenosine	
Sublingual nitroglycerin	
Dopamine	

Adapted from Pina IL, Balady GJ, Hanson P: Guidelines for clinical exercise testing laboratories: A statement for healthcare professionals from the Committee on Exercise and Cardiac Rehabilitation, American Heart Association. Circulation 91:912–921, 1995.

Personnel

The exercise stress team often consists of nurses, physicians, physician assistants, an exercise physiologist or specialist, and a physical therapist as well as electrocardiography and nuclear medicine technicians. Members of the team should have appropriate training and periodic proficiency evaluation in the duties they perform routinely. All staff members should receive training in basic cardiac life support, with at least one member of the team versed in advanced cardiac life support. Stress testing in the outpatient environment is usually conducted under the supervision of a clinic physician who should be available in the immediate area during the conduct of stress testing. A laboratory policy and procedure manual should be established in keeping with the policies of the health care facility and any state or local restrictions. An individual identified as the Medical Director of the testing facility should be active in the formulation of policies and procedures as well as proficiency evaluations of the staff members. Documentation of this duty should be ongoing and available for review. Requirements for physician competency in the exercise stress testing of patients with known or suspected cardiac pathology are well outlined in the American College of Physicians/American College of Cardiology/American Heart Association statement on clinical competence (Schlant et al, 1990).

Procedure for Exercise Stress Testing

Applying Electrodes and Obtaining Resting Electrocardiographic Tracings

1. Remove hair in the testing region of the electrode placement with battery-operated shaving equipment.
2. Remove lotions and skin oil from the area of electrode application with alcohol-saturated gauze. Allow the skin to dry.
3. Place commercially available electrodes in the proper location.

Note: In many laboratories, an abrasive (fine sandpaper or commercially available pads) is used to abrade the superficial layer of skin, thus decreasing skin resistance to 5000 Ω or less.

4. Attach lightweight ECG cables to the electrode array and secure the central module to the patient, usually with a holster-and-belt device around the waist.
5. Apply a flexible tube vest over the patient's trunk to help in decreasing electrical mechanical interference associated with lead bouncing.
6. Perform a baseline ECG in the standard 12-lead configuration.
7. Perform a standard 12-lead ECG with the patient in the supine and standing positions and after 30 seconds of hyperventilation.

Note: ST-segment depression occurring with hyperventilation, although uncommon, should be taken into account before initiation of the exercise test itself.

Procedure for Exercise Stress Testing – *(continued)*

8. Evaluate the tracing for baseline ST-T abnormality or other rhythm disturbances that would prohibit the performance of stress testing.

Note: When using an imaging modality, the baseline ECG is performed at this time. To afford adequate acoustical windows, often leads V_4, V_5, or V_6 must be altered to accommodate ultrasonographic transducer placement.

Data Collection

Note: Average individuals will exercise between 8 and 12 minutes when tested on the appropriate exercise treadmill protocol. There are a variety of protocols available, each with their proponents. Most can be programmed with a typical electrocardiographic-treadmill system. The Bruce protocol is used most commonly, beginning with a low level of stress and increasing in speed and incline every 3 minutes (Bruce, 1977).

9. Demonstrate the proper technique for mounting the treadmill, handgrip placement, and body positioning for performing the exercise protocol.

10. Advise the patient that the protocols start the patient at a slow walking pace with a minor or no incline and then ramp up to the next level of work (speed and incline) at predetermined time intervals.

11. Have monitoring personnel or yourself obtain a 12-lead ECG at least every minute (depending on the patient's symptoms) and a blood pressure check just before advancement to the next stage.

Note: Because of the inaccuracy of data generated by automated systems, manual blood pressure measurement, using a mercury manometer, stethoscope, and trained personnel, remains the preferred technique of monitoring (Froelicher, 1993).

12. Instruct the patient to communicate to the monitoring team his or her perception of exertion.

Note: Often, a hand-held card or sign (in large print), with various descriptions of perceived exertion (Borg scales [Borg, 1982]), is held before the patient by the monitoring team in preparing for test termination (Fig. 11–3).

Note: Symptoms of general fatigue, dyspnea, leg fatigue, and pain are often difficult to quantify, and a system of quantifying perceived exertion can aid in stopping at an appropriate end point.

Modified Borg Scale		Original Borg Scale	
0	Nothing at all	6	
0.5	Very, very weak	7	Very, very light
1	Very weak	8	
2	Weak	9	Very light
3	Moderate	10	
4	Somewhat strong	11	Fairly light
5	Strong	12	
6	Somewhat hard	13	
7	Very strong	14	
8		15	Hard
9		16	
10	Very, very strong	17	Veryhard
	(almost maximum)	18	
		19	Very, very hard
	Maximum	20	

Figure 11–3. Adapted from Pollock ML, Wilmord JH: Exercise in Health and Disease: Evaluation and Prescription for Prevention and Rehabilitation, 2nd ed. Philadelphia, WB Saunders, 1990, p 290.

Procedure for Exercise Stress Testing – *(continued)*

13. Counsel patients not to exit the treadmill while it is going, but rather to signal to the testing team their impending exhaustion so that the test may be terminated in a safe manner.

Note: The test should be stopped as indicated. End points for stress testing include, but are not limited to, the following:

- Progressive angina
- Persistent ventricular tachycardia
- Significant blood pressure blunting or decrease below baseline
- Significant and progressive ST-T depression or any ST-T elevation
- Progressive heart block
- Excessive blood pressure response greater than 250 mm Hg systolic and greater than 120 mm Hg diastolic
- Lightheadedness
- Confusion
- Ataxia
- Cyanosis or evidence of cerebral or peripheral circulatory collapse
- Sincere patient requests to stop the test
- Failure of critical monitoring equipment

14. On completion of the test, assist the patient into a supine position while serial ECGs and blood pressure data are collected every 1 to 2 minutes or until the patient's heart rate approximates baseline by 10%.

Note: Exercise stress testing using imaging requires special patient positioning, such as a left side–lying position (stress ECG), thus resulting in a short delay in vital sign monitoring.

15. Record blood pressure, heart rate, and electrocardiographic data recording continually until patient is asymptomatic and near-baseline vital signs are present.

16. Observe patients manifesting signs or symptoms of cardiac disease during or after testing (angina, hypertension, hypotension, ventricular tachyarrhythmias, or other clinical indications for continued monitoring) until those conditions stabilize.

Note: A typical monitoring period after exercise recovery is between 6 and 12 minutes.

17. While the patient is preparing for exit, review electrocardiographic, hemodynamic, and applicable imaging data before the patient's discharge from the testing facility.

18. Although a final report may require a more detailed analysis, in the interest of patient safety, make a preliminary evaluation of the collected data and inform the patient of these preliminary findings and, if appropriate, the referring provider.

Special Considerations

It is imperative that the test administrator monitor vital signs (blood pressure, heart rate, respiratory rate, and tissue perfusion) throughout the exercise protocol, which includes pre-exercise evaluation and continuous monitoring throughout the exercise test itself and throughout an appropriate recovery period. Symptom evaluation using the BORG scale serves as an important aid in the assessment of functional capacity, as well as dictating appropriateness of test termination. The testing team, directed by the test administrator, must be continuously vigilant for signs of cardiovascular compromise or deteriorating ambulatory ability. Scenarios whereby test termination must occur abruptly should be practiced frequently by the testing team, with provisions for acute intervention in the setting of hemodynamic collapse. Most patients experiencing an abrupt inability to continue will provide adequate warning to the testing team and afford them the opportunity to terminate the test and come to the aid of the patient without resultant injury.

- In the setting of abnormal cardiac rhythm, rapid intravenous cannulation and supplemental oxygen are essential to the patient's positive outcome.
- In patients in whom rhythm abnormality or hemodynamic deterioration is highly suspected, intravenous placement before testing affords the testing team a route for rapid drug administration.
- In the setting of ventricular tachyarrhythmias, immediate termination of the testing protocol and placement of the patient in a supine position with supplemental oxygen and establishment of intravenous access are important.
- Individuals who continue to manifest ventricular or atrial tachycardia, or both, benefit from antiarrhythmic therapy, typically lidocaine or adenosine, but may require elective or even emergent DC cardioversion.
- Individuals manifesting lightheadedness, confusion, pallor, cyanosis, or diaphoresis in the setting of profound ST-T abnormalities may be demonstrating acute ischemia and may benefit from oxygen therapy and nitroglycerin.
- Chronotropic impairment (i.e., relative bradycardia in the setting of increasing metabolic demands) is treated most successfully with termination of cardiac stress and rest.
- Patients manifesting severe bradycardia may benefit from instructions to "cough" until sinus node function returns.
- Patients demonstrating progressive angina on termination of stress testing are best treated with immediate supplemental oxygen therapy, nitroglycerin, and rest.
- Individuals who do not respond to the preceding measures in the setting of significant ST-T abnormality are likely to have multivessel CAD and should be considered unstable angina patients and managed accordingly.

Follow-up Care

- Advise patients on discharge from the testing facility that it is not unusual to feel fatigued for the remainder of the day and counsel against activities that would compound this symptom.

- In individuals with findings suggestive of tachydysrhythmia or ischemia, the referring provider should be involved in making any further recommendations and in initiation of therapy.
- Provide printed literature that addresses findings as well as instructions on activity modifications, monitoring for and response to changes in symptoms, and contacts for further information or evaluation.
- Individuals demonstrating unstable responses to stress testing should be hospitalized (unstable angina; early, marked positive electrocardiographic changes; and hemodynamically unstable rhythms).

References

Borg G: Psycho-physical bases of perceived exertion. Med Sci Sports Exerc 2:100–119, 1982.

Bruce RA: Exercise testing for ventricular function. N EngI J Med 296:671–675, 1977.

Cintron GB: Clinical Exercise Testing. In Chizner MA (ed): Classic Teachings in Clinical Cardiology, vol 1. Michigan, Laennec, 1996, pp 378–392.

Fletcher GF, Blair SN, Blumenthal J, et al: Statement on exercise: Benefits and recommendations for physical activity programs for all Americans: A statement for health professionals by the Committee on Exercise and Cardiac Rehabilitation of the Council on Clinical Cardiology, American Heart Association. Circulation 86:340–344, 1992.

Froelicher VF: Exercise and the Heart, 3rd ed. St. Louis, CV Mosby, 1993.

Gianrossi R, Detrano R, Mulvihill D, et al: Exercise-induced ST depression in the diagnosis of coronary artery disease: A meta-analysis. Circulation 14:87–98, 1989.

Gibbons RJ, Balady GJ, Beasley JW, et al. ACC/AHA guidelines for exercise testing: A report of the American College of Cardiology/American Heart Association Task Force on the Practice Guidelines (Committee on Exercise Testing). J Cardiopulmon Coll Cardiol 30:260–311, 1997.

Gordon NF, Kohl HW: Exercise testing and sudden cardiac death. J Cardiopulmon Rehabil 13:381–386, 1993.

Pate RR, Blair SN, Durstine JL, et al: Guidelines for Exercise Testing and Prescription: American College of Sports Medicine, 4th ed. Philadelphia, Lea & Febiger, 1991.

Pina IL, Balady GJ, Hanson P, et al: Guidelines for clinical exercise testing laboratories: A statement for healthcare professionals from the Committee on Exercise and Cardiac Rehabilitation, American Heart Association. Circulation 91:912–921, 1995.

Schlant RC, Friesinger GC, Leonard JJ: Clinical competence in exercise testing: A statement for physicians from the ACP/ACC/AHA taskforce on clinical privileges in cardiology. J Am Coll Cardiol 16:1061–1065, 1990.

Sox HC, Littenberg B, Garber AM: The role of exercise testing in screening for coronary disease [see comment]. Ann Intern Med 110:456–469, 1989.

Weiner DA, Ryan TJ, McCabe CH, et al: Exercise stress testing: Correlations among history of angina, ST-segment response and prevalence of coronary-artery disease in the Coronary Artery Surgery Study (CASS). N Engl J Med 301:230–235, 1979.

Bibliography

- Darrow MD: Ordering and understanding the exercise stress test. Am Fam Phys 59:401–410, 1999.
- Ladenheim ML, Kotler TS, Pollock BH, et al: Incremental prognostic power of clinical history, exercise electrocardiography and myocardial perfusion scintigraphy in suspected coronary artery disease. Am J Cardiol 59:270–277, 1987.
- Pina IL, Chahine RA: Lead systems: Sensitivity and specificity. Cardiol Clin 2:329–335, 1984.
- Vogel JA, Jones BH, Rock PB: Environmental consideration in exercise testing and training. Resource Manual for Guidelines for Exercise Testing and Prescription. Philadelphia, Lea & Febiger, 1991, p 119.

Chapter 12

Endotracheal Intubation

▷ Shepard B. Stone

Procedure Goals and Objectives

Goal: To successfully insert an endotracheal tube while observing universal precautions and with a minimal degree of risk to the patient.

Objectives: The student will be able to . . .

▶ Describe the indications, contraindications, and rationale for performing endotracheal intubation.

▶ Identify and describe common complications associated with endotracheal intubation.

▶ Describe the essential anatomy and physiology associated with the performance of endotracheal intubation.

▶ Identify the materials necessary for performing endotracheal intubation and their proper use.

▶ Identify the important aspects of patient care after endotracheal intubation.

Background and History

Endotracheal intubation is the process by which a tube is inserted into the trachea. This may be accomplished through the larynx or through the skin of the neck. *Cricothyroidotomy* and *tracheostomy* are the terms for the latter approach. This chapter limits discussion to the former approach and refers to the translaryngeal intubation of the trachea simply as *intubation*.

Intubation is a procedure that is performed daily in many locations around the world—electively in the operating room and urgently in emergency rooms, in clinics, and in the field. Practitioners should be familiar with this lifesaving skill. Proficiency at intubation is a requirement for practitioners whose practices put them in an environment in which advanced cardiac life support, pediatric/neonatal advanced life support, and advanced trauma life support skills are used on a regular basis and in which advanced backup (an anesthesia care provider) is not rapidly accessible.

The technique has been performed since the 18th century (Roberts, 1983). However, its use as we know it became more common in the 1940s. The value of intubation is well established. The ability to place an unobstructed conduit into a patient's airway to assist with ventilation and protect the airway is a skill that may be lifesaving. Conversely, if performed improperly, it may be life threatening. Providing the necessary knowledge and skills to master this technique successfully is the goal of this chapter.

Indications

Intubation, which provides a secure means of maintaining a patent air passage, should be used for the following situations:

- For a patient who has lost the ability to maintain a patent airway if other methods are ineffective or unreliable
- If a patient is at risk of losing the ability to ventilate adequately (e.g., airway edema, decreasing levels of consciousness, respiratory failure)
- For bypassing anatomic obstructions to clear airflow as well as provide a means to suction the lower airways of secretions and foreign materials; positive-pressure ventilation with a self-inflating reservoir bag (e.g., AMBU) is facilitated, as is the use of mechanical ventilators

Contraindications

The only contraindication to translaryngeal intubation is laryngeal disruption itself. Airway compromise must never be tolerated, but intubation through the traumatized larynx may not succeed, may waste precious time, and may exacerbate the injury. In this situation, creation of a surgical airway (e.g., cricothyroidotomy) may be the more prudent choice.

Potential Complications

Complications of intubation may be anatomic, physiologic, or psychological. Anatomic complications, which may result from the intubation itself or from the presence of the tracheal tube, follow:

- Nasal intubations may traumatize the nasal turbinates, the nasal mucosa, or the adenoids or may dissect into the retropharyngeal tissues.
- Oral intubations may cause damage to the lips, teeth, tongue, tonsillar pillars, tonsils, or a combination of these structures. All intubations may damage the epiglottis, the laryngeal cartilages and mucosa, and the vocal cords.
- Esophageal and tracheal perforations have occurred during intubation attempts.
- Cervical spine injuries and ocular injuries have also been reported.
- As in any instrumentation, bleeding may occur.
- Late complications of intubation include vocal cord paralysis and a subsequent increased risk of aspiration, tracheal stenosis, and tracheomalacia.
- The "anatomic" problems of tracheal tube malposition or kinking can also occur.

Physiologic complications of intubation include the following:

- Hypoxia
- Hypercarbia
- Cardiac dysrhythmias (including cardiac arrest)
- Hypertension
- Hypotension
- Intraocular hypertension
- Intracranial hypertension
- Vomiting and aspiration
- Bronchospasm
- Laryngospasm

Late complications include

- Pain
- Sore throat
- Problems with speech
- Swallowing and breathing difficulties
- Sinusitis
- Pneumonia

Psychological complications include

- Post-traumatic stress disorder that may result from intubation of patients who have not been adequately prepared psychologically for the intubation procedure or have not been sufficiently anesthetized or sedated during or after the intubation, or both.

Prevention of all complications in all patients is not possible. However, proper preparations (physical, psychological, and pharmacologic) and gentle manipulations result in both the highest success and the lowest complication rates.

Review of Essential Anatomy and Physiology

The successful performance of any procedure is enhanced by adequate knowledge of the relevant anatomy. Review of the structures of the oropharynx, nasopharynx, and larynx is essential (Fig. 12–1).

The nasotracheal tube traverses the nostrils, passing between the nasal septum and the nasal turbinates and "bending" around the posterior nasopharynx to arrive in the hypopharynx. The nasal mucosa is both friable and sensitive. Efforts must be made to reduce the likelihood of epistaxis before tube insertion.

Orotracheal intubation involves manipulation of the tongue to elevate the epiglottis, exposing the larynx. The lips and teeth are structures to be avoided when manipulating the laryngoscope, as are all other tissues. Epiglottic manipulation is either carried out directly with the laryngoscope blade or indirectly by placing the laryngoscope blade in the vallecula. The vallecula is the point at which the epiglottis attaches to the tongue. Elevation of the tongue at this point causes the epiglottis to rotate anteriorly and expose the larynx.

When the epiglottis is elevated, the larynx is visualized. Note that in pediatric patients (younger than age 3), the epiglottis is relatively long and floppy, and it must be manipulated directly for laryngeal exposure. The key landmark is the glottis, the opening into the larynx itself.

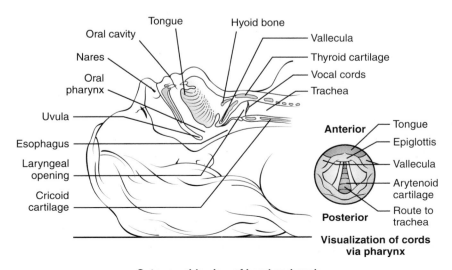

Cutaway side view of head and neck

Visualization of cords via pharynx

Figure 12–1. Anatomy of the oropharynx, nasopharynx, and larynx. (Redrawn from Pfenninger JL, Fowler GC: Procedures for Primary Care Physicians. St. Louis, Mosby-Year Book, 1994, p 456.)

The glottis is bordered laterally by the vocal cords, which are whitish structures originating at the 12 o'clock position and attaching at 5 and 7 o'clock (when the patient is supine). The arytenoid cartilages are the paired posterior laryngeal landmarks from the 3 to 9 o'clock positions. The vocal cords are located in the narrowest portion of the adult larynx. Deep to the larynx (which is formed anteriorly by the thyroid cartilage) is the cricoid cartilage. This is a complete cartilaginous ring attached to the thyroid cartilage via the cricothyroid membrane. This is important to remember when it is desirable to manipulate the larynx during intubation attempts or to occlude the esophagus. Also, the cricoid cartilage is the narrowest part of the pediatric airway. Distal to the cricoid is the trachea itself. The tracheal bifurcation results in the left main stem bronchus taking a more acute deviation to the left than the right main stem bronchus takes to the right. Overly enthusiastic tracheal tube insertion usually results in a right main stem bronchial intubation. The esophagus lies posterior to the airway structures.

The nasopharynx, oropharynx, and larynx are richly innervated by the sphenopalatine ganglion, anterior ethmoidal nerve, glossopharyngeal nerve, superior laryngeal nerve, and the recurrent laryngeal nerve (Sanchez et al, 1996). This must be considered when intubating a patient who is conscious. The placement of a tracheal tube or a laryngoscope, or both, in this circumstance will result in discomfort and autonomic nervous system stimulation. This is the cause of many of the physiologic complications mentioned earlier.

There are certain features assessable on physical examination that may predict difficulties in intubation. Narrow nostrils will make nasal intubation difficult, as will narrow nasal passages. This can be ascertained by occluding one nostril and having the patient breathe in rapidly and deeply through the nonoccluded nostril. If there is occlusion, this will be readily noted by the patient. Limited mouth opening may make laryngoscopy difficult. Limited intraoral visualization (often caused by a large tongue) is a risk factor for difficult laryngoscopy. Limited neck movement, especially extension, may be a predictor of intubation difficulty. A significant overbite or micrognathia may make intubation challenging. If the distance from the chin to the larynx is less than three fingerbreadths, or 6 cm, this is another predictor of possible difficulty. None of these physical examination findings is completely reliable for accurately predicting difficult intubation. Their presence should not be ignored, however, and the presence of multiple risk factors must be considered as an increasing likelihood of difficult intubation (Mallampati, 1996).

Standard Precautions ▷ Practitioners should use Standard Precautions at all times when interacting with patients. Determining the level of precaution necessary requires the practitioner to exercise clinical judgment based on the patient's history and the potential for exposure to body fluids or aerosol-borne pathogens (for further discussion, see Chapter 2).

Patient Preparation

Having a cooperative patient markedly facilitates intubation.

- In the patient who is capable of responding to the environment but requires intubation, it is important to explain why he or she needs to be intubated and what the procedure will entail, both during and after the procedure.

As always, it is important to consider historical information, including the patient's past medical history.

- If possible, query the patient or the patient's family about any prior difficulties with intubation.
- If time permits and previous medical records are available, look for an anesthesia record.
- If it is found that general anesthesia was administered, intubation may have taken place, and if it was difficult, the anesthesia care provider should have noted it.

Pharmacology

Pharmacologic support can be useful. If intubation with the patient awake is desired, the process can be facilitated with the use of topical anesthetics; in fact, intubation may be performed using topical anesthetics alone. Intubation can also be performed without any pharmacologic support; if time is critical, this may be the only option. Providing adequate topical anesthesia requires approximately 10 to 20 minutes of preparation. The anesthetization itself takes no more than 10 minutes, but the drying of the airways that enhances absorption of the local anesthetics takes about 10 minutes after intravenous administration or 20 minutes after intramuscular administration. Glycopyrrolate, 0.2 mg intravenously in adults, is an adequate dose. The advantage of glycopyrrolate over atropine is that it does not cross the blood-brain barrier, decreasing the potential for causing confusion, which can be a major problem when patient cooperation is desired.

Local Anesthetics

Commonly used topical anesthetics include cocaine, benzocaine, tetracaine, lidocaine, or combinations thereof. These drugs are applied to the surfaces that are to be in contact with the laryngoscope and endotracheal tube, but they are not necessary for airway anesthesia. One nerve that must not be blocked is the recurrent laryngeal nerve, because sensory blockade will anesthetize the larynx and part of the epiglottis, and motor blockade will result in vocal cord paralysis. A unilateral block will cause hoarseness, dysphonia, and possible aspiration; a bilateral block will cause complete airway obstruction. One may attain sensory blockade only by topical application of local anesthetics to the larynx and trachea (this may be carried out from above the larynx or by injecting through the cricothyroid membrane). If the patient is at risk for pulmonary aspiration of oral or gastric secretions, it is sometimes argued that anesthesia should not be provided so that the patient will be able to sense the presence of aspirated material and be able to clear it by coughing.

Cocaine

Cocaine offers the unique advantage of also providing topical vasoconstriction. This is useful for reducing epistaxis when performing intubations via the nasal route. If used, no more than 3 mg/kg of body weight of a 4% or 10% solution should be used to avoid toxicity. It should also be avoided when tachycardia and hypertension are a concern. If vasoconstriction is desired, phenylephrine (Neo-Synephrine) or oxymetazoline (Afrin) may be used in conjunction with other local anesthetics.

Benzocaine

Benzocaine has a rapid onset and brief duration of action. The dose limit of 4 mg/kg is readily exceeded, because it comes in high concentrations of 10%, 15%, and 20%. Overdosage can also result in methemoglobinemia.

Tetracaine

Tetracaine has a longer duration of action than benzocaine. It is available in dilute concentrations of 0.5%, 1%, and 2%, and the dose limit is 0.5 mg/kg.

Cetacaine

Cetacaine is a commercially available mixture of 14% benzocaine and 2% tetracaine that has a rapid onset and reasonable duration. Be aware that the toxic effects of local anesthetics are additive. Cocaine, benzocaine, and tetracaine are all members of the amino ester group of local anesthetics. This group has a higher associated incidence of allergic reactions.

Lidocaine

Lidocaine is the most readily available local anesthetic. It is of the amino amide group, and allergic reactions to lidocaine itself are rare. It is available in 0.5%, 1%, 2%, and 4% solutions; 2% viscous solution; 2% jelly; 2.5% and 5% ointments; and a 10% aerosol spray. The dose limit is 5 mg/kg.

Sedatives

The intubation of the patient who is not obtunded (by pathologic or iatrogenic processes) is made easier by sedation. Drugs that have a rapid onset and brief duration of action are best for this purpose. Surprisingly small amounts are necessary in the presence of a well-anesthetized airway; in fact, the anesthetization itself may be facilitated with judicious sedation. The most commonly used drugs are fentanyl and midazolam. These drugs also have the advantage of having an antagonist available — naloxone (Narcan) and flumazenil (Romazicon), respectively. Titrated to effect, they are not likely to produce adverse hemodynamics. Any drug can be used as long as the desired effects are achieved, that is, a patient who breathes and is calm and cooperative. The advantage of intubation performed in an awake patient is that the patient maintains airway patency, spontaneous ventilation, the ability to protect the airway, and the ability to verify neurologic function during and after intubation. This is particularly important with cervical spine injuries (Sanchez et al, 1996). It should always be considered in patients who are known to be difficult to intubate, those who are anticipated to be difficult to intubate, those who have airway or neck trauma, or those who are hemodynamically unstable (Sanchez et al, 1996).

Other Methods of Anesthesia

If intubation while the patient is awake is not required, it is usually faster and easier for both the patient and the practitioner to perform intubation while the patient is unconscious. Psychological stress is reduced, and the intubating conditions may be improved by sedation. The risk of sedated intubation is that it removes the patient's ability to maintain the airway and ventilation and increases the chance that the intubation will not succeed. If the patient cannot be ventilated by face mask or other device and cannot be intubated and the anesthetizing drugs cannot be cleared, the only recourse to save the patient's life is to create a surgical airway, which is not without risk. In the process of performing intubation, it is important to remember to "do no harm."

The practitioner can use the sedatives mentioned earlier in larger doses to obtain unconsciousness, or other drugs can be used. The intravenous agents used most commonly to induce rapid unconsciousness are thiopental, propofol, etomidate, and ketamine. They all work within seconds. Thiopental and propofol may cause hypotension. Propofol and etomidate cause local pain on injection and sometimes cause myoclonic movements. Etomidate has a high incidence of nausea associated with its use. Ketamine is associated with auditory and visual hallucinations during the recovery phase that may be attenuated by benzodiazepines. It also causes bronchodilatation, making it especially useful as an induction agent in status asthmaticus. Both etomidate and ketamine tend to maintain blood pressure and are the preferred induction agents in hemodynamically unstable patients in whom anesthetized intubation is desired. Note that ketamine and etomidate may cause increases in cerebral metabolic rate and are not the agents of choice if cerebral ischemia is of greater concern than is the ability to intubate the anesthetized patient. Usual induction doses are thiopental, 3 to 5 mg/kg; propofol, 2 to 2.5 mg/kg; etomidate, 0.3 to 0.5 mg/kg; and ketamine, 1 to 2 mg/kg. Doses should be decreased in the elderly, the hypovolemic patient, and the hemodynamically unstable patient. There are no reversal agents for these drugs.

Neuromuscular Blocking Drugs

Rendering the patient unconscious may be helpful; providing neuromuscular blockade (NMB) or paralysis may be helpful or it may result in death. By causing all the skeletal muscles to relax, the patient cannot cough or offer any physical resistance to intubation. The jaw muscles will be lax, enabling easier mouth opening and facilitating laryngoscopy. The lack of coughing will prevent movement of an unstable cervical spine. Lack of coughing will also prevent increases in intrathoracic pressure that can increase central venous pressure, which can result in increased intracranial pressure. The life-threatening complication of neuromuscular blockade is cessation of any spontaneous ventilatory efforts. If the patient cannot be intubated and ventilated, and surgical access to the airway is not attained rapidly, the patient may die.

The other problem with neuromuscular blocking drugs is that they paralyze skeletal muscles only. They do nothing to suppress consciousness, pain, or the reception and interpretation of any sensory stimulus. NMB agents administered alone will have the patient as awake as you are, with the ability to feel, hear, smell, taste, and see (if you open their eyelids). The only way that the patient can protest is autonomically by becoming hypertensive, developing arrhythmias, becoming bronchospastic, or increasing intracranial pressure. Subtle clues are pupillary dilatation, tearing, and diaphoresis. Administering sufficient amounts of sedating and anesthetizing drugs can prevent these undesirable effects. If this cannot be carried out because of hemodynamic status, the patient should be informed of this. Let the patient know that he or she will feel and hear everything that goes on.

The desirable characteristics of NMB agents to facilitate intubation include the rapidity of onset and brevity of duration; therefore, if intubation fails, breathing may return sooner. The absence of unwanted hemodynamic and other side effects is also desirable. The NMB agents are of two classes: depolarizers and nondepolarizers. The one depolarizer, succinylcholine, causes muscular depolarization at the neuromuscular junction. This is just like acetylcholine. Unlike acetylcholine, however, it takes minutes rather than seconds to be cleared from the muscle receptor. The depolarizers (all the other NMB agents) are competitive inhibitors of acetylcholine, preventing depolarization by occupying the muscle receptor site where acetylcholine normally triggers the depolarization. Termination of effect takes minutes to hours, depending on the drug and the dose; a greater dose results in a longer duration of action. There are anticholinesterase reversal substances (e.g., neostigmine, pyridostigmine, and edrophonium) that can be used when indicated.

Succinylcholine

Succinylcholine is effective at a dose of 1 mg/kg (in children 1 to 2 mg/kg). Its onset is within 60 seconds, and the duration of action is about 5 to 10 minutes. Increasing the dose increases the duration of action. Its mode of action, skeletal muscle membrane depolarization, results in a transient hyperkalemia of about 0.5 to 1 mEq/L. Patients who are paretic, those who have been burned, those who have sustained crush injuries, or those who are hyperkalemic for any reason may sustain a hyperkalemic increase of 5 to 10 mEq/L, resulting in cardiac arrest. Succinylcholine may also trigger malignant hyperthermia. It may also cause transient increases in intraocular and intracranial pressures, so it should be used with caution if the patient has an open globe injury and closed head injury unless the risk of a failed intubation is greater than the risk of increased intracranial pressure. Succinylcholine may cause bradycardia; therefore, its use in pediatric patients should be preceded by anticholinergic administration. Myalgias sometimes follow succinylcholine use; they may be reduced by administering a small dose of a nondepolarizing agent before administering the succinylcholine. If a nondepolarizing NMB agent is used, the dose of succinylcholine should be increased to 1.5 mg/kg.

Nondepolarizing Neuromuscular Blockade Agents

The nondepolarizing NMB class includes curare, metocurine, pancuronium, vecuronium, atracurium, *cis*-atracurium, doxacurium, pipecuronium, mivacurium, and rocuronium. Rocuronium offers the fastest onset (within 1 minute and maximal effect within 3 minutes, with a duration of 30 minutes) at a dose of 1.2 mg/kg. The others have a slower onset. Increasing the dose enhances the onset of all these drugs, increasing their duration of action. Increasing the dose also increases the likelihood of unwanted side effects. Some of the drugs listed release histamine when given rapidly or in a large dose, which may cause flushing, hypotension, and bronchospasm.

Physical Preparation

Patient positioning is critical.

- Intubation is easiest if the patient is supine with the head as close to the practitioner as possible at the level of the practitioner's xiphoid cartilage.

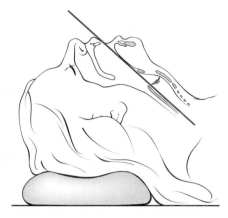

Figure 12-2. Axes in line with "sniffing" position. (Redrawn from Pfenninger JL, Fowler GC: Procedures for Primary Care Physicians. St. Louis, Mosby-Year Book, 1994, p 456.)

- The patient's head should be in the "sniffing" position of cervical flexion with C1-2 extension.
- If cervical spine injury is a possibility, the patient should either be in an appropriate collar or should have axial stabilization maintained by an individual who does nothing else during the intubation sequence.
- In normal adults, the sniffing position is readily attained by placing a support under the head while displacing the occiput toward the patient's feet.
- In children and the obese, the position may be attained by placing support under the shoulders and neck.

Caution: The importance of this maneuver cannot be overstressed. The sniffing position aligns the axes of the oropharynx (mouth), hypopharynx (throat), and larynx, making the shortest distance from the "outside world" to the trachea (Fig. 12-2).

Materials Utilized to Perform Endotracheal Intubation (Fig. 12-3)

Adjuncts
- Emergency support equipment; more frequently than not, tracheal intubation is an urgent, if not an emergent, procedure
- An adequate source of suction to reduce the likelihood of aspiration and to enhance visualization
- Airway adjuncts such as oropharyngeal and nasopharyngeal airways
- An appropriately sized face mask, self-inflating reservoir bag, and oxygen source
- For patients in whom mask ventilation and intubation is unsuccessful, a laryngeal mask airway, which may be a lifesaving aid

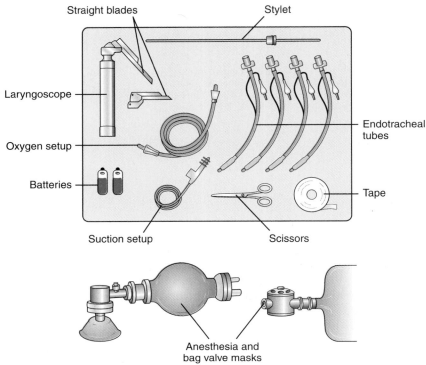

Straight blades

Stylet

Laryngoscope

Oxygen setup

Batteries

Suction setup

Scissors

Endotracheal tubes

Tape

Figure 12–3. Endotracheal intubation equipment. (Redrawn from Pfenninger JL, Fowler GC: Procedures for Primary Care Physicians. St. Louis, Mosby-Year Book, 1994, p 454.)

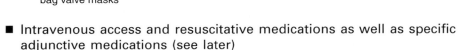

Anesthesia and bag valve masks

- Intravenous access and resuscitative medications as well as specific adjunctive medications (see later)
- Monitors for pulse oximetry, electrocardiography, and blood pressure
- If neuromuscular blocking drugs are to be used, a peripheral nerve stimulator to monitor the onset and duration of action of those drugs

Laryngoscopes
- The laryngoscope is a lighted tongue elevator (rather than depressor) and is a necessity for most oral intubations and some nasal intubations.
  Note: The intubator should confirm that the laryngoscope is functioning. As with a flashlight, if the batteries are exhausted or the bulb is burned out, it will significantly impede the intubation process. Other common causes of malfunction are loose bulbs and impurities between the contacts of the blade and the handle.
- Appropriately sized blades for the patient: for adults, Macintosh No. 3 and No. 4 (curved blades) and Miller No. 2 and No. 3 (straight blades) (Fig. 12–4); for pediatric patients, straight blades in order to directly manipulate the relatively large and floppy epiglottis
- Available backup equipment, such as additional handles, batteries, and blades

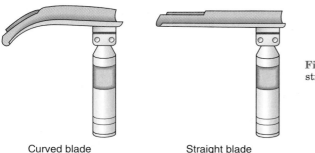

Curved blade   Straight blade

Figure 12–4. Curved and straight laryngoscope blades.

Tracheal Tubes

Tracheal tubes (or endotracheal tubes), constructed of a plastic that has been implant tested to prove it is not harmful to biologic tissues, are needed. They are for single-patient use. The tubes are described by their size, which is determined from the internal diameter in millimeters. Common sizes are from 2.5 to 10 mm. Sizes frequently used in adults are 7 to 8 in women and 7.5 to 8.5 in men (Fig. 12–5).

Note: An often-used formula for calculating tube size in children is 18+ [age in years] / 4; this is a rule of thumb, and adjustments are made as required (see later). Tracheal tubes of the expected size, as well as those a size larger and a size smaller, should be immediately available. The tubes have centimeter markings along the distal length.

Note: Tracheal tubes should be kept in the sterile wrapper until ready for insertion. Preparation of the tube includes confirming that the 15-mm external diameter adapter is securely in place—it is usually loosely in place in the unopened package. If the adapter is lost, conventional ventilation equipment will not be able to "mate" with the tracheal tube, and only

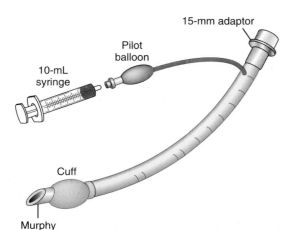

15-mm adaptor

Pilot
balloon

10-mL
syringe

Cuff

Murphy
eye

Figure 12–5. An endotracheal tube.

"mouth-to-tube" ventilation or spontaneous ventilation will be possible.

Note: Other preparation includes confirming that the tube's inflatable cuff and its inflation valve are functional. First injecting a volume of air sufficient to distend the cuff into the inflation valve and then detaching the inflation syringe from the inflation valve accomplishes this. The cuff should be observed to maintain its inflated state. If it does, both the cuff and inflation valve are functional. If the syringe is not removed, the competence of the inflation valve has not been confirmed. It is more common to have a defective inflation valve than a defective cuff on a new tracheal tube.

Note: Tracheal tubes for children younger than age 6 are usually not cuffed (cuffed tubes are manufactured but are not commonly used). This is because of concerns of postextubation airway narrowing. The inflammation after intubation of the narrow pediatric airway can result in obstruction to airflow. Adult airways also develop inflammation, but because they are of much greater diameter, the effect of the inflammation usually is not clinically significant.

■ Lubrication for tracheal tubes

Note: This may be helpful in the presence of dry oral mucosa (oral intubations). Lubrication is essential for nasal intubations to reduce nasal trauma, bleeding, and pain. Water-soluble lubricants (sterile) or local anesthetics (e.g., lidocaine, 2% jelly) are useful. It is of interest to note that lubricating tubes are associated with an increased incidence of sore throat, although the cause is unknown.

Stylets
The final step in tube preparation is preparing a lubricated stylet for the tracheal tube.

■ Stylets are made of a malleable metal, often coated with polymeric silicone (Silastic). They serve to provide a means of modifying the tube's innate mild curve to the shape desired by the intubator.
■ Stylets should be lubricated before insertion into the tracheal tube. The lubricant must not be harmful if inhaled into the lungs. A sterile, water-soluble jelly is used most often. Care should be taken to avoid getting the lubricant on the outside of the 15-mm adapter.
■ It is recommended that a stylet be placed for all oral intubations. During intubation, it is much easier to remove an unneeded stylet than it is to place a needed one.

Magill's Forceps
■ Magill's forceps are used to help pass nasotracheal tubes when laryngoscopes are used to facilitate nasal intubations.

Confirming Tube Placement
■ Tools for confirming correct placement of tracheal tubes must be immediately available.

■ A stethoscope to confirm breath sounds and a carbon dioxide detector (a capnograph is ideal; colorimetric is acceptable) to confirm placement in a perfused, ventilated airway
Note: Other devices are advocated but are not yet in common use.

Medications
■ See "Patient Preparation."

Other Equipment
Note: The equipment described will be sufficient for most intubations. If it is insufficient, it is recommended that specialized assistance be obtained. If this assistance is unavailable, transcricothyroid jet ventilation or cricothyroidotomy should be considered. Tracheostomy specifically is not recommended.

A failed intubation is likely due to anatomic abnormalities such as a short, thick neck; airway edema and bleeding; and cervical immobilization. Emergently "cutting down" into this anatomy to search for the trachea while striving to avoid the carotid arteries, the jugular veins, and the thyroid gland while the patient is becoming increasingly distressed is not recommended. Many patients have died in such a circumstance. The specialist consultant may have more experience, "tricks of the trade," and special equipment. Examples of this equipment include fiberoptic laryngoscopes, fiberoptic bronchoscopes, specialized laryngoscope blades, antegrade and retrograde intubating stylets, and intubating laryngeal mask airways.

Procedure for Oral Endotracheal Intubation

1. Reliable intravenous access should be in place before beginning the procedure. Cardiac and respiratory monitors should be applied. The patient must be breathing 100% oxygen, and suction and intubating equipment must be immediately available in close proximity.
2. On completion of the preceding preparations, open the patient's mouth as wide as possible, with the right thumb displacing the mandible toward the patient's feet and the right index finger pushing against the patient's maxillary teeth.

Note: This is best accomplished at the level of the molar teeth, which are flat and will not injure the fingers as incisors might. Additionally, molars are closer to the temporomandibular joint, so displacement there will yield greater mouth opening, and by having a hand off to the patient's right, there will be ample room to place the laryngoscope in the mouth.

3. Hold the laryngoscope in the left hand and place it in the right side of the open mouth. Slide along the tongue, displacing the tongue anteriorly and to the left.

Procedure for Oral Endotracheal Intubation – *(continued)*

4. Keep the tongue from falling over the right side of the blade, as this obscures visualization.
5. Keep an eye on the tip of the blade as it is being manipulated.

Note: As the blade is advanced, the epiglottis will come into view.

6. When a fair amount of the epiglottis is visualized (curved blade; Fig. 12–6), apply force along the axis of the laryngoscope's handle. This lifts the tongue and rotates the epiglottis, exposing the larynx (Fig. 12–7).

Note: When using a straight blade (Fig. 12–8), the epiglottis is directly elevated with the tip of the blade, again exposing the larynx.

Note: A common mistake is inserting the blade too far. This can be disorienting, as the ensuing esophageal visualization is unanticipated. Another common error is not applying the force vector along the laryngoscope handle's axis but "levering" the laryngoscope. This tends to cause it to pivot on the patient's upper incisor teeth, sometimes breaking them. More importantly (in a lifesaving situation), it makes laryngeal visualization more difficult because it tends to lift the larynx anteriorly out of the view of the intubator. The goal is to raise the structures above the larynx, leaving the larynx in the field of vision. Assistance may be obtained by displacing the cricoid cartilage posteriorly; this will displace the larynx for a better view. A cephalad displacement may also be helpful.

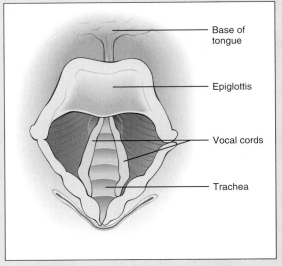

Base of tongue

Epiglottis

Vocal cords

Trachea

Figure 12–7

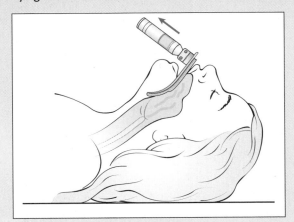

Figure 12–6

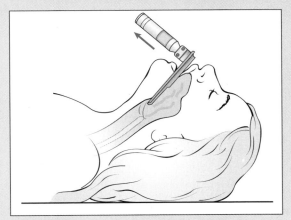

Figure 12–8

Procedure for Oral Endotracheal Intubation – *(continued)*

7. Take tracheal tube in the right hand, held as one would hold a writing instrument, and pass from the right side of the mouth into the laryngeal inlet, medial to the vocal cords and anteromedially to the arytenoid cartilages.

8. If the patient is breathing spontaneously, the vocal cords will be moving. Time the tube insertion to correspond to the end of inspiration. This is when the vocal cords are farthest apart.

Note: Be aware that at the moment of tube insertion, the view into the larynx will be lost. If the tube is not properly aligned with the larynx, it is possible for it to be deflected into the esophagus. The key to this potential problem is to keep one's eye on the larynx during and after the tube insertion. If the tube is visualized between the vocal cords and anterior to the arytenoids after tube insertion, the tube is in the correct position. If it is visualized posteriorly in the esophagus, it is not in the correct position and should be removed and placed properly.

9. Pass the tube so that the cuff just passes the vocal cords; more is neither necessary nor better.

Note: There is a great tendency among practitioners who intubate infrequently to advance the tube much too far. In most adults, the depth of insertion will be in the range of 18 to 24 cm at the level of the upper incisor teeth; the depth will be less in shorter patients and more in taller patients. As long as the cuff is just beyond the vocal cords, tube placement is adequate.

10. Pass the uncuffed pediatric tube so that the heavy black marker line just passes the vocal cords.

11. At this point, remove the laryngoscope from the patient's mouth, holding the tube securely while the stylet is removed.

12. Inflate the cuff at this time with just enough air to cause a seal within the trachea.

Note: The volume of air depends on the size of the tube relative to the size of the trachea: large tube, small trachea, small volume; small tube, large trachea, large volume. It is usually in the range of 5 to 10 mL. More is not better, because excessive pressure will be exerted on the tracheal mucosa. This causes ischemia that may predispose to tracheal scarring and stenosis or tracheomalacia. Just enough air should be administered so that during positive-pressure ventilation, one does not hear air leaking around the tube out of the patient's mouth.

Note: In children, a leak should be heard at 20 cm of water pressure. If there is no leak at this level of positive pressure, replace the tube with a smaller one. If, conversely, the leak is so large that one cannot effectively ventilate the child, replace the tube with a larger one.

Note: A recommended technique to change the tube is to repeat the laryngoscopy and, under direct vision, withdraw the wrong-sized tube and replace it with another.

12. Confirm tube placement by auscultating breath sounds bilaterally at the lung apices (either in the axillae or supraclavicularly)—first the right and then the left. If tube placement is in question, radiographic confirmation may be helpful.

Note: Auscultating the right side first will confirm placement in the airway; if there are sounds, there is either a tracheal or right main stem bronchial intubation. No sounds indicate esophageal intubation. If there are sounds on the left, it confirms tracheal intubation.

13. Assess if the expiratory gas contains the appropriate amount of carbon dioxide.

Note: This is highly desirable, especially if a capnographic waveform is available for analysis. This enables one to rule out a false-positive determination, as is seen when a patient has recently consumed carbonated beverages. False-negative determinations occur when there is a total absence of blood flow to the lungs, as happens during either cardiac arrest or massive pulmonary embolus.

14. Also inspect for symmetrical chest expansion, fogging of the tube with airway moisture, and absence of gastric distention. If the tube is seen in the larynx after tube placement, it is in place (unless it gets displaced afterward). The tube must now be secured.

15. Degrease the patient's skin and prepare the skin with tincture of benzoin or other skin adherent/protector.

Note: The tube can be secured by circumferentially wrapping the tape around the patient's neck and then the tracheal tube. Performed properly, it is almost impossible for the tube to "fall out." The tube can also be secured circumferentially with cloth umbilical tapes.

Procedure for Nasal Endotracheal Intubation

Note: Nasal intubation is most easily performed in the spontaneously breathing patient who is placed in a sitting position. Topical vasoconstrictors are essential to reduce the chance of epistaxis. If both nostrils are equally patent, the right nostril is preferred, as the bevel of the tube is less likely to "scoop" the nasal turbinates as it passes them.

1. Lubricate the tube; an easy way is to place water-soluble jelly or anesthetic jelly in the nostril, and the tube will "pick up" the jelly as it is inserted.

2. Exert firm, steady pressure along the axis of the nasopharyngeal floor (just as one would do with a nasogastric tube).

3. As the tube reaches the posterior nasopharynx, some resistance will be felt; continue the steady pressure, and the resistance will decrease as the tube "turns the corner."

4. As the tube is advanced further, breath sounds will be audible. It may be helpful to occlude the other nostril and the patient's mouth so that all ventilation is via the tube.

5. Advance the tube during inspiration.

Note: If the tube is aligned with the larynx, it will pass into the trachea. This is often marked with a cough and, if the patient is conscious, the loss of the ability to phonate.

6. If alignment is off in the midline, flex the patient's neck and advance the tube. This may attain success.

7. If the tube is misaligned laterally (the tube causes a bulge laterally), rotate to remedy the situation.

Note: Because of the resistance of the tube in the nose, a much greater rotation is necessary than would be expected. It might be necessary to rotate the tube 180 degrees to get 30 degrees of rotation at the tube's tip.

Procedure for Nasal Endotracheal Intubation – *(continued)*

8. If these maneuvers are ineffective, place the patient supine as for oral intubation and perform laryngoscopy and advance the tube under direct vision.
Note: The Magill forceps is often helpful at manipulating the tube into the larynx.

Caution: Do not grab the tube's cuff with the forceps, as it may tear. An assistant should advance the tube as the intubator guides it.
9. Once in place, confirmation should be obtained and the tube secured.

Follow-Up Care and Instructions

Having succeeded in this therapeutic maneuver, the patient must be protected both physically and psychologically.

Physical Protection

- Provide an adequate amount of humidified oxygen.
- Prevent the tube from kinking and becoming dislodged.

Psychological Protection

- Administer sedation and analgesia. If drugs are used to facilitate intubation, the patient will experience pain and anxiety after their effects have dissipated. It is both cruel and dangerous not to treat these symptoms. It is dangerous because self-extubation is likely, and hypertension, tachycardia, arrhythmias, and increased intracranial pressure may occur. NMB agents are an inappropriate means of keeping the tube in place in the absence of sedatives and analgesics.
- There are infrequent circumstances when the patient's hemodynamic status is so precarious that administration of sedatives and analgesics is inadvisable, and the patient must be pharmacologically paralyzed to prevent him or her from self-harm or harming others, to facilitate evaluation and treatment, or to allow mechanical ventilation at safe airway pressures.
- When these circumstances exist, all personnel must remember that the patient is *awake* and *sensate* and must be treated appropriately. Speech must be appropriate, and comfort and explanations offered to the patient. It is my opinion that NMB agents are overused both inside and outside the operating room.

References

Mallampati SR: Recognition of the difficult airway. In Benumof JL (ed): Airway Management: Principles and Practice. St. Louis, CV Mosby, 1996.

Roberts JT: Overview in Fundamentals of Tracheal Intubation. New York, Grune & Stratton, 1983, p 4.

Sanchez A, Trivedi NS, Morrison DE: Preparation of the patient for awake intubation. In Benumof JL: Airway Management: Principles and Practice. St. Louis, CV Mosby, 1996.

Bibliography

- Applebaum EL, Bruce DL: A short history of tracheal intubation. In Tracheal Intubation. Philadelphia, WB Saunders, 1976.
- Benumof JL: Airway Management: Principles and Practice. St. Louis, CV Mosby, 1996.
- Mallampati SR: Airway management. In Barash PG, Cullen BF, Stoelting RK (eds): Clinical Anesthesia, 3rd ed. Philadelphia, Lippincott-Raven, 1997, pp 573–594.

Chapter 13

Office Pulmonary Function Testing

▷ Daniel L. O'Donoghue
▷ Gary R. Sharp
▷ Roger A. Elliott
▷ Daniel L. McNeill

Procedure Goals and Objectives

Goal: To perform office pulmonary function testing (PFT) on a patient successfully.

Objectives: The student will be able to . . .

▶ Describe the indications, contraindications, and rationale for performing office PFT.

▶ Identify and describe common complications associated with office PFT.

▶ Describe the essential anatomy and physiology associated with the performance of office PFT.

▶ Identify the materials necessary for performing office PFT and their proper use.

▶ Identify the important aspects of patient care after office PFT.

Background and History

The first explanation of the working of the body in mechanical terms dates back more than 300 years, and PFT has been used for more than 150 years. Thackrah, in 1832, was the first to present data on lung function in human subjects. He was investigating the effects of occupation on lung size. His initial study revealed that workers who stooped at work tended to have smaller lungs than those who did not. Hutchinson's work, in 1844, is typically identified as the founding work in spirometry and includes the first accurate description of the use of spirometry to measure vital capacity. The first measurement of dynamic lung function was proposed in 1933 by Hermannsen, who recorded maximal voluntary ventilation. Tiffeneau and Pinelli first proposed the measurement of a timed forced expiratory volume (forced expiratory volume in 1 second [FEV_1]) in 1947 (Miller, 1998).

Objective measurements of pulmonary function were initially developed in the 1940s with the advent of spirometry. Improvements in spirometric design, along with the development of complex procedures such as body plethysmography and gas dilution techniques, continue to provide valuable physiologic data on lung function. Because of the complexity of performing and interpreting the techniques, PFT remained within the domain of hospital-based laboratories (Ferguson, 1998). Currently, advances in spirometer design have enabled the primary care provider to conduct PFT testing in the office setting. Office-based spirometry has been made even more reachable by the adoption of standards for testing and interpreting results (American Thoracic Society, 1991, 1995).

When adding PFT to a practice, the provider must determine if it will be used simply to manage or assess disease or if it will be used to quantify pulmonary function for impairment ratings or for meeting Occupational Safety and Health Administration (OSHA) requirements. For impairment or Occupational Safety and Health Administration uses, the examiner must undergo certification training through a National Institute of Occupational Safety and Health–approved course and must adhere to stringent requirements for testing. Because of the governmental regulations that apply to the use of spirometry in occupational medicine, this chapter focuses on using the technique in a primary care setting. In addition, the terms *PFT* and *spirometry* will be used interchangeably.

Indications

It is important to realize that diagnoses are not made singularly with PFT. Spirometry alone does not establish the diagnosis of a specific disease. Spirometry does, however, aid in differentiating pulmonary dysfunction as having an obstructive, restrictive, or mixed cause (Bosse and

Criner, 1993). Knowing the pattern of dysfunction, along with the clinical presentation, allows the provider to make a diagnosis and to assess the degree of impairment (Crapo, 1994; Stephenson et al, 1998). Understanding some basic facts about the respiratory system can enhance an accurate diagnosis. PFTs provide objective measures of respiratory function that aid the provider in establishing a diagnosis, which leads to proper disease management and prognosis (Bosse and Criner, 1993). Common indications for the use of office-based spirometry include the following:

- Evaluating patients with pulmonary complaints such as wheezing and dyspnea
- Determining the degree and reversibility of impairment in airflow
- Assessing preoperative pulmonary risk
- Establishing the impact of related risks on lung function, such as smoking or occupational exposures
- Assessing abnormalities of chest wall motion
- As a component of periodic physical examination testing for individuals requiring certification in respirator use, for example, emergency personnel, carpenters, and many industrial workers

Contraindications

There are no absolute contraindications for performing spirometry. Despite the absence of absolute contraindications, the examiner should exercise common sense and not perform spirometry on a patient unable to tolerate the physical demands of the procedure. Patients with such relative contraindications, as defined by The American Association for Respiratory Care (American Association for Respiratory Care, 1996), follow:

- Hemoptysis of unknown origin
- Pneumothorax
- Unstable cardiovascular status
- Thoracic, abdominal, or cerebral aneurysm
- Recent eye surgery
- Recent surgery involving the thorax or abdomen

Given the number of patients who are encountered routinely with indications for spirometry, each clinic must determine the economic prudence of adding spirometry to the practice or continuing the referral of patients to a PFT laboratory. To aid in this decision, one must realize that the cost of a reliable and completely computerized and automated spirometer starts at about $1500, with replacement mouthpieces costing about $1.50 per test. Generating a spirogram takes approximately 10 minutes. Using Medicare as a "standardized" payment source, reimbursement under Part B for performing spirometry (CPT 94010) is approximately $21.50, and reimbursement for the technical component (e.g., interpretation, CPT 94010TC) is approximately $10.85. Thus, one could anticipate a total reimbursement from Medicare of about $32 per spirometry examination (U.S. Department of Health and Human Services, 1999). Using a nonscientific survey of four clinics in the authors' state, third-party and self-pay reimbursement for performing and interpreting spirometry ranged from $25 to $75 per examination.

Potential Complications

Common complications of spirometry are usually related to the physical condition of the patient.

- Individuals with cardiopulmonary disease, for example, asthma, emphysema, chronic obstructive pulmonary disease (COPD), or unstable angina, may suffer an exacerbation of symptoms when spirometry is performed.
- Paroxysmal coughing, bronchospasm, and chest pain have been reported after spirometry.
- A more commonly occurring untoward effect of the procedure is light-headedness or, on rare occasions, syncope brought on by the momentary change in intrathoracic pressure.
- Patient fatigue or lack of understanding of the test may compromise the results of the procedure.

For optimal results, it is important to have a well-motivated patient who understands that spirometry is a patient effort–dependent procedure. Consequently, providing patient education and instructions before the procedure begins is important. This is particularly useful in avoiding patient fatigue resulting from an incomplete understanding of instructions regarding performing the test. Finally, a well-trained staff is essential for maximizing the quality of the procedure and reliability of the data.

Review of Essential Anatomy and Physiology

From a practical viewpoint, the lungs may be divided into the following:

- Large airways consisting of the trachea and bronchi
- Small airways, which include bronchi and bronchioles less than 2 mm in diameter
- The respiratory component consisting of the alveoli

Although the diameter of the airways becomes progressively smaller over the 23 or so generations of divisions, the total cross-sectional area of the small airways actually increases (Brooks, 1981). Thus, resistance to airflow decreases as one proceeds from the lung hilum to the parenchyma. Because small airways contribute only about 15% to total airway resistance, significant disease must be present before evidence of small airway dysfunction is measurable by spirometry.

Obstructive Disease

Disorders that present with an obstructive pattern by spirometry are noted in Table 13–1. Congenital or mechanical impediments to airflow in the large airways obviously result in an obstructive dysfunction. However, in the smaller airways, the cause of obstructive dysfunction may be due to a decrease in the elastic recoil of the lung or an increase in airway resistance, or both. For example, a decrease in recoil is observed in emphysema, in which breakdown of alveoli and loss of lung stroma contribute to a decrease in elasticity. The increase in airway resistance observed in chronic bronchitis and asthma is produced by a decrease in small airway diameter secondary to mucosal edema, hypersecretion, spasm, or a combination (Brooks, 1981).

Obstructive diseases reduce the ability of the lungs to move air, whereas lung volumes and capacities remain normal or increase. Abnormalities in air movement become most obvious by spirometry during forced expiration (Fig. 13–1). As such, obstructive diseases result in a decrease in the volume of air a patient is able to move during the first second (FEV_1) and in midphase ($FEV_{25\%-75\%}$) of forced expiration (Table 13–2).

Table 13–1

Pulmonary Disorders That Commonly Yield an Abnormal Spirogram

Disorders Resulting in Obstructive Dysfunction	Disorders Resulting in Restrictive Dysfunction
Asthma	Fibrosis
Emphysema	Pneumonitis
Chronic bronchitis	Pneumoconiosis
Neoplasm	Granulomatosis
Foreign body	Pulmonary edema
Tracheal stenosis or malacia	Neoplasm
Vocal cord paralysis	Atelectasis
	Pleural effusion or fibrosis
	Kyphoscoliosis
	Neuromuscular disease
	Obesity
	Abdominal distention

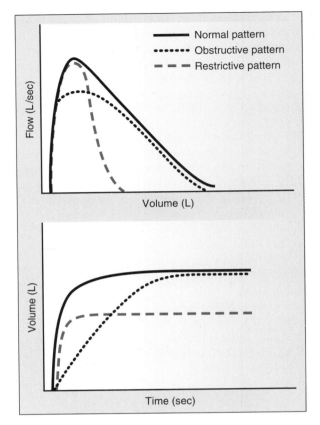

Figure 13–1. Normal and abnormal spirographic patterns.

Restrictive Disease

The pathologic presence of fibrotic tissue in the lungs underlies the basic cause of restrictive diseases. As a result of pulmonary fibrosis, the lungs are stiffened, thus increasing the elastic recoil pressure with a reciprocal decrease in compliance. The net effect is that restrictive disease

Table 13–2

Volumes and Flows in Obstructive and Restrictive Disease

Interpretation	FEV$_1$	Forced Vital Capacity	FEV$_1$/FVC Ratio	Vital Capacity	Total Lung Capacity
Normal	NL	NL	NL	NL	NL
Obstruction	Low	NL/low	Low	NL/low	High
Restriction	NL	Low	NL/high	Low	Low
Mixed	Low	Low	NL/low	Low	Low

NL, normal; FEV$_1$, forced expiratory volume, the volume of air *forcefully* exhaled in 1 second; FVC, forced vital capacity, the volume of air that can be exhaled *forcefully* after full inspiration; vital capacity, the maximal volume of air exhaled from the point of maximal inspiration; total lung capacity, vital capacity plus the total volume of inspired air.

prevents the lungs from expanding fully. Table 13–1 lists disorders that result in a restrictive lung dysfunction pattern.

In pure restrictive disease, there is no obstruction to airflow. Therefore, FEV_1 and other parameters of flow remain relatively normal (see Fig. 13–1 and Table 13–2). Conversely, spirogram tracings from patients with restrictive disease reveal a decrease in lung volumes that may be identified by the forced vital capacity (FVC) (see Fig. 13–1 and Table 13–2).

Mixed Disease

A mixed pattern of obstructive and restrictive disease is typical in patients presenting with more than one disease, for example, asthma and pulmonary edema. More commonly, a mixed pattern is observed in smokers with some degree of chronic obstructive pulmonary disease. Therefore, caution must be exercised when attempting to make a diagnosis of restrictive disease if the comorbid obstructive disease is severe (Brooks, 1981). The reason for caution is that in severe obstructive disease, the FVC may be decreased because of hyperinflation and air trapping from the obstructive process. If severe obstructive disease is suspected, the examiner may rely on other parameters of lung volume, such as vital capacity (VC) without forced effort and total lung capacity (vital capacity plus total volume of inspired air; Milhorn, 1981). In mixed diseases, FEV_1, FVC, VC, and total lung capacity are all decreased (see Table 13–2).

Standard Precautions ▷ Every practitioner should use Standard Precautions at all times when interacting with patients, especially when performing procedures. Determining the level of precaution necessary requires the practitioner to exercise clinical judgment based on the patient's history and the potential for exposure to body fluids or aerosol-borne pathogens (for further discussion, see Chapter 2).

Patient Preparation

- Patient education regarding the procedure is the primary preparation required for spirometry.
- Since the procedure requires the ability to follow instructions and give maximal effort, children younger than age 5 are not good candidates.
- Although a common cold usually will not affect the outcome of the test, individuals with acute bronchitis or pneumonia should wait 3 weeks for recovery in order to perform at their optimal level (Horvath, 1981b).

- Advise the patient to wear loose-fitting clothing and not to eat a meal within an hour of testing.
- If the patient is a smoker, instruct him or her not to smoke for at least 1 hour before spirometry.
- Advise the patient not to use a bronchodilator within several hours of the procedure.
- At the time of the examination, ask the patient to loosen any tight clothing and remove dentures if worn.
- The use of a nose clip during the procedure is optional.
- The patient may be seated or standing for the procedure. If the patient chooses to stand for the test, it is wise to place a chair behind him or her should lightheadedness ensue during the procedure.

Materials Utilized for Performing Pulmonary Function Testing

Spirometers on the market today fall into two main groups. There are those that measure volume, such as a rolling seal or bellows type, and those that measure flow directly, such as a rotating vane, hot wire anemometer, or pneumotachograph. Most instruments today are connected to a computer for data collection and analysis. The spirometer of choice should be one that meets the American Thoracic Society standards. The type of instrument should be selected based on the need to store patient data, load computerized measurements into databases, ability to transmit data, cost per procedure, and maintenance requirements.

Procedure for Pulmonary Function Testing

Note: It is important to read the instructions specific for the operation of each machine, because operation may vary from model to model.

Calibration

1. The rationale for calibration is to provide data to the spirometer that corrects for fluctuations in ambient atmospheric pressure. Therefore, before performing PFT, the machine should be calibrated daily or every 4 hours, or both, if multiple tests are administered in a day.

Note: Calibration involves using a 3-L syringe to blow air through a mouthpiece. The syringe is usually provided with the machine. In addition, results from each patient must be corrected to BTPS (body temperature, ambient pressure, saturated with water). The BTPS correction factor is necessary because volumes change when warm expired air rapidly cools to the lower ambient temperature. Modern machines, fortunately, provide the BTPS correction automatically.

2. To complete the calibration, the altitude above sea level and the temperature must be entered into the machine.

3. For each test, enter the patient's height (without shoes); weight, age, gender, and race are also entered.
4. Many modern instruments are programmed to input patient information on smoking history, presence of chronic cough, and so forth. Although not critical in terms of calculating the results, recording the patient's history may be informative when interpreting the spirogram.

Patient Instructions

Note: Providing patients with instructions and active coaching during the test is critical in obtaining an acceptable spirogram.

5. Instructing the patient that, "I want to see how hard and how fast you can breathe or exhale your air" is usually sufficient. Explain the maneuver by stating, "Take in a deep breath, close your mouth around the mouthpiece, and then blow the air from your lungs into the mouthpiece as hard and as fast as you can" (Fig. 13–2).
6. The preferred patient posture for performing spirometry is standing. A sitting position is acceptable if the patient is unable to stand or if the risk of syncope is a concern.
7. During the maneuver, it is important to provide active coaching. As the patient begins to exhale, enthusiastically say, "Blow, blow, blow!" When it appears that the patient is nearing the end of expiration, say, "Keep blowing!"

Note: Most machines have a signal that identifies when the patient has reached a plateau (a change of 25 mL or less in 2 seconds) or meets the length requirement (between 6 and 15 seconds), or both. A

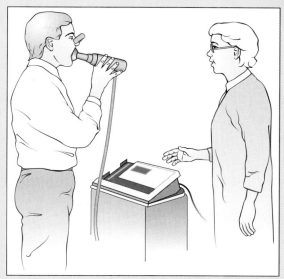

Figure 13–2. Redrawn from Pfenninger JL, Fowler GC: Procedures for Primary Care Physicians. St. Louis, Mosby-Year Book, 1994, p 489.

plateau signifies the end of an acceptable maneuver.

Note: The maneuver may also be ended when the patient cannot or should not continue.

Obtaining a Meaningful Spirogram

Note: An acceptable maneuver is free from coughs, early termination, hesitant starts, or variable effort. Coughs typically show up as spiked notches on the volume-time curve.

- Early termination is defined as an inability of the patient to plateau or have a change of 25 mL or less within 2 seconds.
- A hesitant start is determined by back extrapolation from the volume-time curve.

Procedure for Pulmonary Function Testing – *(continued)*

- Variable effort is an inconsistent curve and is often a sign of poor compliance with the procedure.
- Many computerized instruments have a "built-in" algorithm program that looks for and reports any of the preceding flaws in technique.
- If possible, it is best to save each maneuver, even if flawed.
- An acceptable spirometry test is composed of at least three acceptable maneuvers, with the two best curves for FVC and FEV_1 being within 5% of each other.
- No more that eight maneuvers should be performed at any one session, because fatigue can become a factor in the quality of expiratory effort. Most instruments let the examiner know when an acceptable spirometry test has been accomplished.
- It is important to note that individuals with disease may not fulfill all criteria for an acceptable test. In such circumstances, information gained from at least an attempt may be useful in the management of their disease.

8. Documenting the patient's effort in complying with the procedure aids in interpreting the spirogram and is useful when comparisons are made with subsequent tests as part of monitoring the progression of disease.

9. It is common for errors in technique to occur during spirometry. Frequently, the patient may give up too soon, resulting in a spirogram tracing lacking a plateau. Properly encourage the patient toward the end of the maneuver to correct this.

10. Air leakage around the mouthpiece can give erroneous readings. Have the patient wet his or her lips to obtain a better seal.

11. Look for pursed lips and obstruction with the tongue, which are errors readily correctable by proper technique.

12. At the conclusion of the test, computerized instruments allow you to print the results of the test (Fig. 13–3).

Comparison of Results with Standards

13. Interpreting spirometry involves comparing the patient's actual results with predicted results from an accepted standard.

Note: Many spirometers allow the examiner to choose which standard will be applied. The two standards used predominantly are those of Morris (also referred to as the ATS Standard) (Morris et al, 1971) and Knudson (Knudson et al, 1976). Knudson's is the standard used when performing spirometry to satisfy Occupational Safety and Health Administration requirements. In all other circumstances, at present Morris's is the standard. Another standard, termed National Health and Nutrition Examination Survey III, developed in 1999 from a broad-based study, will probably become a more suitable standard for primary care practice (Hankinson et al, 1999). However, the NHANES III standard as yet is not available on all computerized spirometers.

14. Report the highest values obtained from any of the three maneuvers as the results for the test.

Note: Using the highest values is consistent with the Morris standard. In fact, a principal difference between the two standards is that Morris uses the best of the three maneuvers, whereas the Knudson standard is an average of the three spirogram results.

Procedure for Pulmonary Function Testing – *(continued)*

SPIROMETRY REPORT
PB100 SW Rev: J-J

University Occupational Health
Clinic, OUHSC, OKC, OK, 271-3100

TEST DATE:
TIME: 08:47

Patient Name:_____   PreMed Time: 08:48
Patient ID: Age: 42   Height (in): 72   Weight (lbs): 200   Sex: Male   Race Correction: No   Smoker: No
Barometric Pressure (mmHg): 730   Temp (deg F): 76   BTPS Correction: 1.093   Sensor: FS200   Insp Code: None
Last Cal Date: 03/08/00

FVC TEST DATA - Clinical Format   BEST TEST SUMMARY   Knudson 83 Adult Predicted Normals

Measurement		PreMed	Pred	%Pred	PostMed	%Pred	%Change
FVC	(L)	5.16	5.40	96			
FEV1	(L)	4.29	4.42	97			
%FEV1	(%)	83.13	81.58	102			
FEF25%–75%	(L/S)	4.82	4.55	106			
PEF	(L/S)	13.55	9.73	139			
FEV3	(L)	4.84	4.97	97			
FET	(S)	14.04					

Variability : PreMed: FVC = 0.2%(10 mL) FEV_1 = 0.2%(10 mL)   PEF = 2.6%

PREMED

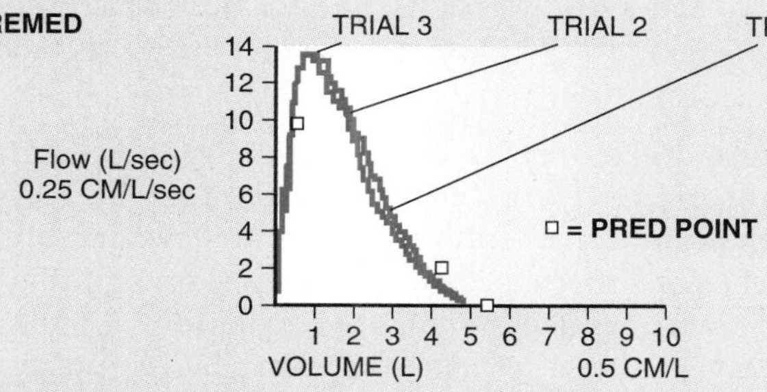

TRIAL 3   TRIAL 2   TRIAL 1

Flow (L/sec)
0.25 CM/L/sec

□ = PRED POINT

VOLUME (L)   0.5 CM/L

PREMED

TRIAL 3   TRIAL 2   TRIAL 1

□ = PRED POINT

Volume (L)
0.5 CM/L

TIME (sec)
1 CM/S

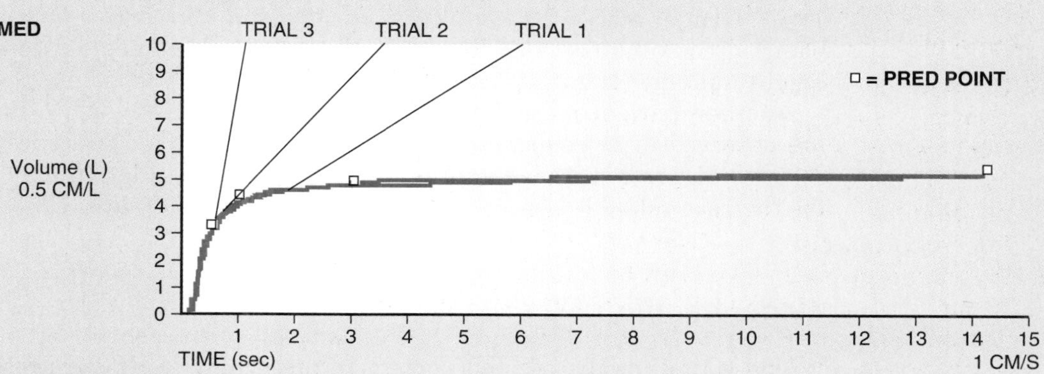

Interpretations:

PREMED: Testing indicates normal spirometry.

Comments:

Figure 13–3

Postbronchodilator Test

Note: A major use of spirometry in the office setting is in determining a patient's response to an inhaled bronchodilator, thus aiding in the diagnosis of asthma.

15. To test for reversibility of pulmonary dysfunction, ask the patient to perform prebronchodilator spirometry.

16. After collecting the results, give the patient two puffs of albuterol by metered dose inhaler.

17. Fifteen minutes after administration of the albuterol, perform postbronchodilator spirometry.

Note: The general agreement is that a 12% to 15% increase in FEV_1 and FVC after bronchodilator use is diagnostic of asthma or reversible airway disease.

Special Considerations

Patient Variability

Normal values for spirometric results vary with body habitus and gender. Height and age are of particular concern and must be considered with all spirometry examinations. Interestingly, airflow in liters per minute increases linearly with increased height. However, age has an opposite effect on airflow, with a decline of approximately 4% to 5% in FEV_1 and FVC occurring every 5 years after age 25 (Knudson et al, 1983). Gender also must be taken into consideration, with FEV_1 and FVC being approximately 10% less in women than in men of comparable height and age (Horvath, 1981a).

Another patient-related variable is race. Specifically, FEV_1 and FVC are observed to be consistently 15% less in nonwhites. Differences in thoracic configuration and diaphragm position are speculative explanations for the race-related decreases in flow and volume (Horvath, 1981a).

Understanding What Is Normal

The actual, predicted, and percent of predicted values are presented in Figure 13–2. Regardless of which standard is applied, there is great variability in the normal values. For example, a patient's FEV_1 and FVC can fall between 80% and 120% of predicted and still be considered normal. This range represents two standard deviations from the mean. Other values frequently reported have an even larger range. One example is the $FEV_{25\%-75\%}$, which has an individual daily variability of 20% versus a 3% daily change in FEV_1 or FVC.

Table 13-3

American Medical Association Guidelines for Determining the Degree of Pulmonary Dysfunction

Characterization	FEV$_1$, Forced Vital Capacity, or Both (Percent of Predicted Values)
Normal	80%
Mild disease	60–79%
Moderate disease	41–59%
Severe disease	40%

From American Medical Association: Guides to the Evaluation of Permanent Impairment, 4th ed. Chicago, American Medical Association, 1993, pp 153–167.

Despite the variability, a workable guideline for identifying the degree of pulmonary dysfunction (American Medical Association, 1993) is described in Table 13-3. Note that when following disease progression by spirometry, it is more prudent to document changes in the patient's actual values than to compare them with predicted values.

Follow-Up Care and Instructions

In the management of pulmonary disease in the outpatient setting, it is crucial to be able to stabilize the airway using various pharmacologic approaches and to have rescue medications available in the event that stabilizing modalities fail.

■ Provide patients with instruction on (1) the mechanism of action for each medication, (2) monitoring the progress of therapy, and (3) follow-up care.
■ Encourage patients to call if they are confused or if they have questions concerning medications. For patients with multiple medications, a simple outline may alleviate confusion and prevent exacerbations due to noncompliance.
■ For patients who smoke, an unambiguous statement of the continued health risks of smoking should be emphasized at every visit.

The success of treating pulmonary disease depends largely on patient compliance with regimens. Providing patients with a peak flowmeter is a useful means of helping them to monitor their lung function at home. Patients will tend to comply better if they understand the different treatment modalities and the central role of monitoring pulmonary function.

Acknowledgment

The authors are grateful to Ms. Cate Stow, R.N., M.Ed. for her input into the preparation of this chapter.

References

American Association for Respiratory Care: Clinical Practice Guideline: Spirometry. Respir Care 41:629–636, 1996.

American Medical Association: Guides to the Evaluation of Permanent Impairment, 4th ed. Chicago, American Medical Association, 1993, pp 153–167.

American Thoracic Society: Standardization of spirometry: 1994 update. Am J Respir Crit Care Med 152:1107–1136, 1995.

American Thoracic Society: Lung function testing: Selection of reference values and interpretative strategies. Am Rev Respir Dis 144:1202–1218, 1991.

Bosse CG, Criner GJ: Using spirometry in the primary care office: A guide to technique and interpretation of results. Postgrad Med 93:122–148, 1993.

Brooks SM: Pulmonary anatomy and physiology. In Horvath EP (ed): Manual of Spirometry in Occupational Medicine. Washington, D.C., U.S. Department of Health and Human Services, 1981, pp 3–11.

Crapo RO: Pulmonary function testing. N Engl J Med 331:25–30, 1994.

Ferguson GT: Screening and early intervention for COPD. Hosp Pract 33: 67–84, 1998.

Hankinson JL, Odencrantz JR, Fedan KB: Spirometric reference values from a sample of the general U.S. population. Am J Respir Crit Care Med 159: 179–187, 1999.

Horvath EP Jr: Calculations. In Horvath EP (ed): Manual of Spirometry in Occupational Medicine. Washington D.C., U.S. Department of Health and Human Services, 1981a, pp 17–33.

Horvath EP Jr: Technique. In Horvath EP (ed): Manual of Spirometry in Occupational Medicine. Washington, D.C., U.S. Department of Health and Human Services, 1981b, pp 13–16.

Knudson RJ, Lebowitz M, Holberg CJ, et al: Changes in the normal maximal respiratory flow-volume curve with aging. Am Rev Respir Dis 127:725–734, 1983.

Knudson RJ, Slatin RC, Lebowitz MD, et al: The maximal expiratory flow-volume curve: Normal standards, variability, and effects of age. Am Rev Respir Dis 113:587–600, 1976.

Milhorn HT Jr: Understanding pulmonary function tests. Am Fam Phys 24: 139–145, 1981.

Miller MR: Chronic obstructive pulmonary disease and 150 years of blowing. Hosp Med 59:719–722, 1998.

Morris JF, Koski A, Johnson LC: Spirometric standards for healthy nonsmoking adults. Am Rev Respir Dis 103:57–67, 1971.

Stephenson N, Morgan R, Abdel-Rahman-Abdel-Wahab E, et al: Hospital doctor's assessment of baseline spirometry. Postgrad Med J 74:537–540, 1998.

U.S. Department of Health and Human Services: Medicare Part B, Participation Program for Physicians. Oklahoma City, Okla, Health Care Financing Administration, 1999.

Bibliography

- Eaton T, Withy S, Garrett JE, et al: Spirometry in primary care practice: The importance of quality assurance and the impact of spirometry workshops. Chest 116:416–423, 1999.
- King D: Asthma diagnosis by spirometry: Sensitive or specific? Aust Fam Phys 27:183–185, 1998.
- Thiadens HA, de Bock GH, Dekker FW, et al: Identifying asthma and chronic obstructive pulmonary disease in patients with persistent cough presenting to general practitioners: Descriptive study. BMJ 316:1286–1290, 1998.

Chapter 14

Nasogastric Tube Placement

▷ Dan Vetrosky

Procedure Goals and Objectives

Goal: To perform nasogastric (NG) tube placement in a patient safely and accurately.

Objectives: The student will be able to . . .

▶ Describe the indications, contraindications, and rationale for performing NG tube placement.

▶ Identify and describe common complications associated with performing NG tube placement.

▶ Describe the essential anatomy and physiology associated with the performance of NG tube placement.

▶ Identify the materials necessary for performing NG tube placement and their proper use.

▶ Describe the steps for correctly inserting an NG tube.

Background and History

The first record of use of a tube for feeding placed into the esophagus was reported by His to have been by Capivacceus in 1598 when he introduced nutrient substances into the esophagus using a hollow tube with a bladder attached to one end. In 1617, Fabricius ab Aquapendente reported using a silver tube passed through the nostril into the nasopharynx for feeding a patient with tetanus. In 1867, Kussmaul introduced a flexible orogastric tube for gastric decompression, and Ewald and Oser introduced the soft rubber tube for gastric intubation in 1874 (Randall, 1990).

The passage of a hollow tube into the stomach has been used for research and medical-surgical purposes for many years. Sampling the gastric contents, decompressing a distended stomach, preventing aspiration during surgery, and performing gastric lavage are just a few of the current and past uses for the NG tube. This chapter covers the indications, rationale, types of NG tubes, insertion techniques, and complications of NG tube placement.

Indications

Indications for the insertion of an NG tube are many and range from severe diverticular disease to unrelenting vomiting. NG tubes are indicated for:

- Sampling gastric contents
- Removing air, blood, ingested substances, and gastric contents
- Providing nutritional support for patients who cannot eat but have a functional gastrointestinal tract (GI) tract

Table 14-1 outlines some of the indications and rationale for the insertion of the NG tube.

Contraindications

NG tube placement is contraindicated when the intended path of the tube is obstructed or any of the structures the NG tube would traverse are damaged, as well as the following situations and conditions.

- Choanal atresia
- Significant facial trauma or basilar skull fracture
- Esophageal stricture or atresia
- Esophageal burn
- Zenker's diverticulum
- Recent surgery on the esophagus or stomach
- History of gastrectomy

■ Table 14–1

Indications and Rationale for Nasogastric Tube Insertion

Indications	Rationale
Diverticulitis—usually severe	To rest the gastrointestinal tract, especially if bowel obstructive symptoms exist; relieves abdominal distention and vomiting if present
Gastric outlet obstruction	As above and can be diagnostic if >200 mL foul-smelling fluid obtained in the presence of obstructive symptoms
Gastrointestinal bleeding	Diagnostic if bright red blood or "coffee grounds" material is aspirated; can intermittently suction to assess presence of active bleeding (should *not* perform lavage in these patients because it may increase the chance of aspiration)
Intestinal obstruction	To relieve abdominal distention and vomiting
Near drowning	Used to empty swallowed water and to prevent aspiration
Vomiting	Prevention of aspiration and in intestinal obstruction, if present
Surgery (stomach, abdominal)	Decompresses stomach and may help lessen the chance for aspiration; can monitor postoperative bowel function return
Severe burns	Patients in the immediate postburn period are prone to develop ileus; nasogastric intubation helps empty the gastric contents and lessen the chance of aspiration
Nutritional support	Used in patients who cannot take in adequate amounts of nutrition orally; must be used only in patients who are able to sit up in bed and can protect the airway; aspiration is a concern
Gastrointestinal lavage-aspiration	Used in patients with suspected or known overdose to lavage and evacuate any residual medication or ingested agents

Potential Complications

- Trauma to the turbinates or nasopharynx, or both, during passage of the tube: Bleeding from the nares and spitting of blood from the mouth are signs of trauma to the nasopharyngeal region caused by NG tube placement. Proper insertion techniques, gentle pressure during the tube's passage, and ensuring patient cooperation will help obviate these problems.
- Erroneously assuming that the tube is in the stomach: Irrigation of an NG tube that is in the lungs can cause serious complications, such as pneumonia.
- Placement of the NG tube into the trachea and lung can result in pneumothorax if the tube is advanced forcefully into the lung tissue.

The best way to avoid complications associated with NG tubes placed in anatomic locations other than the stomach is to obtain radiographic confirmation. If radiography is not available, placing the NG tube in a glass of water once it has been passed can confirm poor placement. If the tube is placed in the lung, submerging the end of the tube in water will reveal bubbles during exhalation. When this occurs the tube must be removed completely and another NG tube reinserted.

Other potential complications follow:

- Gastric erosion with hemorrhage
- Erosion or necrosis of the nasal mucosae
- Aspiration pneumonia
- Sinusitis
- An NG tube passed in a patient with significant head, neck, thoracic, or abdominal trauma: In this setting, the NG tube may traverse a break in the nasopharynx, larynx, esophagus, or stomach. Advancement of the tube in this setting may result in severe damage to the brain, lungs, or peritoneal cavity.

Review of Essential Anatomy and Physiology

Insertion of the NG tube involves passing it through one of the nares into the nasopharynx. It is then passed into the posterior oropharynx and further inferiorly until it reaches the level of the larynx. At the level of the larynx, the tube may pass either anteriorly into the trachea or posteriorly into the esophagus (Fig. 14–1). Having the patient swallow greatly facilitates the passage of the NG tube into the esophagus. With swallowing, the vocal cords of the larynx are strongly approximated and the epiglottis swings backward, covering the opening of the larynx. Both of these factors help prevent the passage of food (or in this case the NG tube) into the trachea.

During swallowing, the entire larynx is pulled upward and forward by the muscles that are attached to the hyoid bone. This movement causes the opening of the esophagus to stretch. Simultaneously, the upper portion of the esophagus (upper 3 to 4 cm) relaxes and thus food moves more easily into the upper esophagus.

The esophagus is a muscular tube that begins at the level of the cricoid cartilage and is an average of 20 cm long and 3 cm in diameter in most adults. It courses through the posterior mediastinum, behind the heart and aorta, and penetrates the esophageal hiatus of the diaphragm. It then joins the cardia portion of the stomach just below the level of the diaphragm. Once the NG tube reaches the upper esophagus, rapid peristaltic waves are initiated, which assist in passing it down the length of the esophagus and facilitating its advancement into the stomach. The esophagus has two sphincters, one at each end, which serve to physically isolate the remainder of the gastrointestinal system from the outside environment. The esophagus, like other organs in the thoracic cavity, undergoes negative pressure during inspiration, and without sphincters, gastric contents would be sucked into the esophagus with each breath.

Anterior flexion of the cervical spine during NG tube insertion also facilitates passage into the esophagus. This occurs by causing the tube to rest or press against the posterior portion of the oropharynx as the NG tube is advanced. Consequently, it is better aligned to pass into the esophagus when it reaches the level of the larynx.

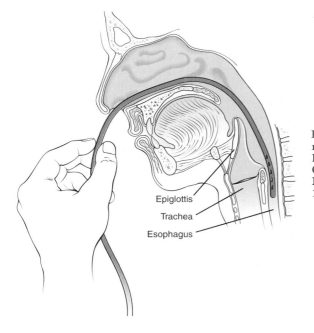

Figure 14–1. Passage of the nasogastric tube. (Adapted from Rosen P, Bankin RM, Sternback GL: Essentials of Emergency Medicine. St. Louis, CV Mosby, 1991, p 615.)

Epiglottis

Trachea

Esophagus

Standard Precautions ▷ Practitioners should use Standard Precautions at all times when interacting with patients. Determining the level of precaution necessary requires the practitioner to exercise clinical judgment based on the patient's history and the potential for exposure to body fluids or aerosol-borne pathogens (for further discussion see Chapter 2).

Patient Preparation

- The patient should be alert and able to cooperate with the procedure.
- Informed consent is not typically required.
- Explanation and discussion of the procedure before beginning helps facilitate patient cooperation.
- Explain to the patient the importance of keeping the neck flexed until the tube is in the esophagus. This is essential to avoid placement of the tube in the trachea.
- Patients should be informed that the introduction of the tube normally produces some degree of gagging.
- Ask the patient to take small sips of water through a straw and swallow to facilitate placement of the tube into the esophagus.

Materials Utilized to Perform Nasogastric Tube Placement

Note: Typical equipment needed for placement of an NG tube can include the following (equipment may vary slightly from setting to setting):

- Nonsterile procedure gloves, goggles, and gown
- Portable or wall suction equipment and connection availability
- Hypoallergenic tape, an occlusive seal dressing, or a premanufactured NG tube holder (some hospitals keep them available)
- Tincture of benzoin
- Emesis basin
- Cup of water and a straw
- Stethoscope
- 20- to 60-mL irrigation syringe (an irrigation-tip Toomey syringe, not a Luer syringe)
- 100 mL of water (tap or sterile) for irrigation
- Towels to protect patient gown and bed linen in case of emesis
- Malleable stylet if small feeding tube is used
- Appropriate size and type of NG (Levin) tube

Note: The most common type of NG tube used today is the Levin tube. These tubes range is size from a 3 French (Fr) to an 18 Fr. Tubes larger than 18 Fr should not be passed nasally because of the increased risk of trauma. Larger tubes, placed through the oral cavity, are reserved for extreme emergency procedures, and can be as large as 26 to 32 Fr.

The size of the NG tube used is dependent on the patient's age and size, purpose of the NG intubation, length of time the tube will be required, the viscosity of the fluids being instilled or evacuated, and disease processes present, if any. Neonates, infants, and patients with sinus or esophageal problems may require very small sizes (3 Fr to 8 Fr), whereas typical, otherwise healthy adult patients require NG tubes from 10 Fr to 18 Fr. Patients who require gastric lavage for medicine overdosage, ingestion of certain toxic substances, or evacuation of blood clots require larger bore NG tubes or may require oral gastric intubation.

Specialized NG tubes, such as those with weighted ends, are used to facilitate passage into the duodenum and small intestine. Double-lumen NG tubes that have one opening at the distal end (for feeding or instillation of fluids) and other openings along the distal sides of the tube allow for gastric decompression as well as jejunal feeding. NG tubes with multiple openings along the distal length, known as sump tubes, are used when it is necessary to irrigate or evacuate large amounts of fluids from the stomach.

Procedure for Performing Nasogastric Tube Insertion

1. Make sure the patient is sitting in a 45-degree angle or greater.
2. Ensure that all necessary materials and personnel are readily available before beginning the procedure.
3. Wash hands and don gloves, goggles, and gown.
4. Place protective sheet in place over patient's chest and abdomen.
5. Check for nasal patency and examine each nasal passageway. Choose the appropriate, most patent nostril for tube placement.
6. Using the tube to be inserted, measure from the tip of the nose to the ear lobe, and from the ear lobe to the patient's xiphoid to determine the appropriate tube insertion length and distance (Fig. 14–2).

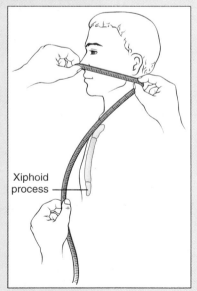

Xiphoid process —

Figure 14–2. Adapted from Potter PA, Perry AG: Fundamentals of Nursing: Concepts, Process, and Practice, 4th ed. St. Louis, CV Mosby, 1997, p 1407.

Note: Either count the premade markings on the tube or place a small piece of tape at the measured insertion length. If the tube is to be placed below the stomach, add an additional 15 to 25 cm to the premeasured mark.

7. Lubricate the first 2 to 3 inches of the tube with lidocaine jelly lubricant.
8. Before inserting the tube, make sure the beveled opening or side of the tube is positioned toward the nasal septum to avoid trauma to the turbinates.
9. Have the patient flex the neck forward, bringing his or her chin toward the chest.
10. Slowly and gently begin inserting the tube into the nostril straight back at a 90-degree angle to the long axis of the head.
11. Have the patient begin taking small sips of water through a straw and swallow as you gently advance the tube. Timing the advancement of the tube in conjunction with the patient swallowing greatly facilitates the passage of the NG tube into the stomach.

Caution: If any obstruction is encountered, *do not* force the tube, because you may cause damage to the turbinates.
Note: If resistance is met, withdraw the tube slightly and try placing the tube again. If continued resistance is met, try the other nostril.

12. If the tube advances without resistance, continue having the patient swallow while gently inserting the tube until the premeasured mark or tape is reached.

Procedure for Performing Nasogastric Tube Insertion – *(continued)*

13. Have the patient slowly begin raising the chin from the chest as the tube passes, because this helps facilitate the tube's passage.

14. If the patient begins to gag, pause and have him or her take some deep breaths until the gagging has stopped or calmed down, and then continue with the insertion as already described.

15. If the tube curls up in the posterior pharynx (which typically causes the patient to gag), gently pull back on the tube until it uncurls.

Caution: *Do not* pull the tube out completely. Wait until the patient has stopped gagging or has calmed down.

16. Make sure the patient takes sips of water and swallows while gently advancing the tube again.

17. Check the position of the tube by:
    • Making sure the tube is inserted the measured or calculated distance
    • Injecting approximately 10 cc of air through the tube while listening over the left upper quadrant of the abdomen with the stethoscope for the "rush of air"
    • Aspirating gastric contents and checking the pH: If the pH reading is less than 3, the tube is in the stomach.
    • Obtaining radiographs: Since there is a radiopaque strip in all Levin tubes, radiography is the gold standard for determining placement of feeding tubes or NG tubes when there is a question of appropriate placement. When radiography is readily available and not contraindicated, all NG tube placements should be confirmed radiographically as soon as conveniently possible.

18. Tape the tube in place; this is important for ensuring maintenance of proper tube placement.

19. Use tincture of benzoin to facilitate the adherence of the tape, pre-manufactured NG tube holder, or occlusive seal dressing.

Caution: **Taping the tube so that no torsion or pressure is placed on the nares while the tube remains in place is paramount (Fig. 14–3).**

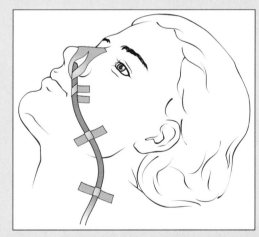

Figure 14–3. Adapted from Rosen P, Bankin RM, Sternback GL: Essentials of Emergency Medicine. St. Louis, CV Mosby, 1991, p 615.

Special Considerations

Patients with impaired mentation or who are comatose and cannot assist with important aspects of the procedure may present technical challenges. In this instance, placing the NG tube in an ice bath before insertion may help by causing the tube to become temporarily somewhat more rigid and less likely to kink. Also it may be necessary to pass the tube to the level of the oropharynx and then pass the tube into the esophagus using a Magill forceps.

Insertion of an NG tube in patients with endotracheal tubes can be challenging. In some instances, deflating the cuff on the endotracheal tube is necessary to pass the NG tube into the esophagus.

Follow-Up Care and Instructions

- Ensure that the NG tube is functioning properly.
- The tubes are ineffective when they are not patent. To ensure the patency, disconnect the tube from the suction device.
- Using a large syringe, inject 20 to 30 cc of air through the NG tube. Free flow of air through the tube indicates that the tube is functioning properly.
- It is important to assess the nares and nasopharynx periodically to ensure that no pressure ulcer or tissue necrosis is occurring from irritation or pressure from the NG tube.
- Remove the NG tube as soon as it is no longer needed or indicated.

References

Randall HT: The history of enteral nutrition. In Rombeau JI, Caldwell MD (eds): Clinical Nutrition. Philadelphia, WB Saunders, 1990.

Bibliography

- Feldman M, Scharschmidt BF, Sleisinger MH (eds): Sleisenger & Fortran's Gastrointestinal and Liver Disease: Pathophysiology, Diagnosis, and Management, 6th ed, vol 1. Philadelphia, WB Saunders, 1998.

Chapter 15

Lumbar Puncture

▷ Virginia F. Schneider

Procedure Goals and Objectives

Goal: To obtain a high-quality sample of cerebrospinal fluid (CSF) while observing universal precautions and with the minimal degree of risk for the patient.

Objectives: The student will be able to . . .

► Describe the indications, contraindications, and rationale for performing a lumbar puncture.

► Identify and describe common complications associated with lumbar punctures.

► Describe the essential anatomy and physiology associated with the performance of a lumbar puncture.

► Identify the necessary materials and their proper use in performing a lumbar puncture.

► Properly perform the actions necessary to collect a sample of cerebrospinal fluid.

► Identify the important aspects of postprocedure care following a lumbar puncture.

Background and History

The first lumbar puncture is attributed to Heinrich Quincke, who performed it in December 1890 on a 21-month old boy with fever, stiff neck, coma, and pneumonia. It was adopted and widely used within a few years as a diagnostic and therapeutic procedure. By 1900, Quincke had also reported the technique of spinal anesthesia using the same procedure with cocaine as a local anesthetic (Evans, 1998). Complications of the procedure quickly became apparent and ranged from self-limited postprocedure headache to tonsillar herniation in the presence of increased intracranial pressure. Recognition of complication risk factors and the development of new equipment and techniques have resulted in a procedure that is relatively simple, safe, and commonly used in the diagnosis of a variety of conditions today.

Indications

- Lumbar puncture is performed in adults, children, and infants to obtain CSF for cell count, glucose, protein, culture, and other specialized analyses.
- It is frequently used in the evaluation of infection of the meninges, subarachnoid hemorrhage, and demyelinating diseases.
- CSF analysis results may also be helpful, although nonspecific, in diagnosing systemic lupus erythematosus with central nervous system involvement, central nervous system malignancy, and subdural or epidural hematoma (Evans, 1998; Martin and Gean, 1986).
- In infants and children, the procedure may be used serially as a way to relieve increased intraventricular pressure from hydrocephalus while the patient is awaiting a more definitive procedure (Hood, 1996).
- Lumbar puncture may serve as a route of administration for various pharmacologic agents, including antibiotics and chemotherapeutic agents for the treatment of disease (Martin, 1986).

*intrathecal admin
Antibx / Chemo*

- Evaluation for bacterial meningitis is the most common reason for lumbar puncture, and characteristically it is suggested by a CSF sample with an elevated white blood cell count, elevated polymorphonuclear cell count, and a low glucose level.
- Organisms may also be tentatively identified by Gram staining the CSF specimen.
- Patients with viral meningitis typically have CSF mononuclear pleocytosis, a normal glucose level, an elevated protein level, and a negative Gram stain.
- Neurosyphilis is a difficult clinical and laboratory diagnosis and is most commonly manifested by a CSF pleocytosis, elevated protein level, and positive treponemal-specific antibody test.

- Fungal meningitis should be suspected in immunocompromised or hospitalized patients on long-term, broad-spectrum antibiotics. In these patients, CSF analysis is usually somewhat abnormal but nonspecific.
- Central nervous system tuberculosis may have similar findings. Identification depends on a high index of suspicion and specific microscopic, serologic, or culture testing for tuberculosis (Martin, 1986).
- Subarachnoid hemorrhage is generally characterized by CSF with a xanthochromic color at the time of the lumbar puncture and an elevated erythrocyte count in the fluid. In contrast, a traumatic lumbar puncture is usually characterized by initially red CSF with subsequent clearing of the fluid as collection progresses (Martin, 1986).
- In the evaluation of demyelinating diseases, lumbar puncture is primarily used in the diagnosis of multiple sclerosis and Guillain-Barré syndrome. In multiple sclerosis, analysis of the proteins by electrophoresis and the identification of specific band patterns is useful as a diagnostic measure. The CSF of patients with Guillain-Barré syndrome has an isolated, very high protein concentration (generally greater than 200 mg/dL), which is specific enough to this condition as to be nearly diagnostic (Martin, 1986).

[handwritten margin note: Bldy tap due to subarch. hemorrhage / Bloody tap due to trauma]

Contraindications

- The primary contraindication for lumbar puncture is increased intracranial pressure. Signs and symptoms of increased intracranial pressure include progressive headache, focal neurologic signs or symptoms, progressive deterioration of mental status over hours to weeks, and papilledema on funduscopic examination. Lumbar puncture and the associated removal of CSF fluid results in a corresponding area of decreased pressure in the spinal column. In patients with increased intracranial pressure, creation of this area of lower pressure may result in herniation of the brain through the foramen magnum. Any patient suspected of having increased intracranial pressure should be evaluated by computed tomography before a lumbar puncture is attempted.
- Lumbar puncture is also contraindicated in the presence of suspected or known coagulation disorders. This may include hemophilia, leukemia, liver disease, or a patient receiving anticoagulant therapy. It is only a relative contraindication in the event of suspected meningitis in a patient with a coagulopathy, because the benefits of the procedure may outweigh its risks.
- Local infection overlying the site of the lumbar puncture risks direct inoculation of organisms into the CSF.
- Abnormalities such as nevi, hair tufts, sinuses, or palpable bony abnormalities may be associated with spinal column structural abnormalities.
- Lumbar puncture is contraindicated in a patient who is severely ill or medically unstable.

Potential Complications

Several potential complications exist for the lumbar puncture procedure. These potential complications follow.

- Postdural puncture headache (PDPH) is the most common complication of lumbar puncture and may occur in as many as 30% to 50% of patients. The headache is always bilateral but varies in location and is usually described as "throbbing" or "pressure." Intensity is increased in the upright position and by movement, coughing, straining, or sneezing. It is relieved by lying supine. Patients may also have neck stiffness, nausea, vomiting, dizziness, or visual symptoms (Evans, 1998). Management of this complication is discussed in the section "Follow-Up Care."
- Herniation into the foramen magnum may occur when lumbar puncture is performed in the presence of increased intracranial pressure. In the presence of tumors or hematoma, herniation is relatively uncommon. It can be difficult to determine if the lumbar puncture or the underlying pathologic condition is ultimately responsible for subsequent neurologic deterioration or death. The absence of papilledema and focal neurologic symptoms does not guarantee normal intracranial pressure. The patient's presentation and differential diagnosis should guide the need for computed tomography or magnetic resonance imaging before lumbar puncture.
- Nerve damage occurs when the needle inadvertently moves laterally, contacting the dura and penetrating a segmental nerve in the extradural space, causing pain, electric shocks, and dysesthesias. Transient cranial nerve dysfunctions have been reported, including cranial nerves III, IV, V, VI, VII, and VIII. Up to a third of patients complain of back pain and discomfort for several days after lumbar puncture because of local trauma. Disk herniation or infection is a rare complication but has been reported.
- Bleeding (e.g., hematoma of the spine and subdural, epidural, or subarachnoid space) is rare and occurs almost exclusively in patients with blood dyscrasias or those receiving anticoagulant therapy. In infants, inquire about a family history of blood dyscrasias, routine vitamin K administration, or signs and symptoms of disorders predisposing to thrombocytopenia, such as cytomegalovirus infection.
- Intraspinal epidermoid tumors are rare but may be induced by lumbar punctures in which epidermal fragments are carried in by the needle and implanted into the spinal canal. Use of a stylet minimizes this risk. Symptoms, occurring months later, consist of pain at the site or neurologic symptoms in the lower extremities.
- Infection may be introduced by improperly preparing the skin, contaminating the needle, performing the procedure through an area of local infection, or introducing blood into the subarachnoid space in the presence of bacteremia. Consequences may range from local cellulitis to meningitis and empyemas of the epidural or subdural space. Sterile technique and selection of an infection-free puncture site significantly reduce the risk of infection.

↑ intracranial pressure always get either CT/MRI B4 doing an LP.

- Needle breakage is an unusual event. If the needle breaks and the fragment is beneath the skin surface, leave the stylet in place, if possible, and use it as a guide to perform a small incision. Once the end is found, it can be removed with a hemostat. If this is not quickly and easily accomplished, a neurosurgeon should be consulted.

Review of Anatomy and Physiology

CSF is produced almost exclusively in the choroid plexuses. Fluid formed in the lateral ventricles flows through the interventricular foramen of Monro and mixes with the fluid produced in the third ventricle. It passes through the aqueduct of Sylvius to the fourth ventricle, where another choroid plexus adds its component, and it flows into the cisterna magna. From there, the fluid is directed anteriorly under the base of the brain and then up over the sulci between the cortical convolutions.

Although the cisterns at the base of the brain communicate freely with the spinal subarachnoid space, the main circulation continues in the cerebral subarachnoid space. The CSF is transferred back into the blood stream by filtration and osmosis chiefly through arachnoid villi and granulations in the supratentorial region.

The spinal cord terminates at the L1 level in an adult (Fig. 15–1). Lumbar puncture is performed usually at the L4–5 or L3–4 interspace by inserting a needle into the subarachnoid space via percutaneous puncture. In the absence of spinal abnormalities, there is little danger of injuring the spinal cord. In infants, however, the spinal cord terminates at the L3 level. More care should be used to ensure appropriate interspace identification, and use of those above L3–4 should never be attempted.

infants spine terminates @ L₃

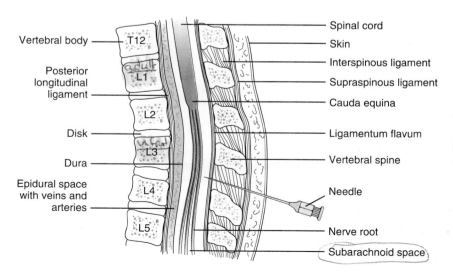

Vertebral body — T12
Posterior longitudinal ligament — L1
— L2
Disk — L3
Dura —
Epidural space with veins and arteries — L4
— L5

— Spinal cord
— Skin
— Interspinous ligament
— Supraspinous ligament
— Cauda equina
— Ligamentum flavum
— Vertebral spine
— Needle
— Nerve root
— Subarachnoid space

Figure 15–1. Anatomic orientation for performing lumbar puncture. (Redrawn from Taft JM, JAAPA 3:473–476, 1990.

Patient Preparation

- Because this procedure involves placing a relatively large-appearing needle into the spinal column, it can be very anxiety-producing for patients and parents. Frequently, patients and families have heard negative anecdotal experiences about the procedure from acquaintances, friends, or family members. Therefore, it is important to establish a good rapport by thoroughly explaining the procedure, answering questions, and addressing any concerns of the patient and family before beginning.
- Explain the steps of the procedure and include the use of drawings to illustrate the anatomy of the spine to emphasize the low risk of spinal cord damage associated with the procedure when properly performed.
- Although complications are possible and may be serious, it is important to emphasize that this is a commonly performed procedure. The risk of complications is low in contrast to the benefit to be gained from the information received from the CSF sample.
- When the procedure is performed on an outpatient basis, the patient is typically retained for observation and monitoring for at least 1 to 2 hours after the procedure has been performed.

Materials Utilized to Perform a Lumbar Puncture in Adults, Children, and Infants

---

The standard lumbar puncture tray contains the following:

- Three sterile skin swabs or sponges
- 1% lidocaine solution
- 20- and 25-gauge skin infiltration needles
- 3-mL syringe
- Four sample collection vials, numbered and capped
- Sterile bandage or dressing
- Sterile gauze pads
- Pressure manometer with three-way stopcock
- 22- or 25-gauge spinal needle, or both, with stylet (Fig. 15–2)
- Spare spinal needle with stylet
- Povidone-iodine solution
- Sterile gloves
- Fenestrated sterile drapes

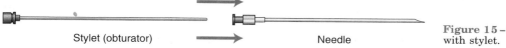

Stylet (obturator)   Needle

Figure 15–2. Spinal needle with stylet.

An assistant is also required (O'Brien, 1999).

Procedure for Lumbar Puncture in Adults

1. Have an assistant present.
2. Position the patient.
   A. Position the patient in the lateral recumbent position with the knees flexed toward the chest and the chin touching the knees.

Note: It is helpful if an assistant gently holds the patient at the upper back and behind the knees in a flexed position. The assistant can help the patient avoid sudden movements during the lumbar puncture. The patient's back should be just at the edge of the table, with the vertical plane of the back perpendicular to the table surface.

   B. For an alternative position, place the patient in an upright sitting position with the legs hanging over the side of the bed and the trunk flexed forward over a pillow or bed table. The head is flexed toward the chest, and the arms are brought forward for support.

Note: Again, it is helpful if the assistant holds the patient in this position during the procedure.

3. Put on sterile gloves.
4. Open the lumbar puncture tray using sterile technique.
5. Pour povidone-iodine solution into the well of the tray or over the skin preparation sponges.
6. Set up the four collection tubes and unscrew the tops. Preassemble the

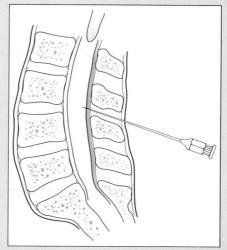

Figure 15–3. Redrawn from Pfenninger JL, Fowler GC: Procedures for Primary Care Physicians. St. Louis, Mosby-Year Book, 1994, p 1112.

manometer and attach the three-way stopcock.

7. Partially remove the stylet from the spinal needle to check for smooth function and then return it to its fully inserted position.
8. Check to make sure all necessary equipment is in the tray before beginning the procedure.
9. Using two sterile drapes, place one under the patient and the second on the table.
10. Clean the patient's back with povidone-iodine solution. Start at approximately

Procedure for Lumbar Puncture in Adults – *(continued)*

the L3 level and work in a circular fashion outward three times, cleansing upward to the lower thoracic spine, downward over the buttocks and sacroiliac area, and sideways over the iliac crests. Repeat this procedure a total of three times.

(margin handwriting: areas to cover in cleaning)

11. Place the fenestrated, sterile drape over the patient's back, with the circular opening centered over the L3–4 area.

Note: The second drape allows you to touch the area around the immediate field while maintaining sterile technique.

12. Identify the level of L4, which is usually lying on an imaginary line created by joining the iliac crests with a straight line. This imaginary line crosses the spine at the level of L4. Anesthetize the skin with 1% lidocaine solution in this area.

13. Once local surface anesthesia has been achieved at the L4 level, slowly insert the spinal needle (see Fig. 15–2) with the stylet into the L3–4 intervertebral space. The needle should be precisely in the midline and directed toward the patient's umbilicus

(Fig. 15–3). Advance the needle slowly.

Note: Removal and replacement of the stylet allows you to determine if the subarachnoid space has been reached. There is usually a "popping" sensation appreciated when the needle passes through the ligamentum flavum. When this occurs, remove the stylet and CSF should flow.

14. Attach the manometer as soon as fluid appears in the hub of the needle and measure the opening pressure. Have the patient gently relax the legs and breathe slowly.

15. Collect approximately 1 mL in each of the four collection bottles provided, using them in numerical order.

16. When sufficient fluid is collected, replace the stylet, and with a quick, smooth motion remove the needle from the spine. Use sterile gauze to apply pressure to the site, holding the pressure for several minutes at a minimum. When no bleeding or fluid leakage can be detected at the lumbar puncture site, cleanse the area and place a sterile bandage over the site (O'Brien, 1999).

Special Considerations

- Traumatic lumbar punctures are extremely common and are estimated to occur in up to 40% of lumbar puncture attempts. If vessels are punctured during needle insertion with a return of bloody fluid, several maneuvers can be attempted. First, rotate the needle 45 degrees from the original orientation. This may move the needle bore away from the site of bleeding and allow clearing of the fluid. Second, be patient and allow a few minutes with the stylet in place to see if the bleeding site will seal over and allow clearing of the fluid. Finally, if these maneuvers are unsuccessful, you may attempt to repeat the lumbar puncture at the next higher interspace if that is an appropriate site within usual guidelines for the patient's age.

- Nerve root pain may occur during insertion if the needle disrupts small nerve fibers in the area. This is usually described by the patient as paresthesias or the sensation of mild shooting pains locally or with radiation down the leg, or both. Repositioning the needle slightly will often eliminate the symptoms.
- Occasionally, no fluid will be obtained at lumbar puncture—a "dry tap." The most common reason for this is that the epidural space was not pierced, and repositioning of the needle is indicated. Other things to consider are dehydration, blockage to fluid circulation, and congenital anomalies.

Procedure for Lumbar Puncture in Children

1. The same precautions and positioning description outlined for adults apply to children (Fig. 15–4).
2. The most important component in performing a successful lumbar puncture in a child is to take the necessary steps to ensure adequate restraint of the patient. With the child in the lateral recumbent position, have an assistant hold the child securely at the knees and shoulders.
3. Depending on the child's clinical state, a mild, short-acting sedative may be administered (Hughes and Buescher, 1996; Rowe, 1994).

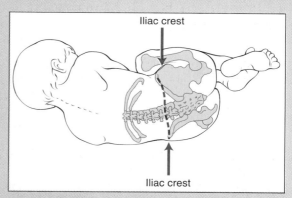

Figure 15–4. Redrawn from Hughes WT, Buescher ES: Pediatric Procedures, 2nd ed, 1980, p 180.

Procedure for Lumbar Puncture in Infants

Note: Maintenance of body temperature, positioning, and maintenance of the airway must be taken into account when performing a lumbar puncture in an infant.

1. Bring the baby to an infant treatment warmer. Attach a skin temperature probe and set the warmer to maintain the baby at normal body temperature during the procedure.
2. Position the infant on the warmer. Two positions can be used. The infant may be placed in the sitting position, with the holder flexing the thighs on the abdomen, allowing him or her to grasp the right knee and elbow with the right hand and the left knee and elbow with the left hand.
3. Gently flex the spine, using care not to cause excessive abdominal pressure or to overflex the neck and occlude the infant's airway (Fig. 15–5). Alternatively, the assistant may place the

Procedure for Lumbar Puncture in Infants – *(continued)*

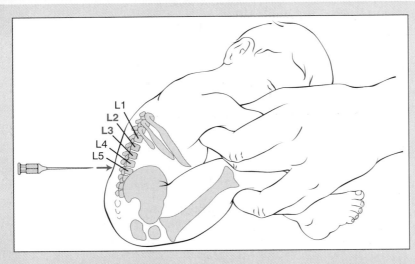

L1
L2
L3
L4
L5

Figure 15–5. Redrawn from Hughes WT, Buescher ES: Pediatric Procedures, 2nd ed. Philadelphia, WB Saunders, 1980, p 181.

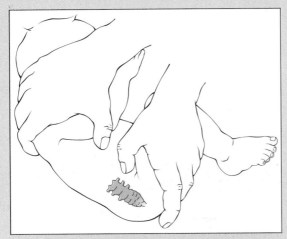

Figure 15–6. Redrawn from Hughes WT, Buescher ES: Pediatric Procedures, 2nd ed. Philadelphia, WB Saunders, 1980, p 181.

infant on his or her side, using one hand to flex the thighs to the abdomen and secure the extremities while the other hand flexes the neck and spine (Fig. 15–6). The second position is useful with small premature and term infants who may not be well enough to tolerate the sitting position.

Note: An infant with a distended abdomen may have difficulty breathing when flexed into a lumbar puncture position and become bradycardic and apneic, requiring cardiopulmonary resuscitation. When performing a lumbar puncture on any ill or premature infant, electronically monitor the heart and respiratory rate during the procedure. Also, be sure an assistant observes the baby during the lumbar puncture for respiratory movements and the development of cyanosis.

Follow-up Care and Instructions

Contrary to conventional wisdom, study data indicate that bed rest and hydration do not reduce the risk of postdural headache, the most common complication of lumbar puncture (Evans, 1998). Follow-up care and instructions should include the following:

- Observation of the patient to ensure that the lumbar puncture site has sealed over, and no leakage of CSF persists.
- Recommendations for treatment of postdural headache:

  - *For initial or mild headache*
    - Bed rest
    - Over-the-counter analgesia
    - Caffeine, 300 mg orally every 6 to 8 hours *or*
    - Theophylline, 300 mg orally every 8 hours
  - *For moderate to severe headache that is present more than 24 hours*
    - Return to the clinic for evaluation
    - Although bed rest does not prevent PDPH, it is a recommended treatment once it has developed. Methylxanthines may relieve PDPH through their action as an intercerebral vasoconstrictor, resulting in decreased cerebral blood flow and intracranial pressure. If the PDPH persists beyond 24 hours, an epidural blood patch is the most effective treatment. This is accomplished by drawing 10 to 20 mL of the patient's blood and then slowly injecting it into the lumbar epidural space near the prior puncture site. The patient should remain in the decubitus position for 1 to 2 hours after the procedure for maximal benefit. The epidural blood patch works by exerting a mass effect and compressing the dural sac, sealing any continued CSF leak (Evans, 1998).

References

Evans RW: Complications of lumbar puncture. Neurol Clin N Am 16:105, 1998.

Hood BR: Lumbar Puncture in Procedures in Infants and Children. Philadelphia, WB Saunders, 1996, pp 202–205.

Hughes WT, Buescher ES: Central Nervous System: Pediatric Procedures. Philadelphia, WB Saunders, 1996, pp 178–185.

Martin KI, Gean AD: The spinal tap: A new look at an old test. Ann Intern Med 1986:104, 840–848.

O'Brien J: Lumbar Puncture in Primary Care Practice Procedures. Philadelphia, WB Saunders, 1999, pp 1109–1114.

Rowe PC: Pediatric Procedures in Principles and Practice of Pediatrics. Philadelphia, JB Lippincott, 1994, pp 2206–2207.

Chapter 16

Urinary Bladder Catheterization

▷ Dan Vetrosky

Procedure Goals and Objectives

Goal: To perform urinary bladder catheterization in a patient safely and accurately.

Objectives: The student will be able to . . .

▶ Describe the indications, contraindications, and rationale for performing urinary bladder catheterization.

▶ Identify and describe common complications associated with performing urinary bladder catheterization.

▶ Describe the essential anatomy and physiology associated with the performance of urinary bladder catheterization.

▶ Identify the materials necessary for performing urinary bladder catheterization and their proper use.

Background and History

Disease processes that require urinary bladder catheterization have existed since ancient times. Urethral strictures, bladder stones, and prostatism are among the first diseases that necessitated urinary bladder decompression by catheterization. The approach to urinary catheterization remains the same today as it was in ancient times. It is the technique of passing a hollow tube through the urethra into the urinary bladder for purposes of circumventing an obstructed urinary bladder or obtaining a sample of urine for analysis, or both.

The first known urologic instruments would be considered somewhat barbaric by today's standards. Ancient and medieval "urologists-lithotomists" used perineal incision and metal and glass tubes to circumvent urinary obstruction. Today's approach often uses a local anesthetic and urethral catheters made of rubber, latex, polytetrafluoroethylene (Teflon), or silicone polymers. Urethral catheterization is currently used for relief of bladder outlet obstruction or when measurement of urinary output must be precise (e.g., in multiple trauma, surgery, intensive care, renal failure).

Indications

Reasons for passing a catheter into the urinary bladder are many. The most common uses of bladder catheterization are the following:

- To obtain a sterile urine sample, especially in the female patient
- To monitor urinary output closely in critically ill patients
- To facilitate urinary drainage in patients who are incapacitated (stroke, advanced Alzheimer's disease, spinal transection, and so on)
- To bypass obstructive processes in the urethra, prostate, or bladder neck caused by disease or trauma until surgical repair can be performed
- To hold urethral skin grafts in place after urethral stricture repair
- To act as a traction device for the purpose of controlling bleeding after prostate surgery
- Specialized 3-way Foley catheters are used after bladder or prostate surgery to allow for continuous bladder irrigation. Continuous irrigation as well as drainage helps prevent the formation of blood clots, which can occlude a catheter and cause bladder obstruction. Three-way Foley catheters also allow for easier evacuation of formed blood clots (Fig. 16–1).

The main reasons for using the "one time," "straight," or Robinson catheter follow:

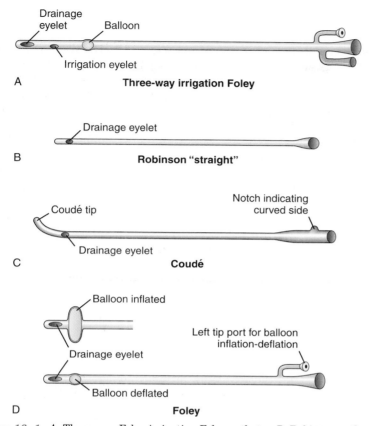

Figure 16–1. *A,* Three-way Foley-irrigation Foley catheter. *B,* Robinson catheter. *C,* Coudé catheter. *D,* Foley catheter.

- To obtain a sterile urine sample or to decompress a distended bladder caused by an acute obstructive process
- As a protocol of intermittent catheterization in persons with neurogenic bladders: Catheterizing patients with neurogenic bladders at regular intervals with the Robinson catheter facilitates complete bladder emptying, routine urine sampling, and "bladder training." Some of these patients may be able to decrease the frequency of their catheterization or may regain complete bladder control, or both, after a time.
- To deliver topical antineoplastic medication to the bladder in patients who have bladder cancer or to deliver medication to patients who suffer from interstitial cystitis

Contraindications

The only contraindication to inserting a catheter (either Robinson or Foley) is the appearance of blood at the urethral meatus in a patient who has sustained pelvic trauma. This finding can be an indication that the urethra has been partially or totally transected. Attempting to pass a catheter in this situation could cause a partial urethral transection to become total. It is advised that a urologist be consulted when blood at the urethral meatus is present in a patient with pelvic trauma. Allergy to materials used in the procedure, such as latex, rubber, tape, and lubricants, is also a contraindication.

Potential Complications

Most of the complications with catheterization are seen in the male patient. Female patients rarely have urethral strictures, and because the urethra is short in this population, false passages are rarely created. Complications can include the following:

- Urinary structural trauma
- Urinary tract infection
- Inflammation of the urinary tract secondary to the procedure
- Catheterizing a male patient with urethral stricture disease, bladder neck contracture, or an enlarged prostate; this may present some technical difficulties for the unsuspecting health care provider
- Passage of a Robinson or Foley catheter in a patient with urethral stricture disease or an enlarged prostate: This increases the danger of creating false passages in the urethra if excessive force is applied when resistance is met during the catheterization. The mechanism of injury occurs when the obstructive process deflects the catheter into the side wall of the urethra. If the clinician meets these types of obstructive processes and continues to apply excessive pressure in an attempt to bypass the blockage, the catheter can act like a drill and undermine the lining of the urethra, thus creating a "false passage." The worst scenario in this situation would be pushing the catheter completely through the urethra into the surrounding tissue. This results in copious bleeding from the urethra and creates the possibility of urine and blood extravasating into the surrounding tissues.
- Having the catheter "double back" or make a "U-turn" at the site of obstruction: It is not uncommon to have the catheter tip reappear at the urethral meatus when there is a significant obstruction or bladder neck spasm.

Review of Essential Anatomy and Physiology

Urine is produced by the kidneys and transported to the bladder by the ureters, where it is stored for transport through the urethra during urination. Bladder catheterization involves the passage of a mechanical device into the bladder through the urethra. To accomplish this without damage requires an understanding of the anatomy of the lower urinary tract. Figure 16–2 illustrates the anatomy in relation to the location at which a urinary catheter would be placed for males and females.

In females, the distance from the distal end of the urethra to the bladder is relatively short (1.5 to 2 inches) and the course through the urethra is relatively unobstructed. Because of this, bladder catheterization in the female patient is typically accomplished faster and with less discomfort than it is in the male patient.

In males, the distance from the distal tip of the urethra to the bladder is longer (typically 6 to 7 inches; however, it can vary considerably) and is more circuitous than in females, thus making catheter insertion potentially more difficult. In males, the path to the bladder typically includes curves that may be encountered while traversing the penis as well as a sharp bend through the prostate. Occasionally, prostatic hypertrophy can make catheter insertion difficult because the pressure of the hypertrophic prostate can add a curvature to the urethra as well as produce urethral obstruction.

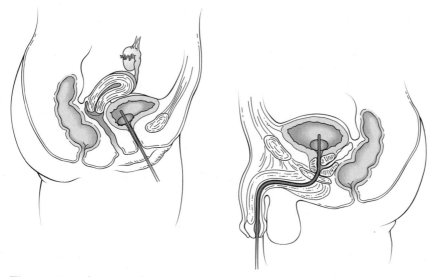

Figure 16–2. Anatomy of the female (*left*) and male (*right*) lower urinary tracts with catheters in place. (Redrawn from Potter P: Fundamentals of Nursing, 4th ed. St. Louis, Mosby-Year Book, 1997, p 1324.)

Standard Precautions ▷ Practitioners should use Standard Precautions at all times when interacting with patients. Determining the level of precaution necessary requires the practitioner to exercise clinical judgment based on the patient's history and the potential for exposure to body fluids or aerosol-borne pathogens (for further discussion see Chapter 2).

Patient Preparation

- Inform the patient before the procedure how the catheterization will be performed and what he or she might expect to feel during the procedure. This will help secure the patient's trust and cooperation. Do not tell the patient that he or she will not feel anything, because this would be untruthful and counterproductive during the procedure. Inform the patient that the passage of the catheter may feel as though he or she must urinate and that it will be slightly uncomfortable.
- Patient comfort must be a primary consideration if a sterile, atraumatic catheterization is to be accomplished.
- Explain to the patient the importance of being reasonably still and not touching your gloved hands or sterile implements.
- Typically, the patient is positioned in the supine position. Drapes should be placed to cover all but the genitalia. The female patient will need to abduct the legs laterally to allow easy access to the urethra.

Materials Utilized to Perform a Urinary Bladder Catheterization

- Sterile tray or working area
- Vessel for collecting urine (sometimes included with tray)
- Sterile gloves
- Sterile lubricant or anesthetic jelly lubricant
- Antiseptic cleansing solution (typically povidone-iodine [Betadine])
- Sterile gauze or cotton balls for cleansing the external exit of the urethra and the surrounding skin
- Sterile forceps
- Syringe filled with sterile water for catheter balloon, 5 mL to 30 mL depending on the balloon capacity of the catheter selected
- Urine collection tubing, bags, hardware, and specimen collection containers
- Sterile drapes to protect the sterile field and nonsterile drapes to maintain patient modesty
- Catheter (see further on)
- Catheterization kits containing the following:
  - Sterile lubricant
  - Sterile drapes

- Sterile gloves
- Sterile cotton swabs
- Povidone-iodine
- Forceps to grasp the cotton swabs
- Sterile specimen container for urinalysis and culture
- Container to catch the urine
- Robinson or Foley catheter, 14, 16, or 18 Fr: If a Foley catheter is used, the kit will also contain a prefilled 10-mL Luer-tipped syringe to inflate the Foley balloon and can contain a preattached drainage bag (attached to the Foley catheter). The advantage of a preattached drainage bag is that once in place, the Foley catheter and the drainage bag are considered a sterile "closed system." The disadvantage is the inability to obtain a specimen or irrigate the bladder without "breaking the seal" and making what was once a sterile closed system a "contaminated" open system.

Types of Catheters

Urinary catheters (Robinson, coudé, and Foley types) are made of various materials and are soft and flexible (see Fig. 16–1). The most common, Robinson or "straight" type, catheter is made of rubber. Catheters can be made of pure rubber, rubber with synthetic coatings such as latex, or pure latex. Pure silicone and silicone-coated catheters are also manufactured, although they are much more expensive than rubber or latex catheters. These coated catheters are more commonly seen in indwelling or Foley catheter lines. The coatings are touted to resist encrustation when left in the bladder for prolonged periods. Patients with latex allergies should not be catheterized with rubber or latex catheters. In such cases, catheters made of pure silicone are an acceptable alternative.

Robinson Catheter

The Robinson catheter is also known as the "straight" catheter and is sterile if the package seal is not broken. It has a soft, rounded tip and one or two drainage eyelets on the tip side walls. The catheter is hollow, and the distal end is flared to facilitate urinary drainage. These catheters are designed for one-time use, hence the term *in-and-out catheter* (see Fig. 16–1).

Coudé Catheter

Coudé catheters have a bend at the distal tip that causes the catheter to follow the anterior surface of the male urethra. This bent tip facilitates the insertion of the catheter in patients with false passages, which typically occur on the posterior surface of the urethra.

Foley Catheter

The Foley catheter is designed to remain in place in the bladder. It too is sterile, and its appearance is similar to the Robinson catheter, with a few exceptions. At the tip, just past the drainage eyelets, is an inflatable balloon. The balloon is inflated after the catheter is properly placed in the bladder to help keep the catheter seated in the bladder. The flared end of the catheter is located at the distal end, and it can be attached to a drainage bag. Also at the distal end is an elbow with a Luer lock cap attached. This elbow is the end of an extremely small lumen, which traverses the length of the catheter and ends in the balloon at the tip. The Luer lock cap allows the balloon to be inflated once the catheter is in place and deflated once the catheter needs to be removed. The balloon is typically inflated with sterile water. Use of saline is discouraged because of the possibility of crystal formation along the balloon's lumen. Should this occur, the balloon might not deflate when the catheter needs to be removed.

There are two sizes of Foley catheter balloons: a 5-mL balloon and a 30-mL balloon. The most common balloon size used is 5 mL, and it is typically inflated with 10 mL of sterile water, which accounts for the lumen volume and the balloon volume; 30-mL balloons are used to ensure that the Foley catheter does not migrate into the prostatic fossa or out of the urinary bladder altogether. In addition, the 30-mL balloon can be inflated with 50 mL of sterile water and used as a traction stent after certain urologic procedures (e.g., radical prostatectomy, transurethral prostatectomy).

Catheter Size Requirements

Urinary catheters come in various sizes and are measured according to the Charrière French scale (0.33 mm equals 1 Fr). A 3 Fr catheter is 1 mm in diameter, whereas a 30 Fr catheter is 10 mm in diameter. The French size of the catheter depends on the patient and the catheter's purpose. As an example, pediatric boys will need a French size between 5 Fr and 12 Fr. Adult men should be catheterized with a 16 Fr or 18 Fr catheter. These sizes are slightly stiffer and will follow the anatomic curvature of the male urethra easier and better than the smaller French catheters will (14 Fr or smaller). Smaller French catheters have a tendency to "turn around" in the male urethra if the slightest resistance is met (especially at the bladder neck). The adult woman should also be catheterized with 16 or 18 Fr catheters, although a 14 Fr should be used most of the time to facilitate comfort. Larger French catheters (20 Fr to 30 Fr) are used to evacuate blood clots in postoperative prostate surgery patients or in patients who are bleeding from the kidney or bladder.

Procedure for Performing a Urinary Bladder Catheterization on a Male Patient

Note: Male patients are more prone to sustaining damage to the urethra during the catheterization procedure. Improper lubrication and excessive force used to "overcome" an obstruction are the most common offending factors causing urethral trauma. The steps outlined here will help reduce the chances of inflicting excessive pain, causing urethral damage, or introducing infection.

1. Obtain the Robinson or Foley catheter that is sized commensurate with the procedure or purpose. Make sure it is sterile (packaging must be intact).
2. Obtain the appropriate catheterization kit or supplies.
3. Follow aseptic techniques and standard precautions by washing hands and putting on sterile gloves.
4. Open the kit in a sterile manner.
5. Prepare the patient by draping him in sterile drapes (found in the kit) and exposing the genital area, making sure to allow for the patient's privacy and comfort.
6. Open the catheter, if not contained in the kit, and place on the sterile drape using sterile technique.
7. Even if a package of sterile lubricant is contained in the kit, it is best to obtain a sterile 15- to 20-mL syringe and place it on the sterile drape.
8. Once the operator is gloved, an assistant is needed to squirt some lubricant into the syringe. Water-soluble lubricant can be substituted for sterile anesthetic jelly (lidocaine [Xylocaine] *jelly, not ointment,* or Anestacon [a prepackaged anesthetic jelly]).

Note: If there is a prefilled sterile syringe with water-soluble lubricant in the kit, this step can be omitted.

9. Open the package of povidone-iodine and pour onto the cotton swabs.
10. Inform the patient that you are going to hold his penis and clean it with the povidone-iodine. Assure him that it will not stain the skin permanently. Swab the head of the penis, making sure to clean the meatal opening first and wiping out to the glans with the povidone-iodine–soaked cotton swabs. (Use your nondominant hand to hold the penis.) Use all the cotton swabs.

Note: If the patient is uncircumcised, the foreskin will need to be drawn back before beginning the cleaning and catheter insertion process.

11. Once the penis is clean, do not let go and position the penis at a 90-degree angle from the abdomen and instill the lubricant or anesthetic agent into the urethra. Gently occlude the urethra so that the lubricant or anesthetic agent will not come back out the urethra. If using anesthetic jelly, wait for approximately 1 minute before proceeding so that the anesthetic jelly has time to work.
12. Position the urine container near the patient's leg or between the patient's legs, as appropriate.
13. Grasp the catheter with your dominant hand about three quarters of the way toward the catheter tip. Inform the patient that you are now going to insert the catheter. Gently begin inserting the catheter into the urethral meatus and continue the insertion without stopping (Fig. 16–3). When the sphincter is encountered, you will feel slight resistance. Ask the patient to take a deep breath,

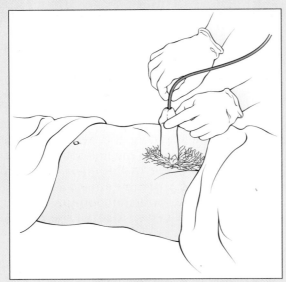

Figure 16-3. Adapted from Potter P: Fundamentals of Nursing, 4th ed. St. Louis, Mosby-Year Book, 1997, p 1323.

which might assist in relaxing him somewhat, but continue to insert the catheter, applying gentle pressure if necessary.

Note: When a stricture or obstruction is encountered during catheterization, the clinician has some techniques and tools that may facilitate atraumatic bladder catheterization. The first technique is to make sure the urethra is well lubricated by instilling sterile, water-soluble lubricating jelly or topical anesthetic jelly into the urethra. Once this is accomplished, a 16 Fr or 18 Fr coudé-tipped catheter (see Fig. 16-1) can be used to facilitate bypassing false passages or bladder neck obstruction. The coudé tip is fashioned to follow the normal curve of the urethra and should be passed with the tip facing the anterior portion of the patient's urethra. If the clinician

continues to meet obstruction and is unsuccessful using the coudé catheter and the techniques outlined, a urologist should be called. The urologist will most likely try using a filiform bougie and followers in order to bypass and dilate urethral structures or bladder neck contractures. If these techniques or tools are not successful, a flexible cystoscope or suprapubic catheterization may be used.

14. Once the sphincter is passed, continue to pass the catheter until almost to the hub of the catheter. Urine should begin to flow, although it may take some time for the lubricant, which will be in the catheter after you pass it into the bladder, to "melt." Place the end of the catheter into the urine container and empty the bladder.
15. Obtain a specimen at this point if needed.
16. Once the bladder is empty, remove the catheter in one continuous motion, making sure to pinch off the distal end so that the column of urine left in the catheter does not pour onto the patient.
17. Make sure to measure the amount of urine obtained and record it.

Note: This is important in any situation, but especially when trying to measure a postvoid residual. Having the patient void immediately before catheterizing him does this. The amount voided must be measured, and then the postvoid residual left in the bladder can be measured during catheterization.

18. If this is a Foley catheter placement, once the catheter is in the bladder and urine begins to flow, get the prefilled syringe (with sterile water) and inflate the Foley balloon.

19. Make sure the Foley catheter is inserted almost to the hub.

Note: This ensures that the balloon is not blown up in the prostate, bladder neck, or urethra.

20. Once the balloon is blown up, pull the Foley catheter out gently until it stops. The Foley catheter is now in the proper position.
21. Attach the drainage bag if it is not already in place.
22. Tape the Foley catheter to the abdomen.

Caution: **Taping the Foley catheter is an important step. The penis should be pointing toward the umbilicus and the catheter taped just below the hub.**

Note: Taping the Foley catheter in this manner prevents it from eroding through the urethra by eliminating the first "S" curve in the male urethra. Maintenance of the Foley catheter includes daily cleaning, retaping in the proper position when necessary, and appropriate meatal care.

23. Apply bacitracin ointment to the urethral meatus one to three times a day as needed. This helps keep the catheter from irritating the meatus excessively and prevents infection.

Note: If the patient is uncircumcised, the foreskin will need to be placed back into its original position.

Procedure for Performing a Urinary Bladder Catheterization on a Female Patient

Note: Females can be difficult to catheterize because of the placement of the urethral meatus. If the female patient has a normal anatomy and is not excessively obese, the urethral meatus should be superior to the vaginal introitus and inferior to the clitoris. Some women's urethral meatus is located just inside the superior aspect of the vaginal introitus. This can make catheterization difficult, as identification of the urethral orifice can be obscured by vaginal tissue.

1. Obtain a Robinson or Foley catheter in a size commensurate with the procedure or purpose, making sure that it is sterile (the packaging must be intact).
2. Obtain the appropriate catheterization kit or supplies.
3. Wash the hands.
4. Open the kit in a sterile manner.
5. Put on sterile gloves.
6. Prepare the patient by draping her in sterile drapes (found in the kit) and exposing the genital area, making sure to allow for the patient's privacy and comfort.
7. Open the catheter, if not contained in the kit, and place on the sterile drape using sterile technique.
8. Instead of instilling lubricant into the female urethra, lubricate the catheter well, about one third of the way from the tip of the catheter up.

Procedure for Performing a Urinary Bladder Catheterization on a Female Patient – *(continued)*

9. Open the package of povidone-iodine and pour onto the cotton swabs.
10. Inform the patient that you are going to swab the urethral opening with povidone-iodine once you separate the labia majora and labia minora. Using the nondominant hand, spread the patient's labia. Wipe the urethral opening with the cotton swabs from an anterior to a posterior direction. If the urethral opening is at or in the vaginal opening, the vaginal opening must be swabbed as well.
11. At this point, you can anesthetize the urethra if desired. To do this, apply lidocaine jelly or aqueous cocaine to a cotton-tipped swab and gently insert it into the urethra. Leave it in place for approximately 1 to 2 minutes before placing the catheter.
12. Place the urine container between the patient's legs.
13. Grasp the catheter with your dominant hand, making sure that the catheter is still well lubricated, and gently insert the tip of the catheter into the urethral opening until urine starts to flow or approximately one third of the catheter has been inserted into the bladder (Fig. 16–4).

Note: If you have missed the urethral opening or inserted the catheter into the vagina, you must obtain a new catheter and try again. A helpful technique is to leave the catheter you missed with temporarily in place. This helps you identify where *not* to place the new catheter.)

14. Once the bladder is empty (and you have obtained your specimen), remove the catheter in one continuous motion, making sure to pinch off the

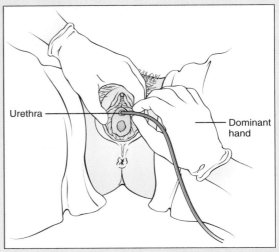

Figure 16–4. Redrawn from Potter P: Fundamentals of Nursing, 4th ed. St. Louis, Mosby-Year Book, 1997, p 1323.

Urethra

Dominant hand

distal end of the catheter so that the column of urine left in it does not pour onto the patient.

15. If this is a Foley catheter placement, once the catheter is in the bladder and urine begins to flow, get the prefilled syringe (with sterile water) and inflate the Foley balloon.
16. Make sure the Foley catheter is inserted at least one third of the way into the bladder.

Note: This ensures that you do not blow the balloon up in the bladder neck or urethra.

17. Once the balloon is blown up, pull the Foley catheter out gently until it stops. The catheter is now in the proper position.
18. Attach the drainage bag if it is not already in place.

Caution: Taping the Foley catheter is an important step.

19. Tape the Foley catheter to the inner thigh. Leave some slack so that it is not taut and pulling against the bladder neck. This can cause bladder spasms. Tape just below the hub.

Note: Maintenance of the Foley catheter includes daily cleaning, retaping in the proper position when necessary, and appropriate meatal care. Typically, povidone-iodine ointment is applied to the urethral meatus one to three times a day as needed. This helps keep the catheter from irritating the meatus excessively and helps prevent infection.

Follow-Up Care and Instructions

Short-Term Catheterization

- Complications are unlikely.
- The most common complications include irritation of the urinary tract and infection.
- Instruct the patient to monitor urination for dysuria, urinary frequency, hematuria, and pyuria, as well as for systemic signs of urinary tract infection such as fever or back pain.

Indwelling Catheterization

- The two major risks associated with an indwelling urinary catheter are trauma and infection. After successful catheter placement, trauma is typically a result of not protecting the catheter properly.
- Instruct the patient that the catheter should be secured with tape at all times and that care should be taken not to snag the tubing on clothing or furniture in a way that would pull on the catheter.

Infection prevention measures include the following:

- Advising the patient always to position the drainage bag below the bladder to prevent urine from flowing back into the bladder.
- Instructing the patient to be careful to avoid kinks in the tubing system.
- Instructing the patient to monitor the bag often to make sure that it is emptied before it becomes full.
- Cautioning the patient to be careful when emptying the bag or manipulating the drainage system, to avoid introducing contaminants.

- Instructing the patient to wash hands frequently and to use latex gloves (if not allergic; if allergic to latex, indicate which type of gloves to obtain).
- Being careful not to have the drainage system come into contact with contaminated objects such as toilet bowls.
- Caution the patient to be aware of signs of infection, such as changes in the appearance of the urine or symptoms of a urinary tract infection and to call the office.

Bibliography

- Potter PA, Perry AG: Fundamentals of Nursing, 4th ed. St. Louis, CV Mosby, 1997.
- Tanagho EM, McAninch JW (eds): Smith's General Urology, 14th ed. Norwalk, Conn, Appleton & Lange, 1995.

Chapter 17

Clinical Breast Examination

▷ Patricia Kelly

Procedure Goals and Objectives

Goal: To perform a thorough breast examination on a female patient in a manner that preserves the patient's modesty while maximizing the likelihood of identifying abnormal findings.

Objectives: The student will be able to . . .

▶ Describe the indications, contraindications, and rationale for performing a breast examination.

▶ Describe the essential anatomy and physiology associated with the performance of the breast examination.

▶ Describe the logical order of the steps used to perform the breast examination.

▶ Describe normal and abnormal findings associated with the breast examination.

Background and History

The clinical breast examination (CBE) is a universally taught ambulatory care skill. As part of a physical examination, CBE complements but does not replace mammography. The CBE is both a screening and diagnostic procedure. As a screening procedure, its purpose is to detect cancer in asymptomatic women. As a diagnostic procedure, it is part of a comprehensive evaluation for patients with symptoms related to the breasts.

Breast cancer is diagnosed in more than 170,000 women annually in the United States. Established risks for breast cancer include age greater than 50, family history of breast cancer in first- and second-degree relatives, a younger age at menarche (<12 years), older age at menopause (>55 years), older age at first birth (>30 years) or nulliparity, benign breast disease (particularly atypical hyperplasia), and hormone replacement therapy. Societal, demographic, and medical trends have markedly increased the number of women at risk.

Before the introduction of cancer screening as an integral part of generalized preventive medical services, most breast cancer was discovered by women themselves or as an incidental finding during the evaluation of other complaints. Frequently, breast cancer was advanced at the time of diagnosis. Specific techniques to increase the sensitivity of the examination, therefore, were not generally thought to be important. In its later stages, the alterations caused by breast cancer were evident on physical examination.

Historically, breast cancer has been a fearful entity. Before 1970, the diagnosis of breast cancer called for "automatic" radical mastectomy, a disfiguring procedure with substantial postoperative morbidity. Because many newly diagnosed women had advanced disease, the prognosis was considered poor. Breast cancer also carried with it a social stigma; therefore, it was not widely discussed. Women were frequently not told of female relatives who had succumbed to the disease. Risk factors for the disease had not been clearly described. Most patients, and many physicians, had incomplete or erroneous knowledge concerning the disease. Adjuvant chemotherapy and hormonal therapy were unavailable until the latter half of the 20th century, and breast cancer generally carried with it an aura of hopelessness. Many women died in excruciating agony. The concepts of palliative therapies or hospice care were not well explored until recent decades.

More recently, societal change and medical progress have correctly imbued us with the notion that breast cancer is a relatively common, although treatable, malignancy. Unfortunately and concomitantly, longevity, decreased rates of childbearing, and younger age at menarche have raised the incidence of this illness. Increased public awareness, along with growing emphasis on screening techniques such as CBE and mammography, have fortunately improved detection efforts as well.

Although breast cancer is still frequently a systemic disease at the time of diagnosis, therapeutic advances and earlier detection have rendered it, in many or most cases, a "curable" entity. More than 60% of breast cancer victims now survive and succumb to other diseases. Less radical surgical interventions, increased consumer knowledge and empowerment, and "gender shift" in the ranks of clinicians have all undoubtedly played an important role in subduing this disease.

Indications

The value of CBE is not universally supported. The American Cancer Society recommends CBE every 3 years in women of reproductive age until age 40 and annually after that. The U.S. Preventive Services Task Force (1996) states that there is insufficient evidence to recommend for or against the examination. The National Cancer Institute recommends annual screening examinations in women age 40 or older.

The following guidelines seem reasonable.

- CBE is performed on an annual basis for women who are age 40 or older.
- Women who have a strong family history of early breast cancer should undergo annual examination at a younger age. Although traditionally performed in all women of reproductive age, it is unclear whether annual examination for women younger than age 40 who are at normal risk confers any survival advantage. The positive predictive value (the chance that an abnormality discovered on examination is malignant) increases with age and with the presence of other risk factors for breast cancer. Barton and coworkers (1999) estimate the specificity and sensitivity of CBE at 54% and 94%, respectively.
- The current legal standard of care strongly suggests that CBE be combined with screening mammography in women age 40 years or older. Neither procedure alone is sufficient. Masses apparent on physical examination require further evaluation even in the face of negative or normal mammographic findings.

The CBE, when used as a screening procedure, has legal as well as medical importance. Failure to diagnose breast cancer is a leading source of malpractice litigation. Providers who fail to perform or document adequate examinations are at high risk for adverse legal consequences.

Contraindications

There are no medical contraindications to the performance of this procedure.

Potential Complications

There are no reported medical complications associated with the performance of this procedure. Legal or practical complications may arise when the examination is omitted or improperly documented. Since this is a sensitive examination, many providers may wish to have the procedure chaperoned or assisted by another clinician or office staff person. Patient education regarding the breast self-examination, necessity of the examination by a clinician, and the presence of any assistants should be documented in the medical record.

Review of Anatomy and Physiology

The average female breast is somewhat "lumpy" to palpation and contains glandular tissue, fibrous tissue, supporting ligaments, and fat. Glandular tissue, intended to produce breast milk, radiates centrally from the nipple. Each glandular lobe terminates in a milk sinus and an excretory duct in the nipple area. The nipple is slightly inferior and lateral to the center of each breast. The skin of the nipple generally extends outward to form the areola. Small sebaceous glands also terminate in the areola. These serve to secrete a protective substance during nursing. Smooth muscles in the subcutaneous tissue under the areola control the erection of the nipple. Small supernumerary nipples, often mistaken for moles, can sometimes be found along the embryological milk lines. These are of no clinical consequence.

Fibrous tissue provides support to the breast, which is connected to the underlying muscle by fascial suspensory structures called Cooper's ligaments. The breasts overlie the pectoral muscles of the chest. Nerves, blood vessels, and lymphatic structures are also contained within the breast. Fatty tissue intermingles with breast tissue in the breast itself. Lymphatic drainage of the breast provides the primary pathway for cancer spread (Fig. 17–1).

The area requiring visual inspection and manual palpation extends inferiorly (vertically) from the clavicle, or second rib, to the seventh rib and laterally from the sternal border to the midaxillary line. The "tail" of the breast extends well into the axilla and must not be omitted during examination. The upper outer quadrant of the breast has the greatest amount of breast tissue and is frequently the site of malignant processes. Peripheral and superficial breast structures are predominantly fatty; deep, central areas contain the greatest percentage of glandular and fibrous tissue. The breasts are usually slightly unequal in size; the left is frequently larger.

The breasts change during maturation and pregnancy and in a cyclic fashion dependent on the menstrual cycle. The glandular breast tissue typically increases in size and tenderness in a pattern conforming to normal

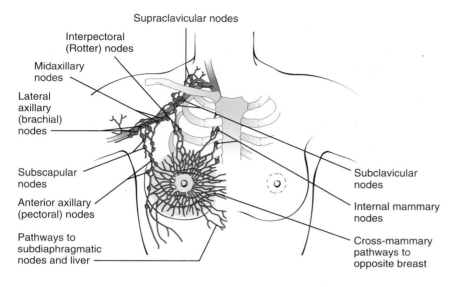

Figure 17–1. Lymphatic drainage of the breast. (Redrawn from Seidel HM: Mosby's Guide to Physical Examination, 4th ed. St. Louis, Mosby-Year Book, 1999.)

hormonal fluctuations. Increased tenderness and engorgement coincide with the immediate premenstrual period and with pregnancy. The premenstrual period, therefore, is not the optimal time for screening CBE.

Women in their reproductive years have "denser" and "lumpier" breasts than postmenopausal women. The latter frequently have some diminution of breast tissue that increases with age. Women who are obese have excess adipose tissue and, hence, larger breasts.

Lactation, or milk production, is influenced by prolactin, which is present secondary to parturition, drug effect, or abnormalities of the pituitary. During nursing, the breasts become markedly engorged.

Abnormalities that are commonly present in the breast may be of the breast tissue itself or of overlying skin. Edema of the skin, characterized by unusually prominent pores (sometimes called peau d'orange because of its orange peel appearance), is an important sign of carcinoma of the breast. Inflammatory breast carcinoma can appear as an eczematous eruption. Erythema can also signify malignancy, although it is more often indicative of infection. Scars may mark the presence of previous biopsies. Retraction or dimpling of skin, although not truly a superficial phenomenon, signifies underlying fibrotic tissue changes that are frequently due to cancer.

Many findings on breast examination are the consequence of stimulating hormones on breast tissue. Both estrogen and progesterone affect breast tissue; progesterone causes more cell division than does estrogen. As previously stated, breast tissue therefore "swells and shrinks" in a relatively predictable fashion during the menstrual cycle. However, sometimes this effect can cause discrete, although benign, abnormalities. Fibroadenomas—characterized by firm, rubbery, nontender, freely moveable but solid masses—can be caused by hormonal influences on one component of breast tissue, the stroma. Breast cysts, which are fluid-filled, tender, benign entities, are also largely due to hormonal fluctuations. As such, they are rare (as initial presentations) in postmenopausal women, who are the group at most risk for breast cancer. Although both these benign entities are fairly characteristic on physical examination, further studies, including ultrasonography, mammography, and tissue cytologic studies, are almost always indicated. The diagnostic evaluation of a breast mass is beyond the scope of this chapter.

Other solitary, nontender breast masses that may be mistaken for carcinoma are chronic abscesses and fat necrosis. These, too, generally must be subjected to biopsy for definitive diagnosis.

Inflammatory breast changes (tender, red) can represent acute mastitis, which generally occurs during lactation or pregnancy. If the cause is not evident (i.e., if this occurs in a 65-year-old, nonlactating woman), inflammatory carcinoma must be ruled out. If not promptly treated, mastitis can lead to an acute abscess, which can present as a localized, fluctuant, exquisitely tender mass.

The classic presentation of breast cancer is a hard, irregular, fixed mass. Evidence of metastatic disease is denoted by enlarged, fixed, hard lymph nodes (pectoral, subscapular, or central groups) in the axilla. If the suspending ligaments are involved, dimpling or retraction may occur. Bloody or clear discharge indicates invasion of the milk ducts. Lymphatic obstruction, as previously stated, can produce skin edema.

Standard Precautions ▷ Practitioners should use Standard Precautions at all times when interacting with patients. Determining the level of precaution necessary requires the practitioner to exercise clinical judgment based on the patient's history and the potential for exposure to body fluids or aerosol-borne pathogens (for further discussion, see Chapter 2).

Patient Preparation

As discussed later, the duration of CBE is important. It is likely that many patients have never received an adequate examination and might be surprised by the length of time required to perform the examination and its thoroughness.

- The examination should be conducted in a room that is climate controlled and ensures privacy. Cold examination rooms deter clinicians and patients; hot rooms cause patients and providers to perspire, inhibiting optimal technique.
- The patient must be relaxed for an adequate examination, and cloth gowns enhance comfort. Pillows provide comfort while improving positioning.

Materials Utilized to Perform a Breast Examination

Note: The CBE can be considered a virtually free examination in that it uses only the time and expertise of the clinician to screen for disease. Basic equipment is listed.

- Powder
- Lotion
- Gloves
- Sufficient light
- Pillow

Procedure for Performing a Breast Examination

Note: Recommendations for performance of the CBE are derived predominantly from Barton and colleagues (1999). These researchers thoroughly reviewed the literature and specified those components of the examination that have been validated in independent investigations.

Note: Some clinicians prefer that a female assistant be present for this sensitive examination.

Inspection

Note: Inspection has been traditionally advised but has not been demonstrated to add additional specificity or sensitivity to an examination with palpatory components alone.

1. Inspect the breasts with the patient sitting, hands by her side (Fig. 17–2).
2. Note the condition of the skin; any eczematous changes, "enlarged pores" (peau d'orange), or erythema.

Note: Tangential light may aid this portion of the examination.

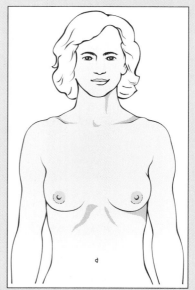

Figure 17–2. Redrawn from Seidel HM: Mosby's Guide to Physical Examination, 4th ed. St. Louis, Mosby-Year Book, 1999.

3. Look for retraction, dimpling, displacement, nipple inversion, or obvious mass defect. Also note scars from previous biopsies.

Procedure for Performing a Breast Examination – *(continued)*

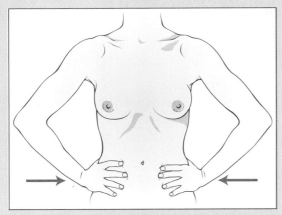

Figure 17–3. Redrawn from Seidel HM: Mosby's Guide to Physical Examination, 4th ed. St. Louis, Mosby-Year Book, 1999.

Note: Since retraction and dimpling are phenomena that result from underlying tissue compression or displacement, the patient may be examined in several different postures. Pressing the hands against the hips contracts the pectoralis muscles (Fig. 17–3); bending at the waist to let the breasts hang free can also be useful (Fig. 17–4).

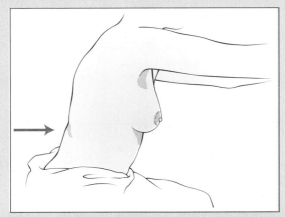

Figure 17–4. Redrawn from Seidel HM: Mosby's Guide to Physical Examination, 4th ed. St. Louis, Mosby-Year Book, 1999.

Palpation in the Axillary Area

4. Palpate the axillae for enlarged nodes (see Fig. 17–1).

Note: Many clinicians conduct this portion of the examination with the patient in a supine position; others support the sitting patient's arm with one hand and examine the axilla with the other. However, palpating the axillae with the patient lying down facilitates a smooth segue into the remainder of the supine breast examination.

Note: Since the axillary areas are frequently damp, the clinician may want to don gloves for this procedure. After the axillary examination, the gloves are removed, leaving a powder residue on the hands. This substance, or lotion, may enhance the ease of the palpatory breast examination.

Palpation of the Breast

Note: Palpation is emphasized because inspection, although traditionally included, has not been demonstrated to substantially increase diagnostic yield.

Note: Most authorities advise that palpation is optimally performed on women who are supine. Some classic references on physical examination technique recommend conducting the examination with the patient sitting and supine. This has not proved to increase sensitivity or yield and would be very time consuming if done with sufficient thoroughness.

Note: Women, especially those with larger breasts, can improve examination efficacy by flattening the breast (raising the ipsilateral hand, rotating the shoulder externally, placing a pillow behind the back, and so on).

Procedure for Performing a Breast Examination – *(continued)*

Technique

5. With the patient supine, and the hands behind the head, use the finger pads of the middle three fingers of the dominant hand to palpate breast tissue. These fingers are held together; the hand may flex slightly at the knuckles.

Note: If the proximal interphalangeal (PIP) joints are flexed, the clinician will examine the patient with the fingertips instead of the fingerpads; this is incorrect and must be avoided. The proximal interphalangeal joints and the distal interphalangeal (DIP) joints should be held in hyperextension for this delicate maneuver (Fig. 17–5).

6. For optimal palpation, "rock" the fingers back and forth in the horizontal and vertical planes, producing an almost circular "rotatory" movement from a central axis located at the fingerpad of the third digit.

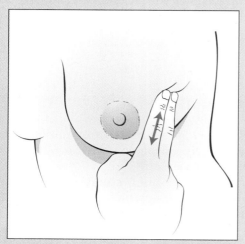

Figure 17–5. Redrawn from Seidel HM: Mosby's Guide to Physical Examination, 4th ed. St. Louis, Mosby-Year Book, 1999.

Note: The diameter of this rotation, as measured from each fingertip, should be no greater than 1.5 cm. Light, medium, and deep palpation are used sequentially.

7. Never lift the fingerpads completely from the skin, but advance very slightly (1 cm or less) by sliding along the skin, still exerting traction, after each area is thoroughly palpated. Again, maintain palpatory pressure at all times.

Note: In order for this maneuver to be successful, the fingerpads and breast tissue must be either powder "dry" or moistened with lotion. Otherwise, the fingerpads stick to the skin surface and cannot be rotated or advanced smoothly.

Note: "Walking" fingertips are to be avoided.

Pattern of Palpation

8. Begin palpation laterally at the midaxillary line and extend inferiorly in a straight line until approximately the level of the seventh rib, where the breast tissue stops.

9. Shift the finger pads medially and continue palpation superiorly, again in a straight line, back to the midaxilla or clavicle, depending on how far medially the examination has progressed.

Note: Some examiners palpate the area around the nipple in exactly this same manner; some, however, also traditionally "squeeze" the nipple to check for fluid. The validity of this technique in cancer detection is uncertain.

Note: This technique, called the *vertical strip pattern,* is analogous to "lawn mowing." Much as in cutting grass, rows need to overlap to avoid skipping areas. The vertical strip pattern has been found to be more thorough and reproducible than the traditional concentric circumferential technique or the radial spoke method (Fig. 17–6). However, it is certain that any uniformly practiced, sequential technique is better than "random" palpation, which is the method unfortunately used by many busy clinicians.

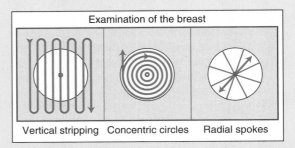

Examination of the breast

Vertical stripping   Concentric circles   Radial spokes

Figure 17–6

Special Considerations

Training and practice enhance diagnostic capability. Silicone breast models, demonstrating common benign and malignant abnormalities as well as the consistency of "normal" breast tissue, have demonstrated efficacy when used with lay and professional populations. Although experience with previous abnormalities does enhance the diagnostic efficacy of a provider, the single most important determinant of examination sensitivity is duration of the procedure. The other vital component is a sequential palpation plan with well-defined landmarks, ensuring that no area of breast tissue is inadvertently overlooked. The attention, thoroughness, and diligence of the examiner are more predictive of screening sensitivity than the examiner's specific professional role (physician assistant, nurse, physician), level of training, or previous experience.

Follow-up Care and Instructions

- A breast examination not recorded is a breast examination not performed. The clinician should clearly document the performance and findings of the CBE and the plan of action.
- If referral for further diagnostic or screening studies is warranted or recommended, "tickler" files or computer reminders to ensure and document patient compliance and the results obtained are essential. Written documentation of all patient contacts regarding referral or recommended further diagnostic or screening studies is vital. Patients who do not keep referral appointments should be contacted by telephone and certified mail.

- Patient education concerning the CBE should include information on the sensitivity and specificity of the examination and information about why the duration of the examination is important.
- Education must also include accurate information concerning breast cancer prevalence.
- Information concerning current recommendations for other breast cancer screening modalities, such as mammography and breast self-examination, should be provided as well.
- The patient education provided must be accurately documented in the medical record.
- Most clinicians include information and education concerning the breast self-examination during the annual CBE. The effect of breast self-examination on breast cancer mortality is uncertain. Self-reported frequency of breast self-examination has never been correlated with improved outcome. Appropriate teaching of technique has, however, been shown to improve the efficacy of breast self-examination in the discovery of smaller, and hence more treatable, masses. Many studies of this practice have provided contradictory results; the evidence is not considered strong enough to make a clear recommendation for or against breast self-examination by many governmental health authorities. Private organizations, however, including the American Cancer Society, recommend this procedure. As a result, women should be instructed in appropriate technique, frequency, and duration of breast self-examination. These examinations, however, should not substitute for CBE.

References

Barton MB, Harris R, Fletcher SW: Does this patient have breast cancer? The screening clinical breast examination: Should it be done? How? JAMA 282:1270–1280, 1999.

US Preventive Services Task Force: Guide to Clinical Preventive Services, 2nd ed. Baltimore, Williams & Wilkins, 1996.

Bibliography

- Armstrong K, Eisen A, Weber B: Primary care: Assessing the risk of breast cancer. N Engl J Med 342:564–571, 2000.
- DeGowin RL, Brown DD: DeGowin's Diagnostic Examination, 7th ed. New York, McGraw-Hill, 2000.
- Fletcher SW, Black W, Harris R, et al: Report of the international workshop on screening for breast cancer. J Natl Cancer Inst 85:1644–1656, 1993.
- Hortobagyi GN: Drug therapy: Treatment of breast cancer. N Engl J Med 339:974–984, 1998.

- National Cancer Institute and American Cancer Society: Joint statement on breast cancer screening for women in their 40s. Press release of March 27, 1997.
- Physician Insurers Association of America Breast Cancer Study: Washington D.C., Physician Insurers of America, 1995.
- Roy JA, Swaka CA, Prichard KI: Hormone replacement therapy in women with breast cancer: Do the risks outweigh the benefits? J Clin Oncol 14:997–1006, 1996.
- Schwartz MH: Textbook of Physical Examination, 3rd ed. Philadelphia, WB Saunders, 1998.

Chapter 18

The Pelvic Examination and Obtaining a Routine Papanicolaou's Smear

▷ L. Gail Curtis

Procedure Goals and Objectives

Goal: To perform a thorough pelvic examination (PVE) in a female patient in a manner that preserves the patient's comfort while maximizing the likelihood of identifying abnormal findings and obtaining a sample for a Papanicolaou (Pap) smear.

Objectives: The student will be able to . . .

▶ Describe the indications, contraindications, and rationale for performing a PVE.

▶ Describe the essential anatomy and physiology associated with the performance of the PVE.

▶ Describe the logical order of the steps used to perform the PVE.

▶ Describe normal and abnormal findings associated with the PVE.

Background and History

Many women dislike having a PVE performed. The lithotomy position makes some women feel vulnerable. In addition, this examination may invoke feelings of embarrassment or even anxiety. It is the examiner's responsibility to put the patient at ease while conveying the importance of the examination. The challenge is to make this experience educational, comfortable, and not to be feared in the future.

The PVE is an extension of the abdominal examination in the female patient. The Pap smear is one aspect of the PVE and was developed in the 1920s by Dr. George Nicolas Papanicolaou, an anatomist and cytologist in the United States. Dr. Papanicolaou identified characteristic cellular changes associated with cervical cancer. The original technology allowed for cytologic evaluation of cervical cells exfoliated from the female genital tract. Approximately 20 years elapsed before the technique named for him, the Papanicolaou smear, was accepted as a cancer screening procedure. The Pap smear was initially used to detect asymptomatic invasive cervical cancer; however, as time passed, the importance of preinvasive disease was recognized. The Pap smear remains a screening test; however, it does not provide a diagnosis. Current standard of care requires further work-up of any abnormality found on a Pap smear. This work-up typically includes a colposcopy and biopsy of cervical samples.

Indications

The indications and rationale for obtaining a routine Pap smear are numerous and worthy of discussion.

Reports of the yearly incidence of cervical cancer in the United States range from 13,500 to 16,000, with an annual mortality rate of 4800 to 6000. American women have a 0.83% chance of developing cervical cancer in their lifetime, and death from the disease is estimated at 0.27%. Pap smear screening has been documented to decrease the incidence and mortality rate of cervical cancer. Despite this, agreement on recommended standards for obtaining a Pap smear, such as age to begin screening, how frequently to screen, and at what age to cease screening, have been difficult to obtain.

Currently, consensus recommendations agreed on by The American Cancer Society (ACS) (1993), the American College of Obstetrics and Gynecology (ACOG), the American Medical Association (AMA), the American Academy of Family Physicians (AAFP), and others state that:

- All women who are or have been sexually active or who have reached age 18 should have annual Pap smears.
- At the discretion of the medical provider, Pap smears may be less frequent after three or more annual smears have been normal.

- The consensus statement does not recommend an age to discontinue ★
  Pap testing.

The current U.S. Preventive Services Task Force guidelines (1996)
follow:

- Regular Pap smears are recommended for all women who are or have
  been sexually active and who have a cervix.
- Testing should begin at the age of first sexual intercourse.
- Pap smears should be performed at least every 3 years. The interval
  between tests should be based on risk factors.
- Insufficient evidence exists to recommend for or against an upper age
  limit for Pap testing. Recommendations can be made on other grounds
  to discontinue regular testing after age 65 in women who have had
  regular previous screening with normal results.
- There is no evidence to support routine screening for human papillomavirus (HPV) infection. *nowadays it's a routine reflex if PAP is >Ascus.*

Many factors are thought to increase the risk for an abnormal Pap
smear result. These can be divided into two broad categories: factors re-
lating to coitus and nonsexual factors. Coitus-related factors include a
young age at first intercourse, multiple sexual partners, sexually transmitted disease, and HPV. Nonsexual factors that can increase risk are to-
bacco smoking, illicit drug use, diet, oral contraceptive use, a prior
history of abnormal Pap smears, poor personal hygiene, and an uncircumcised partner. Although all these factors may play a part, the presence of or exposure to HPV is now accepted as the leading risk factor for
an abnormal smear and development of cervical cancer. HPV types 16
and 18 seem to be the most oncogenic, although the natural history of
how HPV infection progresses to cancer is still poorly understood.

Contraindications

There are no absolute contraindications for performing a routine PVE.
However, care must be exercised to receive explicit permission to perform
the examination.

Potential Complications

False-negative Pap smear results do occur. Common causes of a smear
being interpreted as normal when the cervical epithelium is abnormal
include:

- Sampling error: the lesions are very small or peripherally located so
  that they are missed on sampling

- Lesions that do not shed cells well
- Errors in interpretation

The most common cause is sampling error. However, the error that is most publicized is interpretation. Using the proper technique to obtain the Pap smear can significantly decrease the incidence of false-negative results due to sampling error. New technologies have been developed to decrease the false-negative rate from errors in interpretation, although they are more expensive and therefore not widely used. Other sources of Pap smear screening errors are failure of the clinician to understand or respond appropriately to Pap smear results or failure of the patient to follow the clinician's recommendations. All these issues make routine Pap smear screening less than straightforward for the clinician.

Review of Essential Anatomy and Physiology

External Anatomy (Fig. 18–1)

The vulva consists of the mons pubis, the labia majora, the labia minora, the clitoris, and the glandular structures that open into the vagina. The shape, size, and color of the various structures will vary among individual women and racial groups. Normal hair distribution is in the shape of an inverted triangle centered over the mons pubis.

The labia majora are two mound-shaped structures composed primarily of adipose tissue originating at the mons pubis and terminating in the perineum. They form the lateral boundaries of the vulva. Underlying the skin is a poorly developed muscle layer: the tunica dartos labialis. There are also numerous sweat glands in the labia majora. The internal and external pudendal arteries and a branch of the perineal artery provide the arterial blood supply to the labia majora. The venous drainage is extensive and is provided primarily by the perineal, posterior labial, external pudendal, and saphenous veins. Lymphatics are also extensive and

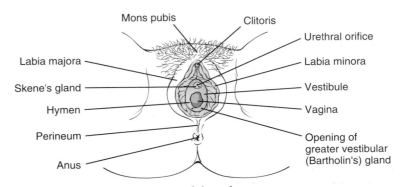

Figure 18–1. External anatomy of the vulva.

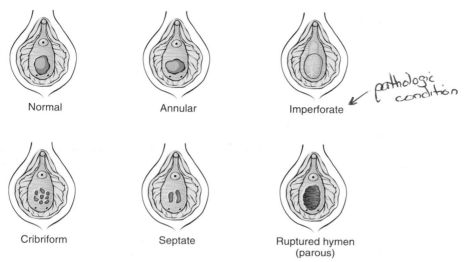

pathologic condition

Figure 18-2. Types of hymens.

use two systems: one superficial and one deep within the subcutaneous tissue primarily draining into the inguinal nodes.

The labia minora are two skin folds medial to the labia majora that begin at the base of the clitoris and extend posteriorly to the introitus. The arterial supply is from the superficial perineal artery. The venous drainage is to the perineal and vaginal veins. Lymphatics pass to the superficial and deep subinguinal nodes. The innervation is supplied from branches of the pudendal nerve, which originates from the perineal nerve.

The clitoris is the homologue of the dorsal aspect of the penis. Blood supply is rich, with the dorsal and pudendal arteries supplying arterial blood. Venous drainage consists of a rich plexus draining into the pudendal vein. The lymphatics coincide primarily with those of the labia minora. Innervation to the clitoris is from the terminal branch of the pudendal nerve. Nerve endings in the clitoris vary, from woman to woman, from total absence to a rich supply.

The vestibule is the space bordered by the labia minora and includes the entrance to the vaginal canal or the introitus. The vaginal opening can be obscured by the hymenal ring or hymen. The hymen is a membrane that partially or wholly occludes the introitus. The shape and opening of the hymen can vary greatly (Fig. 18-2), but only a completely imperforate hymen is pathologic. The arterial supply to the vestibule and hymen is from an extensive capillary plexus from the perineal artery. The venous drainage is also extensive and involves the same areas as the arterial network. The lymphatic drainage terminates in the superficial inguinal nodes and the external iliac chain. The urethra is positioned between the clitoris and the vaginal opening and is not difficult to visualize.

The Skene's glands are posterior to the urethral orifice and are often difficult to locate. The Bartholin's glands lie inferior and lateral to the posterior vestibule, are less superficial, and are usually not visible. The arterial supply and venous drainage is along the pudendal vessels. The lymphatics drain directly via the perineum into the inguinal area. The innervation of Bartholin's glands is a small branch of the perineal nerve.

Internal Anatomy (Fig. 18–3)

The vagina is a muscular canal that is lined with mucosa or rugae and is approximately 7 cm long extending from the uterus to the vestibule. It meets the cervix of the uterus at an angle of 45 to 90 degrees. The cervix projects into the upper portion of the anterior vaginal wall, thereby making the anterior vaginal wall slightly shorter than the posterior vaginal wall. The vaginal arterial supply is from the vaginal branch of the uterine artery, and the veins follow the course of the arteries. The lymphatics drain into the external iliac and inguinal nodes. Both sympathetic and parasympathetic nerves innervate the vagina. The perineum is the tissue between the vaginal opening and the anus.

The uterus is a pear-shaped, thick-walled muscular organ about 7 to 8 cm in length and 4 to 5 cm at its widest in the nonpregnant adult woman. It consists of three parts: the fundus, the body, and the cervix (Fig. 18–4). The uterine cavity opens into the vagina below and into the fallopian tubes above. It is supported by ligamentous attachments to various pelvic structures, including the vagina. The cervix is the portion of the uterus that can be visualized during the PVE and is the structure scraped to obtain the Pap smear. When viewed during the PVE, the cervix appears as a round bagel-like mound with a circular or slit-type opening that varies with parity (Fig. 18–5) and leads to the endocervical canal.

The fallopian tubes extend from the lateral portions of the uterine fundus and terminate in a fringed, cone-shaped conduit that arches toward the ovaries (Fig. 18–6). The ovaries are oval organs measuring about 2.5

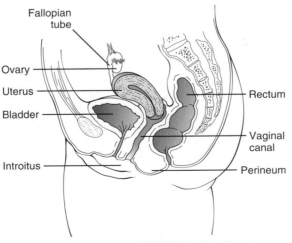

Fallopian
tube

Ovary

Uterus

Bladder

Introitus

Rectum

Vaginal
canal

Perineum

Figure 18–3. Female internal anatomy.

Side view

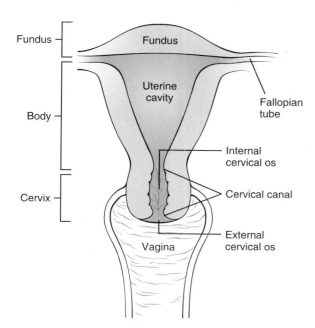

Figure 18–4. The uterus consists of three parts: the fundus, body, and cervix.

to 5 cm in length, 1.5 to 3 cm in breadth, and 0.7 to 1.5 cm in width. The fimbriated ends of the fallopian tubes overhang the upper part of each ovary. The ovarian artery is the chief source of blood for the ovary, and the ovarian veins follow the course of the arteries. Lymphatic channels drain retroperitoneally to the lumbar lymph nodes. The lymphatic channels in the ovaries are extensive and may provide additional fluid to the ovary during periods of preovulatory swelling. The ovaries produce ova and hormones, including estrogen and progesterone.

All the pelvic organs are supported within the lower abdominal cavity by a system of muscles, ligaments, and fascia.

Standard Precautions ▷ Practitioners should use Standard Precautions at all times when interacting with patients. Determining the level of precaution necessary requires the practitioner to exercise clinical judgment based on the patient's history and the potential for exposure to body fluids or aerosol-borne pathogens (for further discussion see Chapter 2).

Patient Preparation

As already noted, some women may be reluctant to have a PVE performed. If a patient has had several previous examinations, she knows

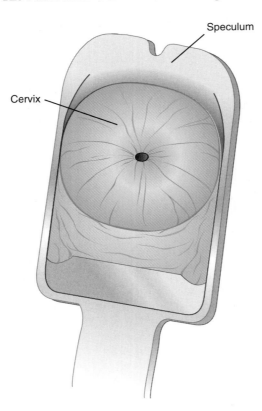

Speculum

Cervix

Figure 18-5. The cervix as viewed during pelvic examination (PVE).

what to expect. If this is her first, she has most likely heard about it from others. Your responsibility as the examiner is to explain what is ahead and provide education in order to decrease anxiety.

First Pelvic Examination Experience

This examination will set the tone for all that follow.

- Schedule enough time to allow a complete explanation of the PVE from beginning to completion.

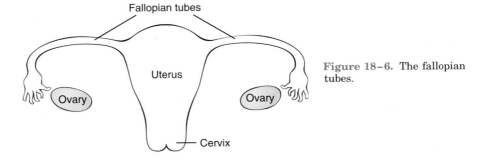

Fallopian tubes

Uterus

Ovary

Ovary

Cervix

Figure 18-6. The fallopian tubes.

- It is helpful to have a diagram or model of the female anatomy to aid the explanation.
- Have the actual equipment to be used on hand to show your patient. Explain all aspects of the PVE and the Pap smear.
- Show your patient, using your closed fist to simulate the cervix, how you will sample her cervical cells (Fig. 18–7). Explain that relaxing her pelvic muscles will ease the insertion of the speculum (again demonstrate with your fist; see Fig. 18–7).
- Allow and encourage your patient to ask questions.
- Explain terms she may have heard and been fearful about such as: "blades," "scraping," and "stirrups."
- Educate her about the lithotomy position: why it is necessary, including how it allows visualization of the cervix.
- Offer opportunities that empower the patient, such as the semisitting position and a hand-held mirror if she desires to observe the examination and visualize her own anatomy while the examination is in progress.
- Assure your patient that this examination is indicated and that the PVE should not be painful. Tell her you will be gentle and that if she wants you to stop at any time during the examination, you will.

The Returning Patient

- Always ask the patient if she has any particular concerns about this examination.

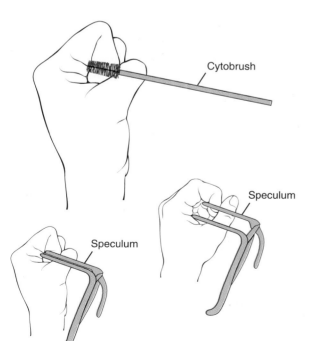

Cytobrush

Speculum

Speculum

Figure 18–7. *Top,* Closed fist, simulating the cervix. Closed fist simulating the vaginal opening for speculum insertion in tensed position (*lower left*) and relaxed position (*lower right*).

- Reassure her that you will be gentle and that there should be no pain associated with the PVE.
- Assure her that she can ask questions at any time during the examination.
- Tell her that if she should experience any discomfort to alert you immediately and you will stop and redirect your attempt.
- Explain every step of the examination as it unfolds.

Chaperone in Attendance for All Patients

Having a chaperone in attendance is important for this examination. This is advised even if the provider is female. In addition to providing assistance with the examination, the presence of another member of the staff helps reduce the likelihood of a patient filing an unfounded accusation regarding inappropriate conduct of the clinician during the examination. Explain that the chaperone is in attendance to assist with any needs during the examination. Avoid statements such as "he or she is here to watch and observe."

> ### Materials Utilized for Performing the Pelvic Examination and Obtaining Cells for a Routine Pap Smear

The Vaginal Speculum (Fig. 18–8)
Several types of speculums are available:

- Pedersen speculum, metal and reusable: This type of speculum comes in short and long sizes. It should be used if at all possible because it has a narrow blade and is more comfortable for most women.
- Graves speculum, metal and reusable: This speculum also comes in short and long sizes. The Graves has a "duckbill-shaped" blade and

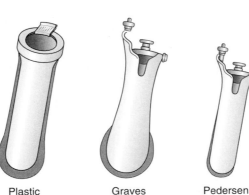

Plastic   Graves   Pedersen

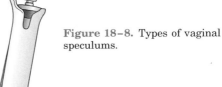

Figure 18–8. Types of vaginal speculums.

is a better choice for viewing the cervix in the following circumstances: The patient is significantly overweight, the patient has a lot of redundant skin surrounding the introitus, or the patient has a severely retroverted uterus. *= Graves' Spec.*

■ Disposable speculum: This type of speculum is made of hard, clear plastic; usually has the Graves-type blades; and makes a loud click when locked into place. Warn patients about the upcoming click, and use great care not to pinch the patient's surrounding skin on insertion.

■ Pediatric speculum: This speculum is useful for children and virginal and geriatric women. The pediatric speculum is also preferable when explaining the PVE to a patient undergoing a first PVE. Its small size reduces undue anxiety and fear of pain about the pending examination.

Note: It is all right to switch speculums during the examination if there is trouble viewing the cervix. Avoid comments such as "I have to get a bigger speculum." Women may feel sensitive to implications that their anatomy is too large. Rather state, "I am having difficulty visualizing your cervix and I don't want to hurt you, so I am going to change speculums to make this examination more comfortable for you."

Note: Whichever speculum is chosen, be sure that you understand how to open it, insert it, and lock it into place before you insert it.

Other equipment needed to complete the examination includes the following:

■ Wooden spatula (Fig. 18–9)
■ Cytobrush (see Fig. 18–9)
■ Cotton swabs (see Fig. 18–9)
■ Pap smear slide or vial of preservative solution
■ Good light source
■ Water-soluble lubricating jelly
■ Latex gloves

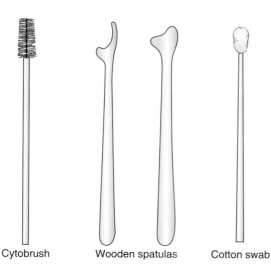

Figure 18–9. Instruments used for gathering cervical cells.

Cytobrush   Wooden spatulas   Cotton swab

Procedure for the Pelvic Examination and Obtaining Cervical Cells

Note: The examination itself is divided into three parts: inspection of the external genitalia; the internal examination, which includes obtaining the Pap smear; and the bimanual examination.

1. Before beginning the examination, have the patient assume the lithotomy position, hips flexed and abducted, feet in stirrups, and buttocks slightly beyond the edge of the examining table.

Note: Many women prefer not to be in the lithotomy position any longer than necessary; therefore, it is important to have all materials set up and ready before positioning the patient for the examination.

2. Extend the foot stirrups and have all your equipment prepared.
3. When ready, ask the patient to lie back in this position and place a sheet as a drape over her. Most women will indicate to you whether they prefer to be fully draped with the sheet to their knees blocking their view of the examination or if they prefer to be able to see you throughout the examination.

Note: Although most examiners have patients lay flat on the examining table, some women prefer to be in a semisitting position (Fig. 18–10). The semisitting position works just as well for the examiner and makes some women feel less vulnerable.

4. After the patient has reclined, ask her to place her feet in the stirrups. If possible, have the stirrups covered with a soft, warm material or allow the patient to keep her socks on.

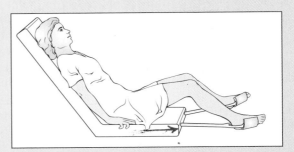

Figure 18–10

5. Have her slide her buttocks toward the end of the table to the appropriate position.

Note: Throughout the examination, be sure to explain each step to the patient as it is being performed. Encourage her to ask any questions she may have. Continue to talk to her, and monitor her status throughout the examination. If she tenses her abdomen or buttocks, ask her to relax them. Once the patient is as comfortable as possible, the examination of the external genitalia should begin.

External Examination

6. Put on gloves and be seated comfortably on a rolling stool at the table end, adjust the light source, and begin by inspecting the external genitalia.
7. First examine the mons pubis, labia, and perineum. Note the pubic hair for its pattern, for any lice or nits, infected hair follicles, or any other abnormality, and then inspect for any lesions, erythema, swelling, nodules, or discharge on the skin.

Procedure for the Pelvic Examination and Obtaining Cervical Cells – (continued)

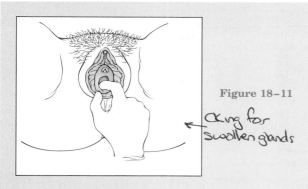

Figure 18–11

cking for swollen glands [handwritten annotation]

8. Expose the clitoris, urethral orifice, and the vaginal opening by gently retracting the labia minora. Inspect for any cysts or other lesions. Inspect the area of the Bartholin's glands. Normal Bartholin's glands cannot be seen or felt.

9. If enlargement or redness is noted, or if indicated by symptoms, examine the Bartholin's glands by inserting your index finger into the vagina and your thumb outside (Fig. 18–11), and palpate the tissue between the internal and external fingers. Check for any discharge from the duct. If discharge is noted, a culture should be obtained using the appropriate medium.

10. Next, ask your patient to perform the Valsalva maneuver or bear down while you check for cystocele, rectocele, or uterine prolapse.

Note: Take care during the external examination to avoid unnecessary contact with the clitoris. [marked with *]

Internal Examination

11. Warm the previously selected vaginal speculum under running water. Water not only will warm the instrument but

also will act as a lubricant to ease insertion. Other lubricants cannot be used because they may interfere with the cytologic studies. *KY generall used* [handwritten annotation]

12. A digital examination performed by inserting a finger into the vaginal canal helps locate the cervix (it has a consistency similar to the end of the nose). Correctly direct the insertion of the speculum for easy visualization of the cervix and comfort of the patient.

13. To insert the speculum, withdraw your internal finger while applying gentle pressure to the perineum in a downward motion. Ask the patient to relax this muscle as you press downward. Insert the speculum over your withdrawing finger with the blades closed and at a 45-degree angle (Fig. 18–12A).

14. Once the blades are fully inserted, rotate the speculum to the appropriate angle (see Fig. 18–12B). Avoid pressure on the more sensitive anterior wall, urethral orifice, or clitoris.

15. If there is a problem locating the cervix, withdraw the speculum and reposition it (usually more posteriorly). Apply gentle pressure to the posterior vaginal wall and try again.

16. Avoid excessive movements of the speculum while searching for the cervix, as this can be uncomfortable.

17. Once the cervix is visualized, lock the speculum in place. Your noncontaminated hand is now free to obtain the Pap smear sample and any other needed cultures or samples.

18. The wooden spatula is used to obtain cells from the cervix and the vaginal wall (Fig. 18–13).
   • Begin with the pointed or longer end of the spatula and insert it into the external cervical os.

Procedure for the Pelvic Examination and Obtaining Cervical Cells – *(continued)*

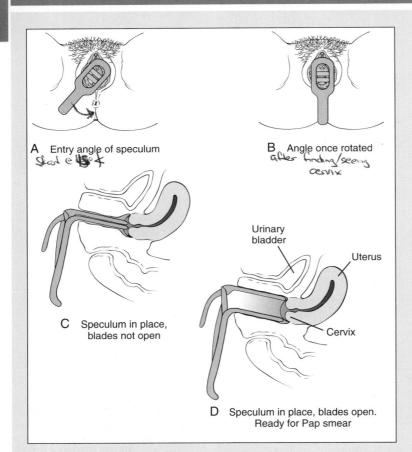

A   Entry angle of speculum
Start @ 45° ↑

B   Angle once rotated
after finding/seeing cervix

C   Speculum in place, blades not open

D   Speculum in place, blades open. Ready for Pap smear

Urinary bladder

Uterus

Cervix

Figure 18–12

- Apply mild pressure while turning the spatula 360 degrees to obtain cells from the squamous-columnar junction or the transformation zone.   *T zone*
- Use the opposite, rounded end of the spatula to sample cells from the vaginal wall.   *opp. end of same spatula →*
19. The cytobrush (see Fig. 18–13) is used next to obtain cells from the endocervical canal.
    - Insert this brush into the cervical os until the bristles are no longer seen and turn two full revolutions.

Note: Always warn the patient that this may induce uterine cramping and mild bleeding.   *※*

20. Next, the cells are collected and are transferred to the appropriate transport medium.
    - Label the Pap smear slide or vial of preservative solution with the patient's name before beginning the examination.
    - Apply the obtained cells to the slide by gently dragging the spatula with

Procedure for the Pelvic Examination and Obtaining Cervical Cells – *(continued)*

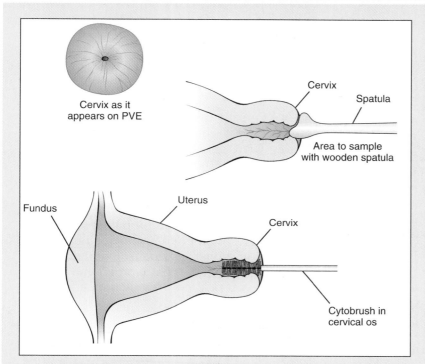

Cervix as it
appears on PVE

Cervix

Spatula

Area to sample
with wooden spatula

Fundus

Uterus

Cervix

Cytobrush in
cervical os

Figure 18–13

the samples from the external cervix and the vaginal wall down the slide.

21. Using the cytobrush, place cells on the slide by rotating the brush counterclockwise while moving the brush from left to right on the slide (Fig. 18–14). Some slides label specific areas for the various samples.

22. After the specimens are placed on the slide, immediately spray the slide with cytologic fixative. There is no specific recommendation for how long to spray the slide, but it is important to cover the entire slide.

23. If using the vial of preservative solution, collect the sample in the same manner, but rather than smearing the cells onto the slide, rinse the collection device into the vial of preservative solution.

[handwritten margin notes: "+ done anymore since Prep's are used"]

Note: If a wet mount or cultures are to be obtained, this should occur only after the Pap smear cells have been obtained.

Note: Be sure to obtain an adequate sample both to avoid having to repeat the examination and to reduce the false-negative rate. In a woman with a uterus,

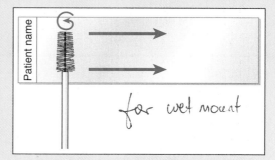

Patient name

[handwritten: for wet mount]

Figure 18–14.

endocervical cells must be obtained. If the cytologic report comes back stating "no endocervical cells seen," this indicates inadequate sampling, and the patient will need to have the examination repeated in order to obtain the adequate sample. Therefore, it is important to sample adequately the first time.

24. After collecting the sample or samples, unlock the speculum and slowly withdraw the instrument while inspecting the vaginal wall for any abnormalities. Allow the speculum blades to close naturally as they are withdrawn.

Once the speculum is removed and the samples are preserved, proceed to the bimanual examination.

Bimanual Examination

25. Inform the patient that you are going to examine her uterus and ovaries. Tell her this will include a digital rectal examination.
Note: Lubricating jelly can be used during this portion of the examination, as the cytologic samples have been procured. This lubricant will make this portion of the PVE more comfortable for your patient.

26. Insert two lubricated fingers into the vagina while applying pressure to the abdomen in a sweeping motion toward the mons pubis.

27. Push upward on the cervix with your internal fingers while pushing downward on the uterine area of the abdomen with the external hand. Palpate the uterine fundus as it rises toward your external fingers.

28. Then palpate the ovaries by moving the internal fingers to the right and left of the cervix while sweeping down on either side of the uterus with the external hand.
Note: Ovaries should be palpable in women until menopause. A palpable ovary in a postmenopausal woman needs further work-up. Most women can tell when you palpate their ovaries and can offer feedback.

29. The rectovaginal examination is the final step in the PVE. Insert your index finger in the vagina and your middle finger in the rectum and repeat the maneuvers of the bimanual examination.
Note: This approach allows assessment of the retroverted uterus and the region behind the cervix.

30. This completes the examination. Remind your patient to push back on the table before trying to sit up. Provide your patient with a towelette to remove any excess lubricant used during the examination.

Special Considerations

Pediatric genital examinations, when necessary, can often be performed using the "frog leg" position (Fig. 18–15). Special attention must be given to semantics and patient education when examining children. Keep in mind that most children have been taught not to allow anyone to touch their genitals.

In the geriatric population, frequency of PVE can often be decreased. Any posthysterectomy patient can receive less frequent examinations, varying from every 3 to 5 years. Some practitioners cease doing examinations altogether unless circumstance dictates. If the ovaries are still present, bimanual examination can still be important. Women not taking hormone replacement therapy (HRT) will have dryer atrophic vaginas. This can make the PVE uncomfortable or painful. Care should be taken to use the smallest possible speculum and not tear the thin tissue.

Follow-up Care and Instructions

- Inform the patient of the results of the examination, taking care not to imply that everything is completely normal until all results are obtained.
- Educate her about when to return for her next screening examination. If anything was noted on examination, explain the possibilities and what follow-up may be necessary.

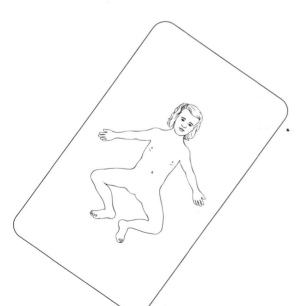

Figure 18–15. Pediatric "frog leg" position.

- Let her know what correspondence to expect from your office and the time period within which to expect it. Specifically tell her how she will receive her Pap smear results (i.e., letter, phone call, report).
- Ask her to call the office requesting her results if she has not heard anything within the specified period.
- Patient education handouts explaining Pap smear results are helpful and should be sent home with the patient. These handouts may increase patient understanding of Pap smears and increase compliance with the recommendations made based on the Pap smear results.

The PVE and the Pap smear are important parts of providing comprehensive well-woman care. Patient education and examiner sensitivity and competence will increase compliance of the female patient in regard to this life-saving examination. For all examiners, competence and sensitivity toward the patient will help make this examination repeatable for the patient and the next provider.

References

American Cancer Society: Guidelines for the cancer-related checkup: An update. Atlanta, American Cancer Society, 1993.
U.S. Preventive Services Task Force: Guide to Clinical Preventive Services, 2nd ed. Washington, DC: US Department of Health and Human Services, Office of Public Health and Science, Office of Disease Prevention and Health Promotion, 1996.

Bibliography

- Agency for Health Care Policy and Research: Evidence Report/Technology Assessment. Rockville, Md, US Department of Health and Human Services, Agency for Health Care Policy and Research, Jan 1, 1999.
- Anderson JE: Grant's Atlas of Anatomy, 7th ed. Baltimore, Williams & Wilkins, 1978.
- Curtis P, Skinner B, Varenholt JJ, et al: Papanicolaou smear quality assurance: Providing feedback to physicians. J Fam Pract 36:309–312, 1993.
- Eddy DM: Screening for cervical cancer. Ann Intern Med 113:214, 1990.
- Goroll AH: Primary Care Medicine, 3rd ed. Philadelphia, Lippincott-Raven, 1995.
- Lundber GD: The 1988 Bethesda system for reporting cervical/vaginal cytological diagnoses. JAMA 262:931, 1989.
- Pfenninger JL, Fowler GC: Procedures for Primary Care Physicians. St. Louis, Mosby-Year Book, 1994.
- Richart RM, Wright TC Jr: Controversies in the management of low-grade cervical intraepithelial neoplasia. Cancer 71:1413–1421, 1993.
- Ryan KJ, Berkowitz RS: Kistner's Gynecology and Women's Health, 7th ed. St. Louis, CV Mosby, 1999.
- Wingo PA, Tong T, Bolden S: Cancer statistics, 1995. CA Cancer J Clin 45:8–30, 1995.

Chapter 19

Examination of the Male Genitalia

▷ Richard Dehn

Procedure Goals and Objectives

Goal: To perform a thorough examination of the male genitalia in a manner that preserves the patient's modesty while maximizing the likelihood of identifying abnormal findings.

Objectives: The student will be able to . . .

▶ Describe the indications, contraindications, and rationale for performing an examination of the male genitalia.

▶ Describe the essential anatomy and physiology associated with the performance of the examination of the male genitalia.

▶ Describe the logical order of the steps used to perform the examination of the male genitalia.

▶ Describe normal and abnormal findings associated with the examination of the male genitalia.

Background and History

Examination of the male genitalia is taught to practitioners as part of the physical examination and should be performed on all patients in whom information derived from the examination is helpful. Although this examination has long been performed for diagnostic purposes, it has gained increasing importance as a screening examination for testicular cancer, prostatic cancer, and colon cancer.

The examination of the male genitalia is typically understood to include the physical examination of the external genitalia, which includes the perineum, penis, and scrotum, as well as a rectal examination in which the prostate is palpated. In addition, the examination often includes an assessment of the presence of an inguinal hernia.

The examination of the penis and scrotum also can have value for early disease detection, particularly if performed by the patient regularly as a self-examination regimen. Self-examination of the penis and urethra can be useful for the early detection of sexually transmitted diseases, and testicular self-examination can lead to early detection of testicular tumors. In young men, testicular tumors are often malignant and aggressive; thus, early detection is a significant factor in increasing survival rates because testicular cancer is the most common malignancy in men 20 to 40 years of age (Kelly, 1998).

The rectal examination and associated prostate examination have also been used for screening directed at the early detection of cancer. A sample of stool is easily obtained during the rectal examination, and the presence of occult blood is correlated with colon cancers. Screening for stool occult blood has been demonstrated to reduce colon cancer mortality, especially in individuals older than age 50, at which time the incidence of colon cancer greatly increases (Towler et al, 1999). The incidence of prostate cancer also increases starting at age 50. Prostate cancer is often discovered by digital rectal examination, although the value of digital rectal examination for detecting cancer before it has spread beyond the prostatic capsule is questionable (Woolf, 1995). Additionally, most examiners can palpate only part of the posterior prostatic surface when performing digital rectal examination; thus, this process will not detect all prostatic lesions.

Indications

The examination of the male genitalia is indicated in the following circumstances:

- For routine preventive screening for testicular cancer
- For routine preventive screening for prostate cancer
- For routine preventive screening for colon cancer

- To derive information concerning the male genital system
- To derive information concerning the male reproductive system

Contraindications

There is no contraindication to performing an examination of the external genitalia. Palpation of the prostate is relatively contraindicated in patients suspected of having acute bacterial prostatitis, as this maneuver can result in septicemia (Dehn, 1998).

Potential Complications

Complications of the male genital examination include the following:

- Temporary discomfort from palpation of the penis and contents of the scrotum.
- Rectal abrasions and fissures from the following:
  - Inadequate digit lubrication
  - Failure to allow the anal sphincter to relax adequately
  - Rectal masses or strictures
- Septicemia from prostatic manipulation if patient has acute bacterial prostatitis

Review of Essential Anatomy and Physiology

Examination of the male genitalia involves structures of the male reproductive system, the lower urinary tract, and the lower gastrointestinal tract (Fig. 19–1). The structures that are accessible by examination include the penis and internal penile structures, the scrotum, and the contents of the scrotal sac. The posterior surface of the prostate is palpable during a digital rectal examination. The anatomy of the rectum is illustrated in Fig. 30–1.

The penis includes structures of both the reproductive system and the lower urinary system. The distal opening of the urethra is located at the glans penis. The urethra travels the corpus spongiosum the length of the penis, passing through the prostate gland to the bladder. The urethra serves as the conduit for both urination and ejaculation from the junction with the ejaculatory duct in the prostate distally. The two corpus cavernosa are located on the dorsum and sides of the penis and expand to produce penile erections when engorged with blood. The skin of the penis is thin and loose to accommodate the changes in size.

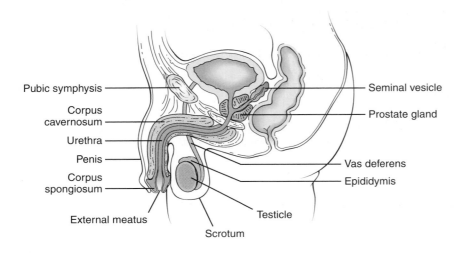

Pubic symphysis

Corpus
cavernosum

Urethra

Penis

Corpus
spongiosum

External meatus

Scrotum

Testicle

Seminal vesicle

Prostate gland

Vas deferens

Epididymis

Figure 19–1. Anatomy of the male genitalia. (Redrawn from Swartz MS: Male genitalia and hernias. In Swartz MS: Textbook of Physical Diagnosis, 3rd ed. Philadelphia, WB Saunders, 1998, p 391.)

The scrotal sac contains the testicles, the epididymis, and the vas deferens. The testicles produce testosterone. Spermatozoa, also produced by the testicles, are transported by the vas deferens to the seminal vesicle at the point where it forms the ejaculatory duct, which then traverses the prostate. The vas deferens, testicular arteries, testicular veins, and associated nerves form the spermatic cord, which traverses the inguinal canal.

Examination of the male genitalia also identifies the presence of inguinal hernias. The inguinal canal, the remnants of where the scrotal sac contents passed through the abdominal wall at about the 12th week of gestation, can present a point of weakness in the abdominal wall. Points of weakness of the abdominal wall include the internal and external rings of the inguinal canal. Occasionally, abdominal contents enter the inguinal canal and can present a strangulation risk. An indirect hernia traverses the inguinal canal from the internal ring to the external ring, sometimes resulting in abdominal contents in the scrotum. A direct hernia traverses the abdominal wall directly through the external ring.

Patient Preparation

- Since the examination of the male genitalia can be embarrassing to the patient, be sure to have the examination take place in an environment where privacy is established and maintained.
- Plan so that enough time can be taken not to rush the examination.
- Take the time to explain carefully to the patient what the examination will involve and make sure the patient understands.
- Ask the patient to remove all clothing, at least from the waist down.
- Provide a hospital gown to ensure protection of the patient's modesty.

Materials Utilized for Performing an Examination of the Male Genitalia

The following materials should be assembled before initiating an examination of the male genitalia:

■ Draping sheet and hospital gown (as noted in "Patient Preparation")
■ An examination table for the patient to support himself during the rectal examination
■ Nonsterile gloves
■ Water-soluble lubricant
■ Sample collection apparatus and Hemoccult (diagnostic aid for occult blood) collection cards if needed
■ A flashlight or penlight for transillumination
■ Facial tissues

Note: Depending on the patient's presenting symptoms and clinical circumstances, samples may be needed for laboratory analysis. The urethra may be sampled with a urethral brush, and the skin and rectal mucosa may be swabbed with cotton applicators. Prostatic secretions may be collected on a microscope slide for cell analysis or collected for culture. Materials for appropriately collecting and transporting the necessary samples should be assembled before starting the examination if possible.

Performing the Procedure of Examining the Male Genitalia

Examination of the External Genitalia

1. Ask the patient to stand. If support is necessary, have the patient stand next to the examining table, using it for support.
2. Sit on an examination stool in front of the patient at approximate eye level with the patient's genitalia.

Note: If the patient is unable to stand, the examination can be performed with the patient in the supine position.

3. Put on nonsterile examination gloves.
4. Expose the patient's genitalia fully.

5. Inspect the external genitalia, including the surrounding skin, penis, and scrotum. Note the hair distribution, the quality of the skin, the structures of the penis, and the structures of the scrotum. Also note any urethral discharge, lesions of the skin and hair, and structural deviations of the penis and scrotum, which should be investigated.

Note: If the patient is uncircumcised, the foreskin should be carefully pulled back for inspection and then returned to its original position when inspection is completed. Some patients prefer to do the foreskin manipulation themselves.

6. Palpate the meatus, penile shaft, and scrotum for abnormal structures and tenderness.
7. Palpate the internal structures of each side of the scrotal sac for masses and tenderness (Fig. 19–2).
8. Palpate symmetrical structures such as the testicles, epididymis, and vas deferens.
9. Insert the index finger into each external inguinal ring, then ask the patient to turn his head to the side and cough (turning the head avoids coughing on the examiner). If a hernia is present, it should be felt at this time.
10. Cover the patient's external genitalia area with the gown or drape.

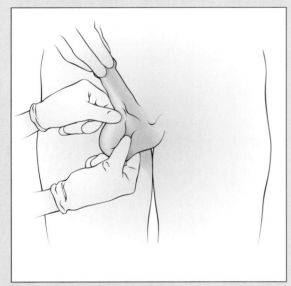

Figure 19–2. Redrawn from Seidel HM, Benedict GW, Ball JW, et al: Male genitalia. In Mosby's Guide to Physical Examination, 4th ed. St. Louis, CV Mosby, 1999, p 654.

Examination Of The Rectum And Prostate

1. Ask the patient to flex forward at the waist, supporting his upper body with an examination table. Instruct the patient to spread his legs shoulder width apart and to place most of his weight on his upper extremities, which are supported by leaning on the examination table.
2. Sit on a stool facing the patient's rectal area.

Note: If the patient is unable to stand, the examination can be performed in the knee-to-chest position or the left lateral decubitus position with the hips and knees flexed.

3. Put on nonsterile examination gloves if the gloves that were used for the first part of the examination were removed.
4. Inspect the area of the anus and surrounding structures. Note hair distribution and skin characteristics in the perineum and perianal region, and any lesions and areas of abnormal coloration.
5. Inspect the anus for lesions, fissures, hemorrhoids, and deviations from normal structure. Spread the patient's buttocks apart to facilitate the inspection process.

Note: Clock numbers define the geography of the anus, with the sacral surface at 12 o'clock. Findings from the examination should use this convention in descriptions and documentation.

6. Liberally lubricate the gloved index finger of the dominant hand.
7. Gently press the lubricated gloved index finger into the anal opening.

Performing the Procedure of Examining the Male Genitalia – *(continued)*

8. Instruct the patient to bear down in a manner similar to having a bowel movement to facilitate the relaxation of the rectal sphincter.
9. When the anal sphincter feels relaxed, gently advance your index finger into the anal canal.
10. Ask the patient to tighten the sphincter around the index finger; the muscle tone should be evaluated in this manner.
11. Rotate your finger using 360-degree motions, and use the pad of the distal finger to palpate for defects in the mucosa. Palpate the entire surface of the anal canal in this fashion by repeating the rotation at progressively deeper finger depths.
12. Advance the examining digit as far as is comfortably possible and palpate the anterior rectum to examine the posterior surface of the prostate (Fig. 19–3).

Note: Firm but gentle palpation should allow determination of the size, shape, consistency, mobility, and tenderness of the prostate.

Note: Palpation of the prostate may cause prostatic secretions to exit the urethra. If clinically indicated, these should be collected for laboratory analysis.

13. Slowly and carefully withdraw your finger.
14. Transfer residual stool on the examination glove to testing medium for occult blood if indicated.
15. Wipe the external anal area clean of lubricating jelly.
16. Provide the patient with toilet paper or tissue to clean the lubricating jelly from his anal area, redrape the patient, and give him privacy to clean up and get dressed.

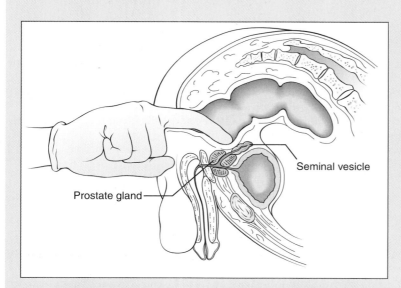

Prostate gland

Seminal vesicle

Figure 19–3. Redrawn from Seidel HM, Benedict GW, Ball JW, et al: Anus, Rectum, and Prostate. In Mosby's Guide to Physical Examination, 4*th* ed. St. Louis, CV Mosby, 1999, p 678.

Special Considerations

- Patients presenting with anatomy that deviates from normal because of past trauma, congenital defects, or past disease may be difficult to examine.
- Examination of young children requires patience and gentle technique.
- Rectal examinations and hernia examinations in children should be performed with the examiner's smallest digit.

Follow-Up Care and Instructions

- Inform the patient before and during the examination that self-examination of the scrotal sac is useful for the early detection of testicular cancer.
- Instruct the patient in the technique for self-examination during the examination in a way that the patient would be able to perform self-examination in the future. The patient should be encouraged to establish a self-examination routine on a monthly basis.
- It is uncommon for the examination of the male genitalia to cause adverse effects. However, after the examination, instruct the patient to report any rectal tenderness, rectal bleeding, back pain, scrotal masses or tenderness, dysuria, pyuria, hematuria, hematospermia, fever, penile discomfort, or penile lesions.

References

Dehn R: Prostatitis. In Moser RL (ed): Primary Care for Physician Assistants. New York, McGraw-Hill, 1998, pp 604–605.

Kelly P: Testicular cancer. In Moser RL (ed): Primary Care for Physician Assistants. New York, McGraw-Hill, 1998, pp 480–482.

Towler BP, Irwig L, Glasziou P, et al: Review: Fecal occult blood test screening reduces colorectal cancer mortality. APC J Club 130:13, 1999.

Woolf SH: Screening for prostatic cancer with prostate-specific antigen. N Engl J Med 333:1401–1405, 1995.

Bibliography

- Seidel HM, Benedict, GW, Ball JW, et al: Male genitalia and anus, rectum, and prostate. In Mosby's Guide to Physical Examination, 4th ed. St. Louis, CV Mosby, 1999, pp 644–688.
- Swartz MS: Male genitalia and hernias. In Textbook of Physical Diagnosis, 3rd ed. Philadelphia, WB Saunders, 1998, pp 390–417.

Chapter 20

Joint and Bursal Aspiration

▷ M.F. Winegardner

Procedure Goals and Objectives

Goal: The goal of this procedure is to aspirate a knee joint or olecranon bursa successfully while observing universal precautions and with the minimal degree of risk to the patient.

Objectives: The student will be able to . . .

► Describe the indications, contraindications, and rationale for performing knee joint or olecranon bursa aspiration.

► Identify and describe common complications associated with knee joint or olecranon bursa aspiration.

► Describe the essential anatomy and physiology associated with the performance of a knee joint or olecranon bursa aspiration.

► Identify the materials necessary for performing a knee joint or olecranon bursa aspiration and their proper use.

► Identify the important aspects of care after a knee joint or olecranon bursa aspiration.

Background and History

Joint aspiration offers both diagnostic and therapeutic benefits when managing joint effusion or inflammation. Diagnostically, the procedure permits acquisition of synovial fluid for analysis. Therapeutically, joint aspiration in the face of painful effusion relieves the patient's discomfort and may facilitate a more accurate joint examination. The same technique can be used for the administration of intra-articular medications. Aspiration of bursal distention relieves discomfort and restriction of motion and decreases the risk of chronic recurrence, spontaneous drainage, or infection within the stagnant bursal fluid (Snider, 1997).

Despite the benefits, joint aspiration is an invasive procedure with the potential for grave injury if not carried out under strict sterile conditions. The procedure always necessitates careful, sterile preparation and sterile technique.

Each joint has specific anatomic landmarks by which the joint space is outlined and the needle can be placed for aspiration. The general steps in a joint aspiration procedure are the same, regardless of the joint. For the purposes of this chapter, knee joint aspiration is described.

Both traumatic and rheumatic processes affect the knee joint, although relatively more aspirations are performed at the knee for traumatic effusion than at other joints, where inflammation and effusion are more likely to be rheumatic in nature. A significant volume of joint effusion can collect within the knee joint. When assembling equipment for a therapeutic knee tap, it is important to recognize that there may be a significant volume of fluid to be aspirated and to plan accordingly.

Indications

Joint aspiration is indicated for the following situations:

- When there is a painful effusion of a joint, a monoarticular inflammation of a joint, or suspicion of a systemic rheumatic disorder of uncertain cause. In the mature patient, trauma can result in painful joint effusion, which can be remedied easily by joint aspiration.
- In the case of articular inflammation of unknown cause, the synovial fluid analysis—including viscosity, crystal examination, cell count, bacterial culture, and Gram stain—may be the most accurate diagnostic tool (Weinstein and Buckwalter, 1994).

Bursal aspiration is indicated for the following situations:

- When painful bursal swelling persists despite conservative treatment or when questions arise about cause
- When olecranon bursitis occurs, necessitating aspiration

Like joint aspiration, strict sterile technique is indicated for bursal aspiration.

Contraindications

- Joint aspiration is contraindicated whenever circumstances exist by which entering the joint facilitates the seeding of bacteria into the joint. Introduction of a needle into the joint space through burns, infected skin, or infected subcutaneous tissue is contraindicated. Aspiration increases the risk of introducing bacteria into the joint when there is concern for overlying soft tissue cellulitis or impetigo, and joint aspiration should not be performed in this situation.
- Aspiration of a bursa is likewise contraindicated when risks for introducing bacteria outweigh the benefits of aspiration.
- Joint aspiration by the generalist is contraindicated after total joint arthroplasty except under the supervision of an orthopedic specialist. Should effusion or inflammation occur any time after joint replacement, the patient must be returned to the care of an orthopedist.
- In the rare circumstance in which aspiration of a hemarthrosis is undertaken in a hemophiliac patient, the hemarthrosis will reaccumulate if bleeding has not been controlled before the procedure. Similarly, aspiration is relatively contraindicated in the patient who has undergone anticoagulation and has a significantly prolonged bleeding time.

Potential Complications

Joint Aspiration

- The most common complications of joint aspiration include bleeding, infection, pain, intra-articular injury, and reaccumulation of fluid. When providing patients with adequate information for informed consent, these complications should be outlined.
- Inadvertent injury to vascular or neural structures near joint spaces can occur, as can a scoring injury of the intra-articular joint surface from the needle. Awareness of the proximity of nerves, arteries, or veins is necessary, as is caution when introducing a needle or infiltrating medications. As with any injection procedure, drawing back on the syringe plunger before administering medication is recommended to confirm that the needle is not within the lumen of a blood vessel.
- Careful history taking concerning topical and systemic allergic reactions, with specific focus on iodine and anesthetic drug sensitivities, further minimizes complications associated with the procedure. With any parenterally administered medication, there must be prompt access to epinephrine 1:1000 for subcutaneous administration, and resuscitation equipment must be available in the advent of a severe adverse reaction. Using a minimal volume of anesthetic is reasonable, and some authors recommend injecting no more than 5 mL of anesthetic solution within 30 minutes (Steinberg et al, 1999). When adequately anesthetizing the needle track for a joint aspiration, it is not difficult

to exceed 5 mL of administered anesthetic. By respecting the land-marks and anatomy unique to each joint, one can minimize complications associated with an aspiration procedure.

Bursal Aspiration

- The most common complications of bursal aspiration are infection, pain, chronic recurrence, chronic drainage via a sinus tract, and acute recurrent swelling. For bursal aspirations, keep in mind that some bursae communicate directly with the joint space.
- Baker's cysts, or popliteal bursae, are actually herniations of the joint capsule.
- Communication between the olecranon bursa and elbow joint may develop in rheumatoid arthritis. When aspirating the olecranon bursa, a lateral aspiration approach is recommended to prevent subsequent development of a chronic sinus tract that can result from introducing a needle directly into the tip of the elbow bursa (Steinberg et al, 1999). Despite the best technique, recurrence of olecranon bursitis with chronic painful inflammatory changes may necessitate definitive orthopedic resection of the bursa.

Review of Essential Anatomy and Pathophysiology for Joint Aspiration

Pathophysiology

The knee is representative of diarthrodial joints, with a synovial lining containing secretory cells and a fine capillary system from which synovial fluid is derived. Plasma transudation and mucin production within the joint combine to give synovial fluid its viscous, lubricating quality that reduces joint surface friction. Synovial fluid diffusion is an important factor in providing nutrition to the intra-articular structures (Weinstein and Buckwalter, 1994). Noninfectious effusions do not generally develop in fibrocartilaginous joints, such as the sacroiliac joint, because of the absence of synovial lining, but effusions do develop within bursae, which are cavities lined with secretory cells that function much like synovial cells (Weinstein and Buckwalter, 1994).

When trauma, inflammation, or infection occurs within the joint, the synovial fluid is characteristically altered, and sampling of the synovial fluid can be diagnostic. In the case of inflammatory reaction, the synovium produces increased synovial volume as a response to mechanical trauma or crystalline precipitants within the joint. Traumatically induced bleeding within the synovial fluid directly damages the synovial cartilage through the release of destructive proteolytic enzymes from blood cells.

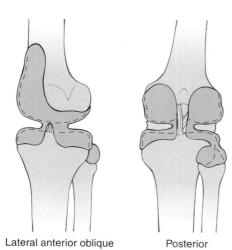

Figure 20–1. Synovial surfaces of knee joint.

Lateral anterior oblique   Posterior

Hemarthrosis management should include aspiration to eliminate biochemical injury to the joint in addition to decreasing discomfort from mechanical distention.

Aspiration of a bloody synovial effusion is best attempted within the first couple of days after swelling develops. The clotting process makes aspiration nearly impossible between 3 and 7 days after injury, but aspiration becomes possible again 7 days after injury because of the breakdown of intra-articular clot. However, some cartilaginous damage is likely to have occurred by the time there is liquefaction of the intra-articular clot.

The synovial surface can also be transformed by chronic inflammatory changes that lead to proliferative changes on the synovial surface (Steinberg et al, 1999). This tissue proliferation can make aspiration techniques difficult or ineffective when the proliferative tissues obstruct the intra-articular needle and prevent aspiration of the joint fluid. Proper placement of the needle can reduce the likelihood of obstruction by avoiding areas commonly affected by synovial proliferation (Fig. 20–1).

Anatomy and Pathomechanics

The knee joint is formed between the distal femur and proximal tibia, with the synovium covering the femur in a saddle configuration and reflecting anteriorly and superiorly on the femur behind the patella and draping inferiorly and posteriorly on the caudad surface of the femur, medially and inferiorly over the lateral surfaces of the cruciate ligaments, and down to the tibial articular surfaces. A small synovial draping also occurs over the proximal fibula. The pommel of the synovial saddle lies on the anterior distal femur behind the patella, reflecting at

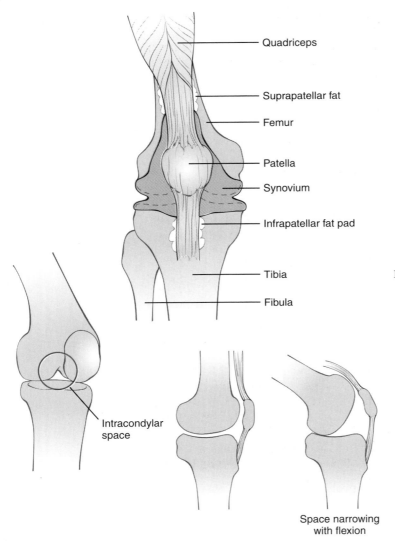

Figure 20–2. Anatomy of knee joint.

the upper margin anteriorly toward the patella. The space medially between the femoral condyles and behind the patella generally permits better synovial aspiration because the probability of encountering synovial
proliferation or abutting a bony surface is less, particularly when the
knee is extended (Fig. 20–2).

Patient Preparation for Joint Aspiration

• Informed consent is appropriate for any invasive procedure. Whether
using a formal written consent form or simply documenting the risks
and benefits discussed, patients should be apprised of the risks for

infection, bleeding, adverse reactions to anesthesia, joint surface injury, ongoing pain, and reaccumulation of fluid.

- For some patients whose effusion has stabilized the knee, the removal of the fluid may uncover previously unnoticed knee instability. It is helpful to prepare patients for this by discussing the possibility before tapping the joint.
- Let patients know that additional management after aspiration may include immobilization of the joint, antibiotic or anti-inflammatory therapy, hospitalization, or referral to a specialist, depending on the findings on aspiration.
- Inform the patient that the procedure will take about 5 to 10 minutes after a 10-minute scrub of the joint area to ensure asepsis.
- Patients must be reminded that once the preparation has begun, it is essential that the patient refrain from touching, pointing, or reaching over the area being prepared. Patients do well with this when told not to touch anywhere within the "covered area," when drapes are used, or where the "soap" was applied until the procedure is completed.
- Patients should be prepared for a brief episode of stinging discomfort when the lidocaine anesthetic is administered subcutaneously. The "bee-sting" sensation lasts less than 30 seconds for most patients.
- Considering overall safety for the patient as well as the position for optimal access of the effusion, it is preferable to have the patient in a supine position with the knee extended as much as the effusion permits. Knee flexion allows the patella to ride more closely to the femur, narrowing the retropatellar space. The widest patellofemoral space is afforded by placing the knee at the fullest extension allowable. Because the tension on the anterior cruciate ligament (ACL) is greatest when the knee is in full extension or deep flexion, the patient may prefer to maintain a 30- to 70-degree flexion to maintain laxity of the anterior cruciate ligament and allow for comfort. Likewise, effusive distention of the joint may prevent full extension.

Materials Utilized for Performing Joint and Bursal Aspiration

- Tray table
- Sterile drapes
- Sterile gloves
- Povidone-iodine solution (unless contraindicated by allergy)
- 1% lidocaine (unless contraindicated by allergy)
- Sterile 1-inch, 25-gauge needles; sterile $1^1/_2$-inch, 19-gauge needles
- Three sterile 20- or 30-mL syringes, sterile 5- or 10-mL syringe
- Sterile hemostat
- Green-top sodium heparin tube or other Vacutainer tubes as indicated (Table 20–1).

Table 20–1

Synovial Fluid Testing

Test	Collection Tube/Container	Amount of Fluid Needed	Special Considerations*
Crystals	Red- or green-top tube	0.5 mL	Caution with other tubes containing EDTA—may be mistaken for joint fluid crystals
RA latex	Red-top tube	0.5 mL minimum	
Total protein	Red-top tube	0.5 mL minimum	
Glucose	Red- or gray-top tube*	0.5 mL minimum	
Mucin clot	Red-top tube	0.5 mL minimum	
Cell count	Purple-top tube	1.0 mL minimum	
Routine culture	Sterile syringe*	0.5 mL minimum	Send to laboratory in syringe
Gram stain	Sterile syringe*	0.5 mL minimum	Send to laboratory in syringe
TB culture	Sterile syringe*	0.5 mL minimum	Send to laboratory in syringe
Fungal culture	Sterile syringe*	0.5 mL minimum	Send to laboratory in syringe

* Individual microbiology and chemistry laboratories may have specific criteria for tests; confirm the laboratory's preference for the tests you are running.

RA, rheumatoid arthritis; TB, tuberculosis; EDTA, ethylenediaminetetra-acetic acid.

Procedure for Joint Aspiration

1. Determine the position that will allow the patient to be most comfortable and the effusion to be most easily accessed.
2. Perform a 10-minute scrub of the knee with povidone-iodine solution. The preparation must encircle the knee and extend 2 to 3 inches above and below the knee.
3. Draping of the knee is not essential but will reduce the risk of infection. If performed, the draping should allow adequate visualization of the joint space for the ballottement of fluid and determination of landmarks.
4. Prepare a sterile field on which to assemble all needed sterile equipment including syringes, needles, hemostat, and sterile cup.
5. Once prepared, don sterile gloves, drape if desired, and define the superior pole of the patella. Identify the joint spaces lateral to the patella by ballottement of fluid beneath the patella (Fig. 20–3A–C).
6. Draw up 1% lidocaine in a 5- or 10-mL syringe.
7. Identify the landmarks to determine the location for needle placement.
Note: The needle may be introduced into the joint space either anteromedially or anterolaterally.

8. Draw a visual line along either lateral margin of the patella to intersect with the line of the superior patellar margin and, entering the skin at that point or slightly more laterally and superiorly, administer a small amount of

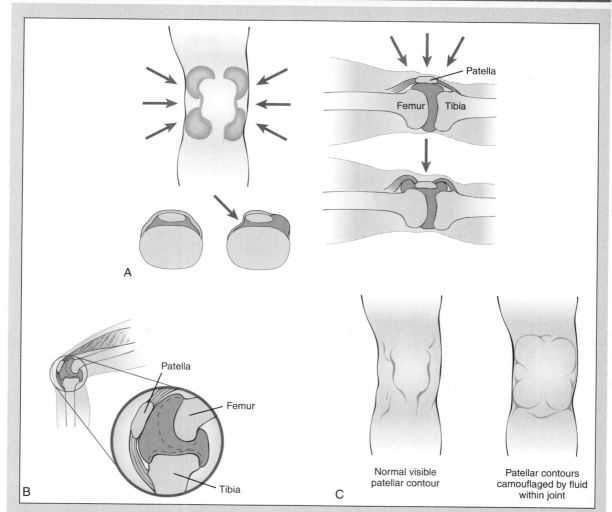

Figure 20-3

the anesthetic subcutaneously. Angle 45 degrees off the sagittal plane and 30 degrees off the frontal plane, directing the needle caudally.

9. Advance the needle as deep as anesthesia is desired, aspirating for blood.

Note: When advancing to the joint capsule, resistance is encountered at the level of the joint capsule.

10. While withdrawing the needle, administer the anesthetic along the track from the joint capsule out to the skin (Fig. 20–4).

11. Remove the smaller gauge needle and syringe and assemble the 18-gauge needle on a 20- or 30-mL syringe. Hold the needle-syringe like a pencil and align to advance medially

Procedure for Joint Aspiration – *(continued)*

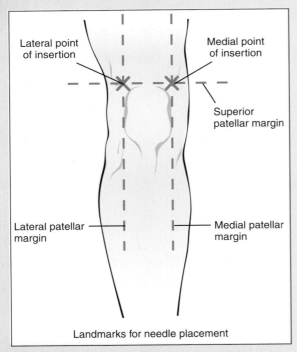

Lateral point
of insertion

Medial point
of insertion

Superior
patellar margin

Lateral patellar
margin

Medial patellar
margin

Landmarks for needle placement

Figure 20–4

and caudally into the joint space behind the patella.

12. Introduce the 18-gauge needle into the anesthetized track angled 45 degrees laterally and directed 30 degrees caudally. Place gentle pressure on the syringe plunger while advancing and aspirate the synovial fluid on entering the joint space as the needle is directed medially and downward behind the patella (Fig. 20–5).

Note: Entering the joint space is painful briefly for the patient.

13. When the syringe is full, place the hemostat on the needle hub, remove the syringe, and replace it with an empty syringe or discharge the synovial fluid into a sterile cup. Repeat this step until the knee joint is no longer visibly distended or fluid can no longer be aspirated.

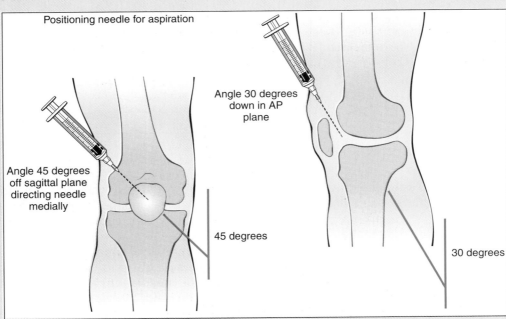

Positioning needle for aspiration

Angle 45 degrees
off sagittal plane
directing needle
medially

45 degrees

Angle 30 degrees
down in AP
plane

30 degrees

Figure 20–5

Procedure for Joint Aspiration – *(continued)*

Note: Pressure applied above the knee joint can "milk" additional fluid centrally for aspiration. Caution must be exercised not to compromise sterile conditions.

14. Intra-articular medication can be administered after the aspiration if indicated.
15. Withdraw the needle from the joint space and apply direct pressure with sterile dressing over the puncture site for several minutes.
16. Confirm that the wound site is dry and active bleeding has stopped and then dress with sterile adhesive dressing.
17. Maintaining sterile conditions, observe the synovial fluid for evidence of a cloudy appearance and obtain Gram stain, cell counts, and cultures if there is suspicion of infection.

Note: Gram stain and cultures are usually collected in sterile syringes and transported promptly to the laboratory. Rapid transport and inoculation on special medium are essential for growth of fastidious bacteria such as *Neisseria gonorrhoeae*. Specimens sent for crystal analysis should not be drawn into an ethylenediaminetetra-acetic acid (EDTA) tube because the EDTA crystals can be confused with intra-articular crystals. See Table 20–1 for guidelines on acquiring samples for the laboratory.

Follow-Up Care and Instructions for Joint Aspiration

- Advise patients to avoid use of the joint for at least 1 day. If traumatic injury preceded the effusion, longer immobilization or avoidance of weight bearing may be indicated. When aspiration eliminates internal splinting, the instability of the joint may become apparent and should be managed as would otherwise be indicated.
- Instruct the patient to call the office in the event of sudden reaccumulation of fluid, increased heat at the joint, fever, chills, or a severe increase in pain, which would necessitate the patient's prompt return for further evaluation (Snider, 1997).
- Evidence or strong suspicion of infection at the time of tapping necessitates an immediate referral to an orthopedist.

Review of Essential Anatomy and Physiology for Bursal Aspiration

Numerous bursae are found around the joints, many of which may accumulate excessive fluid as part of an inflammatory process. The olecranon bursa is one that can become visibly distended because of inflammation. This easily accessible bursa may swell slowly over time or accumulate suddenly from trauma or infection. Because of the relatively

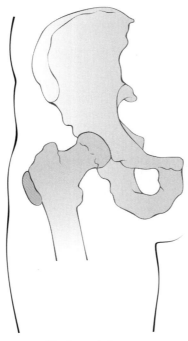

Figure 20–6. Trochanteric bursae are difficult to isolate because of overlying structures.

Trochanteric bursa

exposed and superficial anatomy of the bursa, external mechanical irritation plays a significant role in the initiation and perpetuation of olecranon bursitis. Other differential considerations include ulnar fracture, gout, acute rheumatoid arthritis, or a synovial cyst of the elbow joint (Snider, 1997).

Intrabursal scar tissue, which feels like small nodules within the bursa, can develop rather early as a sequela to olecranon bursitis. These "nodules" may result in chronic pain and tenderness when the elbow is mechanically aggravated.

The general approach to aspirating an olecranon bursitis can be applied to other bursae. Few others have such easily accessible anatomy. Some, such as the trochanteric bursae, are difficult to isolate anatomically because of overlying structures (Fig. 20–6). Others, such as the prepatellar bursae, are nearly as accessible as the olecranon bursae (Fig. 20–7).

Patient Preparation for Bursal Aspiration

- Apprise the patient of the risks of infection, bleeding, adverse reactions to anesthesia, ongoing pain, and reaccumulation of fluid.
- Let the patient know that additional management after aspiration includes resting and protecting the elbow, antibiotic or anti-inflammatory

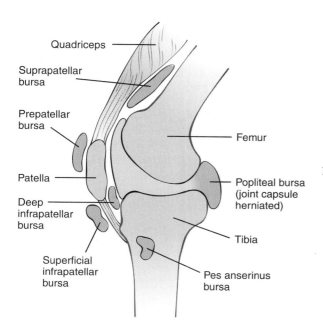

Figure 20–7. Knee bursae.

therapy if indicated, or hospitalization or referral to a specialist, depending on the findings.

- Inform the patient that the procedure will take about 5 to 10 minutes after a 10-minute scrub of the joint area to ensure asepsis. Patients must be reminded that once the preparation has begun, it is essential that the patient refrain from touching, pointing, or reaching over the area being prepared.
- Warn the patient to be prepared for a brief episode of stinging discomfort when the lidocaine is administered subcutaneously. The "bee-sting" sensation will last less than 30 seconds for most patients.

Procedure for Performing Bursal Aspiration

1. Have the patient sit well supported or lying down prone for the procedure. If sitting, the arm must be supported on a Mayo stand flexed at the elbow to 90 degrees. If lying down prone, have the patient rest the arm on the examination table with elbow flexed and shoulder comfortably abducted to allow access to the lateral olecranon bursa.

2. Prepare a sterile field on which to assemble all needed sterile equipment, including syringes, needles, hemostat, and sterile cup.

3. Perform a 10-minute scrub with povidone-iodine solution. Cover the entire olecranon process as well as the lateral elbow surface. Patient may sit well supported or lie down prone for the

Procedure for Performing Bursal Aspiration – *(continued)*

procedure. If sitting, the arm should be supported on a Mayo stand and flexed at the elbow to 90 degrees. If lying prone, the arm should rest on the examination table, with the elbow flexed and the shoulder comfortably abducted to allow access to the lateral olecranon bursa.

4. Once the patient is prepared, don sterile gloves and drape the area so that the bursa is easily accessible but sterility is maintained.

5. Draw up 1 mL of 1% lidocaine in a syringe. Identify the landmarks to determine the location for needle placement.

Note: The olecranon bursa is usually readily visible and distended beyond the typical elbow contour. Anesthesia to the skin and subcutaneous tissues may be administered as desired using a 25- to 27-gauge needle.

6. Administer the anesthetic under the skin of the elbow, centering the needle over the lateral surface of the distended bursa (Fig. 20–8).

7. With the elbow flexed to 90 degrees and resting comfortably, switch to an 18-gauge needle and syringe. Enter into the distended olecranon bursa at 90 degrees to the plane of the arm. Aspirate the fluid slowly until the bursal sac is flat.

8. Apply direct pressure over the puncture site. Dress with an adhesive bandage and wrap the elbow with an

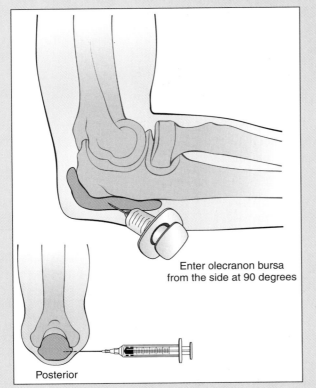

Enter olecranon bursa from the side at 90 degrees

Posterior

Figure 20–8

Procedure for Performing Bursal Aspiration – *(continued)*

elastic compression bandage to retard the reaccumulation of fluid.

9. Observe the synovial fluid for evidence of a cloudy appearance and obtain a Gram stain, cell counts, and cultures if there is suspicion of infection. Tests for crystals or other rheumatoid parameters should proceed as was described in the joint aspiration section (see Table 20-1).

Follow-Up Care and Instructions for Bursal Aspiration

- Advise the patient to avoid general use of the joint for at least 2 days. Recurrence of bursal effusion is more likely with persistent mechanical irritation of the bursa. Avoiding resting the elbow on tables, automobile arm rests, and chair arms decreases irritation. For some patients, these activities are so habitual that the elbow is inevitably chronically irritated and an elbow protector may be indicated. Another option is the placement of a posterior plaster splint after aspiration to limit elbow motion for the first week after the procedure. For those who go on to develop chronic bursitis, surgical excision may become necessary.

- Instruct the patient to call the office in the event of the development of a warm elbow, fever, chills, or severe increase in pain, which would necessitate prompt return for further evaluation (Snider, 1997). Recurrence of olecranon bursitis more than three times probably indicates a need for surgical bursal excision, as does the development of a draining sinus tract.

References

Snider R (ed): Essentials of Musculoskeletal Care. Rosemont, Ill, American Academy of Orthopaedic Surgeons, 1997.

Steinberg G, Akins C, Baran D (eds): Orthopaedics in Primary Care, 3rd ed. Philadelphia, Lippincott Williams & Wilkins, 1999.

Weinstein SL, Buckwalter JA (eds): Turek's Orthopaedics: Principles and their Application, 5th ed. Philadelphia, JB Lippincott, 1994.

Bibliography

- Cailliet R: Knee Pain and Disability, 3rd ed. Philadelphia, FA Davis, 1992.
- Hertling D, Kessler R: Management of Common Musculoskeletal Disorders: Physical Therapy Principles and Methods, 3rd ed. Philadelphia, JB Lippincott, 1996.

- Hertling D, Kessler R: The knee. In: Hertling D, Kessler R (eds): Management of Common Musculoskeletal Disorders: Physical Therapy Principles and Methods, 3rd ed. Philadelphia, JB Lippincott, 1996.
- Kessler RM, Hertling D: Arthrology. In: Hertling D, Kessler R (eds): Management of Common Musculoskeletal Disorders: Physical Therapy Principles and Methods, 3rd ed. Philadelphia, JB Lippincott, 1996.
- Merrill K, Knetsche R, Friedman R: Sports medicine. In: Skinner H (ed): Current Diagnosis and Treatment in Orthopedics. Norwalk, Conn, Appleton & Lange, 1995.

Chapter 21

Casting and Splinting

▷ Donald Frosch
▷ Patrick Knott

Procedure Goals and Objectives

Goal: To apply casts and splints to extremities successfully with the minimal degree of risk to the patient.

Objectives: The student will be able to . . .

▶ Describe the indications, contraindications, and rationale for casting and splinting extremities.

▶ Identify and describe common complications associated with casting and splinting extremities.

▶ Describe the essential anatomy and physiology associated with casting and splinting extremities.

▶ Identify the materials necessary for performing casting and splinting of extremities and their proper use.

▶ Identify the important aspects of care after a casting and splinting application.

Background and History

Immobilization of the extremities in casts and splints is a practice that dates back to nearly 3000 BC when tree bark was used to splint injured forearms. In the 1920s, plaster of Paris was commercially introduced to medicine as a powder that was impregnated into rolls of cloth. Since the 1970s, synthetic materials like fiberglass and plastic have been used to make casts and splints, but throughout time, the principles of immobilization have remained remarkably constant.

There are many different types of casts and splints used by orthopedic specialists to treat an even greater number of specific fractures and soft tissue injuries. Describing each of these special types of immobilization is beyond the scope of this chapter, and the use of many of these specialized types of casts and splints may be inappropriate in the primary care setting. What follows is an explanation of the basic principles of casting and splinting, and their use in the treatment of several straightforward primary care problems.

Two types of casts—the short arm (Fig. 21–1) and the short leg (Fig. 21–2)—are explained in this chapter. The short arm cast is often used for hand, distal radius, and distal forearm fractures. The short leg cast is most often used for ankle fractures or severe ankle sprains. These types of casts are made from rigid materials and are placed completely around the circumference of the arm or leg. Splints, in contrast, use rigid material around only part of the circumference of an extremity. The splints discussed in this chapter are the short arm ulnar "gutter" splint, which is used for fractures of the fifth metacarpal joint ("boxer fracture); posterior mold, which is often used to immobilize ankle sprains and fractures initially (Fig. 21–3); and the sugar-tong splint, which is an alternative to the posterior mold when splinting the lower leg (Figs. 21–4 and 21–5). These splints give less mechanical support and protection than a full

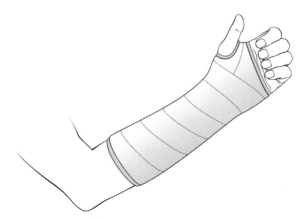

Figure 21–1. Short arm cast.

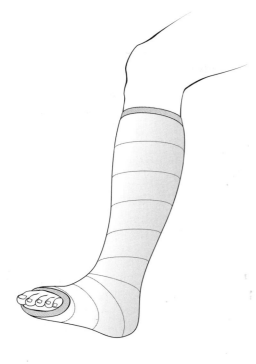

Figure 21-2. Short leg cast.

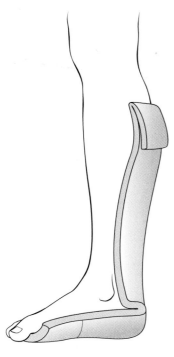

Figure 21-3. Posterior mold splint.

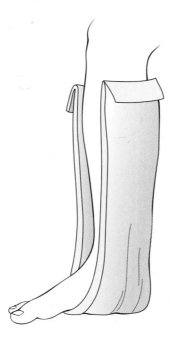

Figure 21–4. Sugar-tong splint for the lower leg.

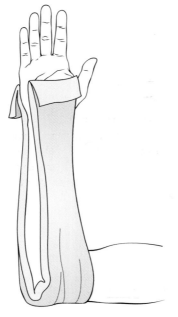

Figure 21–5. Sugar-tong splint for the lower arm.

cast but allow for swelling of the soft tissues in the acute phase of an injury.

There are two primary materials used to make casts and splints today: plaster and fiberglass. Several other synthetic materials are gaining in popularity, but in the primary care setting plaster and fiberglass continue to be the mainstay of treatment. Each material has inherent benefits and drawbacks that make it the best choice in different situations.

Plaster is easy to mold, giving it an advantage when a snug-fitting cast or a cast with many bumps and curves is needed. The chubby, cone-shaped arms and legs of toddlers are perfect examples of places where a well-molded plaster cast is far superior to fiberglass. The drawback of plaster is that it is much heavier than fiberglass and not as durable. It is also messy to apply and gives off quite a bit of heat as it cures, making it uncomfortable for the acutely injured patient. Plaster is considered a greater risk in the patient who cannot indicate whether the temperature is getting too hot.

Fiberglass is popular because of its light weight, ease of application, and excellent durability. It is also water-resistant (although the padding underneath must still be kept dry) and cures rapidly. For all these reasons, it is clearly the material of choice for a walking cast. Fiberglass is several times more expensive than plaster, but if it lasts longer and requires fewer repairs and replacements during the period of immobilization, its higher initial cost is justified.

Indications

Casts and splints are used in the primary care setting to:

- Treat simple, acute, nondisplaced fractures
- Immobilize a dislocation after it has been reduced
- Treat soft tissue injuries, such as ligament sprains and muscle strains

Immobilization is necessary for comfort and healing after a bone fracture and also is beneficial in the short term after soft tissue injury. Long periods of immobilization cause disuse atrophy and stiffness in the affected limb, so the benefits of immobilization must be weighed against these predictable side effects. The length of immobilization is usually adjusted accordingly.

Contraindications

Cast immobilization (circumferential) should be avoided in the following areas:

* • Acute injury where immediate swelling is expected
* • Skin or soft tissue infections
* • Open wounds, where infection may occur

In these situations, a noncircumferential splint is much safer than a cast, because it allows the extremity to expand with swelling and provides access to the skin so that it can be checked for wound healing and signs of infection.

Potential Complications

A circumferential cast on an injured extremity can be a potentially dangerous form of treatment, and the primary care provider must be vigilant to signs of potential complications.

Compartment Syndrome

The most serious complication after the application of a cast is the development of a compartment syndrome. This build-up of pressure within the soft tissues can impede or cut off blood supply to the extremity, causing permanent damage to muscles and nerves. Volkmann's ischemic contracture is the classic example of this type of complication; it results in muscle necrosis and loss of use of the affected arm and hand.

A compartment syndrome typically follows an injury to a large bone or an area where there is a closed compartment formed by fascial layers (e.g., the forearm or lower leg). It is also more likely after a crush injury or arterial laceration, but it is important to remember that a compartment syndrome can occur without any of these predisposing factors.

Symptoms

The most predictive symptom of a compartment syndrome is pain that is increasing with time and is out of proportion to the severity of the injury. The pain is much worse with passive motion of the distal extremity and usually prevents active motion altogether. Additional, but less reliable, signs and symptoms include paresthesias in the limb, decreased two-point discrimination, decreased capillary refill, pallor, and finally pulselessness. Because soft tissue levels of just 30 to 60 mm Hg can cause irreversible damage, counting on decreased capillary refill or changes in the arterial pulse as signs of compartment syndrome is ill advised.

Normal is 0 mmHg

Treatment

Treatment for a suspected compartment syndrome requires immediate loosening of the cast. This is accomplished by splitting the cast down both sides (called *bivalving*) and separating the two halves right down to the patient's skin. Leaving the underlying padding or stockinette layers intact may cause inadequate relief of pressure. If symptoms do not resolve within a few minutes, the compartment pressures should be measured, and surgical decompression should be undertaken if necessary.

Measurement of compartment pressure was originally performed using the Whiteside technique, using a mercury manometer, intravenous tubing, a Luer-Lok syringe, a needle, and a four-way stopcock. Today this technique is seldom used because electronic hand-held devices that accomplish the same task have become readily available.

Other Complications

* Dermatitis: Cast dermatitis occurs because of the lack of air circulation inside the cast. Residual moisture from cast application and a resulting pruritus can cause patients to try to relieve their symptoms by mechanical scratching. If they insert coat hangers, pencils, or other long objects to scratch inside their cast, the objects can cause small abrasions on the skin that can become secondarily infected.
* Pressure sores: These can be caused by increased cast pressure under finger indentations left during cast application. Inadequate padding over bony prominences can also put undue pressure on the skin and cause a pressure ulceration. If not detected early, they may require surgical débridement and skin grafting.
* Nerve injuries: Pressure over superficial nerves, especially the ulnar nerve at the elbow and the peroneal nerve at the fibular head, can cause a temporary nerve palsy or even a permanent paralysis if left untreated.
* Deep venous thrombosis: In addition to lack of ambulation, long periods of immobilization of the lower extremities can lead to formation of deep venous thrombi or pulmonary emboli.

Review of Essential Anatomy and Physiology

A rule of thumb when casting an injured extremity is that the immobilization should include the joint above and the joint below that injury. This rule is frequently broken if the length of the limb above the injury is adequate to allow the cast to gain good fixation. For example, in a fracture of the wrist, the cast may stop below the elbow if the length of cast along the forearm is felt to allow for adequate immobilization of the wrist joint. It should be remembered, however, that [a short arm cast will never completely immobilize the wrist joint, because it does not prevent pronation and supination.] When uncertain about the length of cast required, an orthopedic specialist should be consulted.

Standard Precautions ▷ Practitioners should use Standard Precautions at all times when interacting with patients. Determining the level of precaution necessary requires the practitioner to exercise clinical judgment based on the patient's history and the potential for exposure to body fluids or aerosol-borne pathogens (for further discussion see Chapter 2).

Patient Preparation

1 • Inform the patient about the procedure and answer any questions.
2 • Place the extremity in a position of function. For the short arm cast, the elbow should be flexed to 90 degrees and the forearm should be in neutral pronation-supination, with the wrist in slight extension and the fingers slightly curled. Note that the metacarpophalangeal (MCP) joints of the hand must be able to be flexed to 90 degrees after cast application. Improper immobilization of the MCP joints in extension will cause stiffness in the hand. For the short leg cast, the ankle should be maintained in neutral dorsiflexion at 90 degrees.
3 • It is difficult to keep the patient in proper position during casting, especially when it comes to the ankle, and it may be useful to have an assistant hold the fingers or toes to maintain proper positioning.
4 • When applying a short leg cast, having the patient lie prone with the knee flexed makes application much easier. An ankle that is allowed to drift into plantarflexion during cast application will result in a cast that is plantarflexed and impossible to walk on.

Materials Utilized for Applying a Short Arm or Short Leg Cast

■ Stockinette
   Note: This is a stretchable material that comes on a roll and is cut to the desired length. It is available in 2-, 2½-, 3-, 4-, 5-, and 6-inch widths so that the most appropriate size can be selected, based on the limb involved, the size of the patient, and the degree of swelling of the limb. It serves several pur-

poses. First, it acts as a barrier between the skin and the sometimes itchy cast padding. Second, after the first layer of fiberglass is placed, the stockinette can be pulled down over the cast, thereby pulling cast padding over the rough edge of the fiberglass cast.

■ Cast padding

Note: This comes in 2-, 3-, 4-, and 5-inch widths. Two- or 3-inch padding is usually used on the arms. Three- or 4-inch padding is usually used on the lower leg. Four- or 5-inch padding is usually used on the upper leg. Two types of padding are available: cotton and synthetic. Cotton was the type of cast padding originally used when plaster was the only type of casting material available. When fiberglass casting materials became available, synthetic cast padding was developed. An advantage of synthetic padding is that it absorbs less water than does cotton if it gets wet. Most individuals now use cotton padding with plaster and synthetic padding with fiberglass.

■ Cast Material

Note: This comes in 2-, 3-, 4-, and 6-inch widths. Narrow widths are used more distally, around hands and feet, whereas wider widths are used on longer cylinders. Fiberglass should be kept in the airtight package until it is ready to be applied, because the moisture in the air will initiate the curing process.

■ Large basin or bucket

Note: This is used to immerse the casting material fully under water.

■ Apron and gloves

Note: These are used to protect the clinician from the resin in the casting material and to avoid permanent staining of clothes and hands.

■ Rigid scissors

Note: These are used to cut the padding and casting materials.

■ Cast saw and additional blades

Note: These are used to remove the cast if necessary or to reshape portions of the cast after it becomes set, or both.

General Procedures for Applying the Cast

1. Apply the appropriate size of stockinette (Fig. 21–6).
2. Cut the stockinette so that 3 to 4 extra inches remain on either end. Smooth out so that no wrinkles are in contact with the skin.
3. Apply cast padding. Roll the padding on smoothly, overlapping each time by

General Procedures for Applying the Cast — *(continued)*

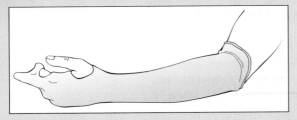

Figure 21-6

about 50%. Take the padding out to 1 to 2 inches beyond the edges of where the cast material will be.
4. Pad well at the top and bottom borders of the cast so that when the stockinette is pulled back, it brings the padding with it, thereby covering the rough edge of the cast.
5. Pad well over bony prominences and in areas of potential cast friction (Fig. 21-7.

Plaster

1. Dip in cool water until "sloppy wet" so that the water can help disperse the heat from the exothermic curing process.
2. It is important to apply the first rolls of material smoothly so that no wrinkles are against the skin.
3. The rolls should overlap about 50% each time around and should traverse the entire length of the planned cast.
4. Avoid bunching or wrinkling the plaster by occasionally folding over and tucking the plaster roll.
5. Mold each layer by gently rubbing the cast with the palms of the hands.

Fiberglass

1. Immerse the fiberglass tape in a bucket of water, wait about 10 seconds, and squeeze once gently to remove the bulk of the water, and then start rolling on.
2. It is important to apply the first rolls of material smoothly so that no wrinkles are against the skin.
3. Overlap each turn of fiberglass tape by about 50% and traverse the entire length of the planned cast.
4. Avoid bunching or wrinkling while rolling by making occasional cuts in the fiberglass roll.

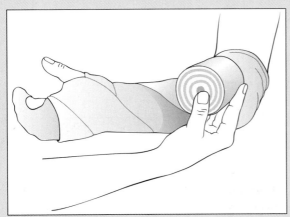

Figure 21-7

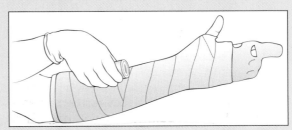

Figure 21-8

General Procedures for Applying the Cast — *(continued)*

5. Start and finish fiberglass about 1 inch from the borders of the padding so that there will be enough padding to roll over the edge of the cast (Fig. 21–8).

6. Pull down the stockinette–cast padding over the cast edges and put on the final layer of fiberglass.

Materials Utilized for Applying a Short Arm Cast

■ Two- to 3-inch stockinette
■ Roll of 3-inch cast padding
■ Two rolls of 3-inch fiberglass casting tape

Procedure for Applying a Short Arm Cast

Note: The cast should extend from about two fingerbreadths distal to the olecranon fossa to just proximal to the MCP joints of all fingers. If properly applied, it should allow for full flexion at the elbow and full range of motion of all the MCP joints, including the thumb. Remember to cut an extra (distal) hole in the stockinette for the thumb when the stockinette is pulled down before the final layer of fiberglass. The patient should be able to perform a thumb-index pinch. The arm and hand are usually cast in the position of function, with the thumb pointing upward, the hand cupped as if it were holding a can of soda, and the wrist in slight extension.

1. Start applying the fiberglass tape at the elbow and work your way down to the hand. After each roll of fiberglass is applied, mold the cast to the extremity using the palms, not the fingertips (Fig. 21–9).

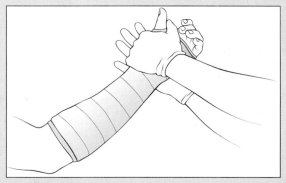

Figure 21–9

2. When rolling through the palm area, pinch or twist the tape to make a narrow pass so that thumb or finger movement is not compromised (Figs. 21–10 and 21–11).

Note: Figure 21–12 illustrates the key features of a properly applied short arm cast.

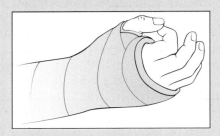

Figure 21–10

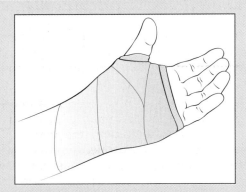

Figure 21–11

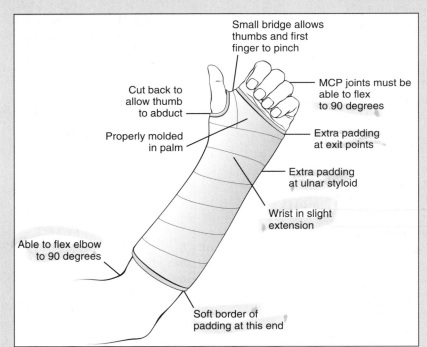

Small bridge allows thumbs and first finger to pinch

Cut back to allow thumb to abduct

MCP joints must be able to flex to 90 degrees

Properly molded in palm

Extra padding at exit points

Extra padding at ulnar styloid

Wrist in slight extension

Able to flex elbow to 90 degrees

Soft border of padding at this end

Figure 21–12

Materials Utilized for Applying a Short Leg Cast

- Three- to 4-inch stockinette
- Three rolls of 4-inch padding
- Three rolls of 4-inch fiberglass tape

Procedure for Applying a Short Leg Cast

Note: If properly applied, the cast should allow full flexion at the knee and full range of motion of all the metatarsophalangeal (MTP) joints, including the little toe.

1. Cast the leg with the ankle in a neutral position (at 90 degrees), with the help of an assistant holding the toes or by laying the patient prone.

Note: The 90-degree angle must be maintained during casting to prevent the cast from hardening with the foot in plantarflexion, making it difficult for the patient to walk and allowing for hamstring and Achilles tendon stiffening. Casting the leg with the knee bent helps avoid the mistake of casting too high into the knee area and restricting knee flexion.

Note: Apply heavy padding at the proximal end of the cast (at the tibial tubercle), over the metatarsal pad area, over the head of the fifth metatarsal, and especially over the heel.

2. To apply heavy padding to the heel, tear strips and lay them over the heel.

Caution: Do not pad the heel by wrapping circumferentially because it will bulk up at the dorsal ankle area.

3. Be sure to pad all the way to the tips of the toes so that the padding can be folded back later to protect the metatarsal areas.

4. Extend the cast from the tibial tubercle to just proximal to the MTP joints of all the toes.

5. If the cast is to be used for walking, one can apply extra layers of reinforcement to the bottom surface and the heel area for increased strength and durability.

6. Apply a cast boot over the finished cast, but do not allow the patient to stand on the cast for 1 to 2 hours for fiberglass or 4 to 6 hours for plaster, until the material completely cures.

Note: Weight bearing before this time can cause cracking and denting of the cast. Figure 21–13 illustrates the essential features of a properly applied short leg cast.

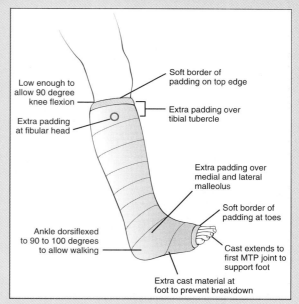

Low enough to allow 90 degree knee flexion

Extra padding at fibular head

Soft border of padding on top edge

Extra padding over tibial tubercle

Extra padding over medial and lateral malleolus

Soft border of padding at toes

Ankle dorsiflexed to 90 to 100 degrees to allow walking

Cast extends to first MTP joint to support foot

Extra cast material at foot to prevent breakdown

Figure 21–13

Materials Utilized for Applying a Short Arm Ulnar "Gutter" Splint

- One-Step cast material by 3M
- Bucket of cool water
- Dry towel
- Ace wrap

Procedure for Applying a Short Arm Ulnar "Gutter" Splint

Note: Gutter splints can be constructed from strips of fiberglass between an upper and lower row of cast padding (without stockinette), or a ready-made splint material can be used.

Note: The splint extends from the tip of the little finger to just below the elbow and like a U-shaped gutter. It runs along the ulnar border of the hand and forearm. The arm is splinted with the forearm in the neutral position (thumb pointing up) and the hand cupped as if it were holding a can of soda.

1. Immerse the splint material in a bucket of cool water.

Note: The ready-made splint material consists of an outer paper shell overlying fiberglass strips containing foam padding on one side. Use the 3 inch × 12 inch material for short arm-hand ulnar gutter splints and for short arm splinting (i.e., midforearm to mid–upper arm).

2. Roll it up tightly or roll it like a jelly roll in a dry towel to ring it out.
3. With the help of an assistant, position it on the patient's arm and wrap it with an elastic wrap.

Caution: **You must remember to place the foam-padded side of the splint against the patient's arm.**

Note: No stockinette is used for splints such as this because of the risk of constriction from acute swelling.

Note: Be sure to free the thumb, index, and middle fingers, excluding them from the final wrapping in order to permit their mobility.

4. Gently mold it around the ulnar aspect of the arm and hand.
5. After it hardens sufficiently, remove the wrap and neatly rewrap it.

Materials Utilized for Applying a Lower Leg Posterior Mold

■ Two or three rolls of 4-inch cast padding
■ 6 inch × 30 inch ready made splint material

Procedure for Applying a Lower Leg Posterior Mold

Note: This type of splint is often used to immobilize ankle sprains and fractures initially. Again, no stockinette is used.

1. Apply generous amounts of padding over the bony prominences, especially at the medial and lateral malleolar and calcaneal areas.

2. To prevent water pooling at the heel of the splint, which risks subsequent skin breakdown, remove as much water from the splint as possible before applying. This is accomplished by placing the splint material on a towel before applying it to the patient's leg.

3. Wrap the splint material in an elastic wrap, starting just below the knee and working to the foot. If the splint ends up being too long, simply fold it back on itself, away from the body, at the foot end. To prevent pressure sores, be sure that the folds in the splint at the ankle area are directed outward and are not pointing in toward the skin.

Note: The "sugar-tong" splint is an alternative to the posterior mold when splinting the lower leg. A longer and narrower piece of splint material (i.e., 3 inch x 45 inch) is placed along the medial side, under the heel, and along the lateral side of the lower leg. The sugar-tong splint gives great mediolateral support to the ankle and can also be used to immobilize fractures of the humerus or forearm.

Follow-Up Care and Instructions

Evaluation after Casting

- Carefully check the final cast before sending the patient out of the casting room.
- Check to make sure that the cast extends to the proper boundaries, yet does not interfere with the range of motion of necessary joints.
- Check for finger indentations and sharp edges. Trim back the cast and repad, or recast if necessary.
- Remember to ask the patient how the cast feels, and allow a few minutes so that he or she can tell whether there are areas of increased pressure or sharp edges that are abrading the skin. If not given an adequate evaluation, many unhappy patients will return hours later for cast modification.

Cast Aftercare

- A sling can be useful to help elevate and cradle the short arm cast. However, patients should be instructed to remove the sling three to four times each day and to perform range-of-motion exercises for the shoulder and elbow to avoid excessive stiffness and loss of function.
- A cast shoe is usually applied to protect the short leg cast. Most lower extremity casts are non–weight bearing initially, until healing progresses over the first few days or weeks.
- Advise patients that when showering, they must wrap a towel around the top of the cast, followed by a plastic bag, tightly secured with tape. If a cast is damaged, it can be reinforced with additional fiberglass, or it may need to be removed and redone.

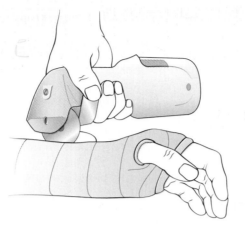

Figure 21–14. Oscillating cast saw.

Cast Removal

- Oscillating cast saws are designed to cut rigid cast material, but not the padding, stockinette, or the underlying skin (Fig. 21–14). Inform the patient of this and demonstrate on your hand.
- Avoid using the saw over a bony prominence because this is where skin injuries occur most often. A long strip of rigid plastic (marketed by the name *Zip Strip)* is sometimes used to slip inside the cast and form a barrier between the saw blade and the patient's skin. This is especially useful in removing a cast from anxious patients, both adults and children.
- Care should be taken not to drag or pull along the cast because this may result in abrasions to the underlying tissues.
- Exercise care not to let the cast become excessively warm while sawing.
- The cast should be cut down both sides. The cut can be widened and separated with a cast spreader. The two shells can be peeled away, and the underlying stockinette can be cut with a bandage scissors.

Bibliography

- Rockwood CA, Wilkins KE, Beaty JH (eds): Rockwood and Greene's Fractures in Adults. Philadelphia, Lippincott Williams & Wilkins, 2001.
- Mercier LR: Practical Orthopedics, 3rd ed. St. Louis, CV Mosby 1991.

Chapter 22

Local Anesthesia

▷ Michelle DiBaise

Procedure Goals and Objectives

Goal: To perform local anesthesia successfully while observing standard precautions and with the minimal degree of risk to the patient.

Objectives: The student will be able to . . .

▶ Describe the indications, contraindications, and rationale for administering local anesthesia.

▶ Identify and describe common complications associated with administering local anesthesia.

▶ Describe the essential anatomy and physiology associated with administering local anesthesia.

▶ Identify the materials necessary for the administration of local anesthesia and their proper use.

▶ Identify the important aspects of care after administration of local anesthesia.

Background and History

Local anesthesia provides reversible blockade of nerves, leading to loss of sensation of pain. Topical application and direct infiltration will anesthetize the immediate area. Regional blocks are designed to anesthetize larger areas via a nerve or field block. Local anesthesia is used for a variety of reasons, including but not limited to elimination of pain so that the following can be carried out: repair of lacerations, skin surgery, treatment of painful oral or genital lesions, and the removal of superficial lesions by chemical or physical means.

Nearly painless anesthesia may be achieved in wound repair or skin surgery when the location, surface area involved, and estimated length of time for the procedure is considered. A patient's emotional response is also critical in ensuring nearly painless anesthesia, as most patients fear that the injection will be painful. Throughout this chapter, a combination of certain anesthetics and procedural techniques are discussed that can help lessen the patient's pain and anxiety.

Review of Essential Anatomy and Physiology

Local anesthetics act to block the conduction of nerve impulses by selectively binding to voltage-dependent sodium channels. The vast majority of local anesthetics may be divided into two main categories: esters and amides. Local anesthetics contain a hydrophobic and a hydrophilic end joined together by an ester or amide linkage (Strichartz 1998; Page et al, 1997). The hydrophilic portion allows the anesthetic to be water-soluble so that it can be injected in solution and diffuse to the nerves requiring blockade. The hydrophobic portion allows the anesthetic to be lipid-soluble and enter the neuronal membrane. It is the hydrophilic end that subsequently binds to the voltage-dependent sodium channel. The ester anesthetics include benzocaine (e.g., Anbesol), cocaine, procaine (Novocain), and tetracaine (Cetacaine, Pontocaine). The amide anesthetics include lidocaine (e.g., ELA-Max, Xylocaine), mepivacaine (Carbocaine), bupivacaine (Marcaine), dibucaine (Nupercaine), and prilocaine (EMLA, Citanest) (Table 22–1).

When proper concentrations of anesthetic are used, the conduction of action potentials is blocked. This effect is reversible and nonspecific. Once anesthetics are absorbed by the local circulation and metabolized or excreted, nerve function returns to normal. Because local anesthetics are nonspecific, they can act on all sensory nerves, depending on the dose administered. A number of factors affect the rate of onset, intensity, and duration of sensory nerve anesthesia. After reading this section and reviewing the multiple variables that affect the quality of local anesthesia, it can be understood that sensory nerve impulses are lost in the order of temperature sensation, pain, touch, deep pressure and, finally, motor.

Table 22-1

Drugs for Local Anesthesia

	Drug Class	Trade Name	Concentration Available (%)	Onset of Local	Onset of Nerve Block	Duration	Maximal Dose	Maximal Dose with Epinephrine
Topical Agents								
Benzocaine	Ester	Anbesol	2–11.8	Rapid		Short		
Cocaine	Ester			2–10 min		45–180 min	3 mg/kg	
Tetracaine	Ester	Cetacaine	0.25, 0.5, 1.0	Rapid		Short		
Proparacaine	Ester	Ophthaine		Rapid		Short		
Dibucaine	Amide	Nupercainal		Rapid		Short		
Lidocaine	Amide	ELA-Max/ LAT/TLE	4.0–5.0	5–30 min		20–60 min	2–5 mL of mixture	
Prilocaine + lidocaine	Amide	EMLA	50/50	30–120 min		20–60 min	2–5 mL of mixture	
Injectable Agents								
Lidocaine	Amide	Xylocaine	0.5, 1, 2	Rapid	4–10 min	20–120 min*	4.5 mg/kg of 1%	7 mg/kg of 1%
Mepivacaine	Amide	Carbocaine	1, 2	1–3 min	6–10 min	30–180 min	4.5 mg/kg of 1%	5.5 mg/kg of 1%
Prilocaine	Amide	Citanest	1, 2, 3	2–6 min		90–240 min	5.5 mg/kg of 1%	8.5 mg/kg of 1%
Bupivacaine	Amide	Marcaine	0.25, 0.5, 0.75	3–10 min	8–12 min	120–480 min	2 mg/kg of 0.25%	3.5 mg/kg of 0.25%
Procaine	Ester	Novocain	0.5, 1, 2	5 min		60–90 min	7 mg/kg	
Tetracaine	Ester	Pontocaine	0.1, 0.25	7 min		120–180 min	0.3–1.4 mg/kg	8.5 mg/kg

* Epinephrine added to lidocaine doubles the duration of action.

Rate of Conduction. Local anesthetics are much more likely to bind to sodium channels that have rapid action potentials (such as those that carry pain impulses) than those with slower action potentials.

Presence of Myelin. Unmyelinated nerve fibers (such as C-type pain and temperature fibers) are more easily blocked by local anesthetics because they are smaller in diameter and lack the lipid barrier of the myelin sheath. Pressure, touch, and motor conduction are transmitted by larger diameter, A-type myelinated fibers. The lipophilic local anesthetics become bound by the highly lipid myelin sheath, which slows the amount of drug at the node, leading to slower onset but longer duration.

Nerve Fiber Diameter. Larger doses of drug are needed to anesthetize larger nerve trunks, such as digital nerves, and the onset of action is slower.

Vascularity of the Location Anesthetized. In highly vascular areas, drug is rapidly removed from the area that requires anesthesia, leading to the need for more drug or a vasoconstricting agent. A shorter duration of action also results. All the local anesthetics are vasodilatory in nature, except cocaine, which is a vasoconstrictor.

Use of Epinephrine. Adding a vasoconstricting agent such as epinephrine decreases blood flow, reduces systemic absorption, shortens onset, and extends duration of action. Epinephrine tends to be more effective with the less lipid-soluble agents (lidocaine and mepivacaine) than with the more lipid-soluble agents (bupivacaine) (Strichartz, 1998; Gage, 1997). As a general rule, the use of epinephrine doubles the duration of anesthesia achieved with lidocaine (Gonzalez del Rey and DiGiulo, 1997). Caution must be exercised in using vasoconstrictive agents in regions of the body supplied by a single vascular source, because tissue necrosis may result.

Anesthetic Solution and Tissue pH. Most anesthetic solutions are acidic in order to maintain their stability or shelf life. Once injected, however, they equilibrate to the pH of normal tissues. This leads to the sensation of burning on injection. Buffering the anesthetic solution with sodium bicarbonate can effectively eliminate this undesirable side effect. Although buffering decreases the onset of action and increases the effectiveness of the blockade, it decreases the shelf life. Plain lidocaine buffered with bicarbonate has a shelf life of approximately 7 days (Usatine and Moy, 1998; Gonzalez del Rey and DiGiulo, 1997). In addition, buffering can degrade epinephrine if it is kept in a container exposed to light (Gonzalez del Rey and DiGiulo, 1997). It is unknown what the shelf lives of buffered mepivacaine and bupivacaine are because studies have not been performed.

Because anesthetic solutions work best at physiologic pH, they are less effective in infected tissues than in normal tissues because of the resultant metabolic acidosis, which decreases pH (Strichartz, 1998).

Method and Technique of Injection. The nerve fibers are present at the junction of the dermis and the subcutaneous fat. Direct infiltration of an open wound at this level provides immediate blockade (Gonzalez del Rey and DiGiulo, 1997). Direct infiltration of intact skin, if started at the junction of the dermis and the subcutaneous fat, also provides immediate and nearly painless anesthesia. If the injection is started higher in the epidermis or at the dermal-epidermal junction, the blockade is slightly slower and more painful. Digital nerve block is slower in onset because of the larger nerve fibers. Technique is important because placement of anesthetic immediately adjacent to a digital nerve can lead to blockade within minutes, whereas delivery that is further from the nerve trunk can delay onset and can lead to inadequate blockade and the possible need for repeat injections.

Concentration of Solution. Solutions of higher concentration may lead to a slightly shorter onset of action when compared with solutions of lower concentration, but this difference is not markedly significant. For example, adding epinephrine to 1% lidocaine achieves the same effect as using 2% lidocaine (Gonzalez del Rey and DiGiulo, 1997).

Total Dose Provided. Increasing the dose leads to more effective blockade; however, too much can lead to side effects. Maximal doses of anesthetic solutions are provided in Table 22–1.

Rate of Metabolism. The ester anesthetics undergo metabolism by first being hydrolyzed by plasma cholinesterases and liver esterases and then being excreted by the kidneys (Hruza, 1999; Strichartz, 1998). They tend to have a shorter half-life than the amide anesthetics (Strichartz, 1998). Amide anesthetics are metabolized by first being N-dealkylated and then being hydrolyzed by the liver's endoplasmic reticulum. Because bupivacaine is highly bound to plasma proteins and tissue at the injection site, it is more likely to cause side effects in patients with severe liver disease (Strichartz, 1998). This is because of reduced liver metabolism and a decreased concentration of plasma proteins, which are made in the liver.

Indications

Local anesthesia in any procedure can be confined to one area of the body in which pain or discomfort associated with the procedure can be anticipated. The most common indication is in minor surgical procedures, including repair of lacerations, incision and drainage of abscesses, removal of lesions, biopsies, and nail removal.

Contraindications

Topical Anesthetics

• Cocaine-containing products are occasionally used to anesthetize adult nasal mucosa; however, contact with these agents should be avoided in infants and neonates. Unless used by a provider skilled in the use of cocaine-containing products on the nasal mucosa, these products should not be administered on the conjunctiva or nasal or oral mucosa. There is a case report of an infant death associated with the use of a cocaine-containing solution that accidentally came into contact with the nasal and oral mucosa (Dailey, 1988). Cocaine-containing products should also not be administered on the fingers, toes, penis, nose, and pinna of the ear because of their vasoconstricting properties.

- There are a few relative contraindications to the use of non–cocaine-containing topical anesthetics in premature infants. Studies are mixed concerning the possibility of the development of methemoglobinemia in premature infants who were given a topical eutectic mixture of lidocaine anesthetics (EMLA), but overall EMLA appears to be safe and effective in most infants and children (Frey and Kehrer, 1999; Essink-Tjebbes et al, 1999).

Local Anesthetics

Listed contraindications to the use of local anesthetics include the following:

- Severely unstable blood pressure
- True allergy
- Severe liver disease when amide anesthetics are being considered
- Severe renal disease when ester anesthetics are being considered (esters are renally excreted) and mental instability (which might mask the symptoms of adverse effects of lidocaine) (Hruza, 1999; Gonzalez del Rey and DiGiulo, 1997).

Epinephrine

Absolute contraindications to the use of epinephrine include the following:

- Untreated hyperthyroidism or untreated pheochromocytoma
- Administration to locations of the body that have a single, dependent blood supply—such as the fingers, toes, penis, nose, and pinna of the ear—or for use in a digital block

Relative contraindications to the use of epinephrine include the following:

- Untreated hypertension
- Severe coronary artery or peripheral vascular disease
- Pregnancy

- Narrow-angle glaucoma
- Use in patients taking beta blockers, phenothiazines, monoamine oxidase (MAO) inhibitors, or tricyclic antidepressants

Epinephrine should be used cautiously in patients with relative contraindications by diluting the epinephrine in half or using it sparingly, or determining not to use it at all.

Potential Complications

The most common complication seen with injection of anesthesia follows:

- Development of anxiety over the impending injection and a subsequent vasovagal reaction demonstrated by hypotension, bradycardia, and syncope (Hruza, 1999; Gonzalez del Rey and DiGiulo, 1997)

Local complications of injection are not as common and include the following:

- Bruising
- Edema
- Infection
- Prolonged or permanent nerve damage
- Temporary motor nerve paralysis (Hruza, 1999; Gonzalez del Rey and DiGiulo, 1997)

Systemic complications are uncommon; when they occur it is usually because anesthetic is inadvertently injected into a vessel. This complication can be avoided by making sure that blood cannot be aspirated before injecting the anesthetic. Systemic reactions include the following:

- Hypotension
- Bradycardia
- Central nervous system depression or stimulation, leading to slurred speech, drowsiness, disorientation, tremor, restlessness, weakness, seizures, paralysis, coma, respiratory failure, and cardiac dysrhythmias

This last complication is more common with bupivacaine than with the other anesthetics. Prilocaine in large doses can lead to methemoglobinemia (Hruza, 1999).

Epinephrine can lead to a number of side effects such as the following:

- Cardiac dysrhythmias
- Increased blood pressure
- Anxiety
- Cardiac arrest

- Cerebral hemorrhage
- Ischemia if used in areas of end artery flow such as the digits, penis, nose, and pinna of the ear, leading to skin necrosis especially in patients with poor circulation

Treatment of complications tends to be supportive. The patient should be placed in the Trendelenburg position, which usually reverses hypotension and bradycardia (Hruza, 1999; Gonzalez del Rey and DiGiulo, 1997). If hypotension continues, an intravenous infusion of normal saline can be started, an airway maintained, supplemental oxygen administered, and cardiac monitoring with frequent vital signs begun (Gonzalez del Rey and DiGiulo, 1997). Seizures are generally controlled by administration of intravenous diazepam (Valium).

Benzocaine is a para-aminobenzoic acid (PABA) derivative that has a tendency to cause allergic contact dermatitis. The literature cites that patients sensitive to benzocaine may also be sensitive to thiazide diuretics, sulfonylureas, sulfonamides, paraphenylenediamine, and para-aminobenzoic acid–based preparations. Because benzocaine is an ester anesthetic, patients hypersensitive to this agent may also be sensitive to other ester anesthetics such as procaine (Novocain), which is rarely used because of the rate of true allergic reactions, and tetracaine, but they will not be sensitive to the amide anesthetics.

True allergic reactions are rare among amide anesthetics but are more frequent with the older ester anesthetics. Allergic reactions may be caused by the preservative methylparaben or bisulfites, which are used in the multiple-dose vials. True allergy is characterized by a skin rash, localized or general urticaria, angioedema and, rarely, anaphylaxis with hypotension and bradycardia. Only 1% of all patients receiving local anesthesia demonstrate a true allergic response (Gonzalez del Rey and DiGiulo, 1997).

Allergic reactions are managed with airway management and administration of supplemental oxygen, IV access, and administration of epinephrine, diphenhydramine and corticosteroids as needed (Hruza 1999, Gonzalez del Rey and DiGiulo, 1997).

Assessment of patients with a reported allergy to local anesthetics should include determining the offending anesthetic and substituting it with a different class (i.e., if allergy to an ester, use an amide and vice versa) or skin test the patient with a preservative-free anesthetic. If the patient has a true anesthetic allergy, Benadryl, normal saline, no anesthetic or conscious sedation are all accepted alternatives.

Standard Precautions ▷ Practitioners should use Standard Precautions at all times when interacting with patients. Determining the level of precaution necessary requires the practitioner to exercise clinical judgment based on the patient's history and the potential for exposure to body fluids or aerosol-borne pathogens (for further discussion see Chapter 2).

Patient Preparation

Several techniques have been offered to decrease the pain and anxiety accompanying an injection of anesthetic.

- Because of the way local anesthesia affects the sensory nerve impulses (see Essential Anatomy and Physiology), an anxious patient may perceive touch as if it were pain. Therefore, reassuring the patient and explaining the expectations of the procedure are key to ensuring nearly painless anesthesia.
- Because the most common reaction to local anesthesia is a vasovagal response or syncope, the patient needs to be in the supine position, placed so that he or she cannot see the injection being administered.
- Engaging in conversation should distract the patient.
- Inform the patient what is being done at each step.
- Encourage the patient to take deep, slow breaths to avoid hyperventilation.
- Continue to reassure the patient throughout the procedure of injection.
- For anxious patients or children, conscious sedation with a benzodiazepine may be necessary; however, detailing its use is beyond the scope of this chapter.
- Use cryoanesthetic, such as ice, ethyl chloride, tetrafluoroethane (Medi-Frig), fluoroethyl (25% ethyl chloride, 75% dichlorotetrafluoroethane), or liquid nitrogen before an injection. This technique can also be used for anesthesia before curettage of superficial lesions as described in Chapter 24. Cryoanesthetics provide short periods of decreased pain sensation. For purposes of anesthesia before injection, liquid nitrogen is not preferred because it can be painful and may lead to unwanted tissue destruction.
- Warming the local anesthetic: This has not been known to reduce the pain of anesthetic injection significantly and requires time and effort to warm the vial or syringe to 37°C to 40°C and then rapidly inject the anesthetic before it cools (Gonzales del Rey and DiGiulo, 1997).

Materials Utilized for Administering Anesthetics

Topical Anesthesia

Note: There are a number of benefits to topical anesthesia compared with injection and include lack of injection (therefore, no discomfort), ease of administration, decreased need for physical restraints, and no distortion of the anatomy. Topical anesthesia tends to work better on the highly vascular face and scalp than on the trunk or proximal extremities (Gonzalez del Rey and DiGiulo, 1997; Trott, 1997). When using topical anesthesia for wound closure, it should be limited to lacerations of 5 cm or less in order to avoid the complication of systemic absorption (Gonzalez del Rey and DiGiulo, 1997; Trott, 1997).

Note: Topical anesthetics are divided into amides (lidocaine, prilocaine), esters (benzocaine, tetracaine), and nonamides, nonesters (dimethisoquin, dyclonine, pramoxine). Each specialty tends to have one topical anesthetic that is preferred over others. Anesthesia of the conjunctiva can be accomplished by the use of proparacaine or tetracaine eyedrops (Hruza, 1999). Topical benzocaine is commonly added as an agent for sunburn relief. It is, however, a common contact sensitizer and should generally be avoided. Anesthetics available for use on the superficial mucous membranes include dyclonine (Dyclone), benzocaine (Anbesol and others), tetracaine (Cetacaine), viscous lidocaine, and lidocaine jelly. Deeper anesthesia of the mucous membranes can be accomplished with a 4% to 10% solution of cocaine. Cocaine-containing products increase the cost of the anesthetic and need to be stored and disposed of under strict protocols. Cocaine-containing products may also be used to anesthetize lacerations. Examples of cocaine-containing products include:

- TAC: tetracaine 0.5%, epinephrine 1:2000, and cocaine 11.8%
- TAC, ½ strength: tetracaine 1%, epinephrine 1:2000, and cocaine 4%
- *or* tetracaine 0.25%, epinephrine 1:4000, and cocaine 5.9%

Other topical agents without cocaine used for wound repair include:

- LAT: Lidocaine 4%, epinephrine 1:2000, tetracaine 1%
- TLE: Lidocaine 5% and epinephrine 1:2000

Note: All these products can be prepared by a pharmacist as a liquid or gel; however, although gels decrease the risk of mucosal exposure, they may also decrease the amount of total dose delivered (Usatine and Moy, 1998; Gonzalez del Rey and DiGiulo, 1997). Some authors have stated that TAC/LAT/TLE combinations provide inconsistent anesthesia for lacerations on the extremities, leading to the need for supplemental anesthetic injection (Gonzalez del Rey and DiGiulo, 1997).

Note: For intact skin, superficial anesthesia can be achieved with EMLA (eutectic mixture of lidocaine anesthetics) or ELA-Max (4% lidocaine). EMLA is 50% lidocaine and 50% prilocaine in an acid-mantle cream. Neither cream should be used on mucous membranes or conjunctiva because of the risk of greater absorption leading to potential systemic side effects.

- Other equipment
  - Cotton-tipped applicators or gauze pads
  - Materials to clean the wound or anesthesia site

Injection Anesthesia

The most commonly used agents follow:

- Lidocaine (Xylocaine 1% and 2%, with and without epinephrine)

- Rapid onset of action
- Readily penetrates nerve sheaths, leading to an almost immediate anesthesia with local infiltration
- For direct wound infiltration, the duration of action is approximately 20 to 30 minutes and is approximately 60 to 120 minutes for nerve blocks

Caution: There is a subset of patients who metabolize lidocaine quickly and require repeat injections.

Note: The use of epinephrine with lidocaine increases the duration of action and improves local hemostasis.

- Method of buffering lidocaine: 1 mL of bicarbonate + 9 mL of 1% lidocaine

Note: Buffering of 2% solutions may cause precipitation.

Note: The shelf-life of buffered lidocaine is 7 days.

- Mepivacaine (Carbocaine 1% and 2%)
  - Slightly longer onset of action with direct infiltration (6 to 10 minutes), but the duration of action is longer, approximately 30 to 60 minutes
  - Does not cause as much vasodilation as lidocaine; therefore, does not require epinephrine for hemostasis
  - Method of buffering mepivacaine: 0.5 to 1 mL of bicarbonate + 9 mL of mepivacaine
  - Shelf life unknown, therefore, do not use after 24 hours
- Bupivacaine (Marcaine 0.25% and 0.5%)
  - Slow onset of action (8 to 12 minutes) with direct infiltration, but the duration of action is much longer than with either lidocaine or mepivacaine. It lasts approximately four times longer than lidocaine, offering significant postsurgical relief from pain.
  - Method of buffering bupivacaine: 0.1 mL of bicarbonate + 20 mL of bupivacaine

Note: The shelf life is unknown; therefore, do not use after 24 hours.

- Diphenhydramine (Benadryl)
  - For allergic reaction to amide or ester anesthetics, or both, alternatives include Benadryl and normal saline or no anesthesia.
  - Provide adequate anesthesia for at least 30 minutes.
  - Benadryl should be diluted to 12.5 mg/mL with normal saline.

Note: The technique for direct infiltration with Benadryl is the same as with other anesthetics. Benadryl, however, is more painful to inject than lidocaine and is not reduced by buffering.

- Other equipment
  - Materials to clean the site or wound
  - Materials to ensure sterile technique
  - 27- or 30-gauge needle $1/2$- to $1\frac{1}{4}$-inch length
  - A syringe, size dependent on the quantity of anesthetic to be injected
  - The injectable anesthetic

Procedure for Using Topical Anesthesia

1. For intact skin, achieve superficial anesthesia with EMLA (50% lidocaine and 50% prilocaine in an acid-mantle cream) or ELA-Max (4% lidocaine).

Note: Neither cream should be used on mucous membranes or conjunctivae because of the risk of greater absorption leading to potential systemic side effects. Young children should be watched closely to avoid accidental ingestion.

2. When applying ELA-Max, do not keep on skin for greater than 2 hours at a time.

Note: Anesthesia with EMLA and ELA-Max works best for removal of superficial skin lesions, for some laser procedures, and before injection of anesthetic. With both creams, the depth of anesthesia is directly proportional to the duration of application and lasts for several hours. ELA-Max appears to have a more rapid onset of action than does EMLA. Neither cream appears to cause irritating effects or hypersensitivity reactions with repeated or prolonged use.

3. Gently remove blood clots from the area.

4. For wound repair, saturate a gauze sponge or cotton swab with anesthetic.

5. Fold the anesthetic-saturated sponge into and around the wound and tape into place.

6. Have the parent or assistant or yourself apply constant, gentle pressure for 15 to 20 minutes.

Note: The person applying pressure should wear gloves in order to avoid absorption.

Note: Anesthesia is complete when blanching is observed around the wound. One report stated that about 5% of wounds require supplemental injection of local anesthetic to achieve complete anesthesia. Studies have also shown that about 2 to 3 mL of topical anesthetic is sufficient to provide anesthesia for most wound repairs (Gonzalez del Rey and DiGiulo, 1997).

7. If administering EMLA or ELA-Max, cover the area requiring treatment with a $\frac{1}{4}$-inch-thick layer of cream.

Note: EMLA is then occluded with a plastic adhesive dressing 1 hour before the procedure. ELA-Max does not require occlusion, although this may be performed.

8. Remove both creams before the start of the procedure.

Procedure for Administering Local Anesthetic by Injection

Note: Nearly painless anesthesia is more likely with the use of a 27- or 30-gauge needle. This occurs not only because the caliber of the needle is smaller but also because it decreases the speed with which anesthetic is injected. Rapid tissue expansion is more uncomfortable for the patient, so the provider should aim for a slow injection technique, which will be facilitated by selecting a 1- to 3-mL syringe.

Procedure for Administering Local Anesthetic by Injection – *(continued)*

Note: Needle length varies from ½ to 1¼ inch. The shorter length is adequate for small punch biopsies, whereas longer needles are better for larger excisions, wound infiltration, and field and digital blocks.

Direct Infiltration of Wounds

1. Initiate the injection on the side where sensory innervation originates and then proceed distally.

Note: Direct wound infiltration is recommended in most minimally contaminated wounds. The injection should be located between the dermis and the subcutaneous fat. Tissue resistance is less and the sensory nerves are rapidly affected by the anesthetic at this level.

2. Once the needle is inserted, aspirate to ensure that the needle is not in a vessel. If no blood is withdrawn, inject a small amount of anesthetic.
3. Reposition the needle adjacent to, but still within, the area where anesthetic was placed.
4. Aspirate and proceed to inject if no blood is withdrawn.
5. Continue to repeat the preceding steps until all edges of the wound are anesthetized.
6. If at any time bloody aspirate is obtained, withdraw the needle slightly and aspirate until clear. A 3- to 4-cm laceration should require about 3 to 5 mL of anesthetic (Hruza, 1999; Gonzalez del Rey and DiGiulo, 1997) (Fig. 22–1).

Local Infiltration of Intact Skin

1. Clean the intended procedure site with an alcohol wipe or alternative antiseptic.

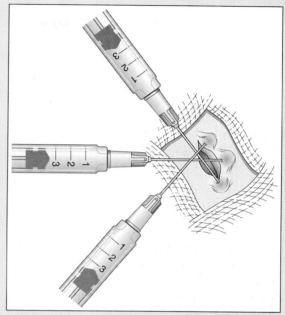

Figure 22–1.

2. Pinch the skin in the vicinity of the injection site. This will decrease the sensation of pain from the injection.
3. Infiltrate at the junction of the dermis and subcutaneous fat and then reposition the needle to the level of the epidermis and inject a small amount of anesthetic.

Note: Always remember to aspirate before injection. For punch biopsies, only 1 to 2 mL of anesthetic is generally required.

Field Block

Note: Field block is an alternative to direct wound infiltration when a larger area requires treatment or in wounds that are grossly contaminated to avoid bacterial spread. It has the advantage of fewer injections than direct wound infiltration.

Procedure for Administering Local Anesthetic by Injection – *(continued)*

1. Start the injection in the same plane as described in local infiltration of intact skin; however, a larger bore (25- to 27-gauge), $1\frac{1}{4}$- to 2-inch needle is required.
2. Insert the needle into the skin and advance to the hub parallel to the dermis and subcutaneous fat. After aspiration, a slow injection of anesthetic is left as the needle is withdrawn to the insertion site.
3. Reinsert the needle at the end of the first track and repeat the procedure until a wall of anesthesia surrounds the area to be treated (Usatine and Moy, 1998; Gonzalez del Rey and DiGiulo, 1997) (Fig. 22–2).

Digital Block

Note: 1% lidocaine or 1% mepivacaine without epinephrine, with or without bicarbonate, and 2% lidocaine without epinephrine or bicarbonate, are commonly used for digital blocks (Stroichartz, 1998; Page et al, 1997; Gage, 1997). Lidocaine with bupivacaine is an alternative. Bupivacaine's onset of action is too slow to use alone. It does accord longer duration of action for extended procedures as well as significant postoperative relief from discomfort for the patient.

Note: A digital block is generally recommended for procedures distal to the mid-proximal phalanx of the digit and is preferred for nail avulsion, paronychial drainage, and repair of lacerations of the digits.

1. A digital nerve block is accomplished by injecting anesthetic just distal to the web space in the middle of the digit.
2. After aspirating, inject 0.1 of anesthetic locally into the epidermis.
3. Advance the needle to the bone, withdraw slightly, and then move dorsally, where 0.5 mL of anesthetic is injected after aspiration.
4. Withdraw the needle again to the midline, advance to bone, and move ventrally where another 0.5 to 1 mL of anesthetic is injected after aspiration.
5. Withdraw the needle and repeat the whole procedure on the other side of the digit (Fig. 22–3).

Note: Larger volumes of anesthetic are not required if injected near the nerve. The needle should always be withdrawn between dorsal and ventral injections to avoid nerve and vessel damage. Anesthesia is reported to occur anywhere from 4 to 20 minutes after injection, depending on the anesthetic and technique used.

Note: There are alternatives to the method described for performing a digital block.

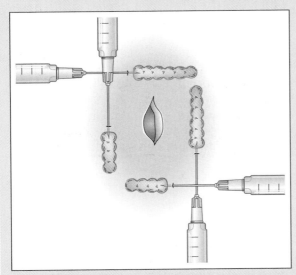

Figure 22–2. Adapted from Pfenninger JL, Fowler JC: Procedures for Primary Care Physicians. St. Louis, Mosby-Year Book, 1994, p 147.

Procedure for Administering Local Anesthetic by Injection – *(continued)*

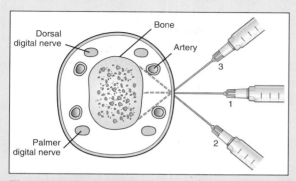

Figure 22-3. Adapted from Pfenninger JL, Fowler JC: Procedures for Primary Care Physicians. St. Louis, Mosby-Year Book, 1994, p 149.

Alternatives To Performing A Digital Block

1. Since the second to fifth toes are small, one technique uses a dorsal midline injection. Anesthetic is then deposited on one side of the toe.

2. Withdraw the needle and move to the opposite side without completely withdrawing the needle from the skin (Gonzalez del Rey and DiGiulo, 1997).
Caution: **This technique is not recommended for the great toe.**
Note: For surgery on the distal nail unit, periungual administration may be performed. It is essentially a field block technique of the nail unit (see Chapter 28). It

is more painful than a digital block but is more rapid in onset.

1. It is completed by injecting first along one lateral nail fold, then perpendicularly along the proximal nail fold, and then along the opposite lateral nail fold. Lastly, anesthetic is administered in the hyponychial area (Gonzalez del Rey and DiGiulo, 1997).
2. Another alternative is to inject at a 30-degree angle into the middle of the proximal nail fold, where the needle is then advanced distally under the nail matrix.
3. After aspiration, inject anesthetic as the needle pierces the nail plate, the nail matrix, and the nail bed.
Note: The nail matrix and nail bed will blanch with injection of anesthetic. It is painful, but anesthesia is immediate. This type of anesthesia can be used for most procedures performed on the proximal half of the nail unit, but not for removal of the nail matrix or complete nail avulsion (Gonzalez del Rey and DiGiulo, 1997).
Note: Other digital blocks used include supraorbital, supratrochlear, infraorbital, mental, auricular, median, ulnar, radial, sural, and tibial. These are used for procedures or repair of lacerations covering a large surface area; however, their description is beyond the scope of this book.

Follow-Up Care and Instructions

- Complications from local anesthesia are uncommon. Occasionally a patient exhibits sensitivity to a component of the anesthetic, which may later present as a rash or inflammatory reaction. Instruct the patient to notify the office if there is any unusual skin color, itching, or pain in the area where the anesthetic was injected, or if sensation does not return promptly after the anesthesia was to have worn off.

References

Dailey RH: Fatality secondary to misuse of TAC solution. Ann Emerg Med 17:159–160, 1988.

Essink-Tjebbes CM, Hekster YA, Liem KD, et al: Topical use of local anesthetics in neonates. Pharm World Sci 21:173–176, 1999.

Frey B, Kehrer B: Toxic methaemoglobin concentrations in premature infants after application of a prilocaine-containing cream and peridural prilocaine. Eur J Pediatr 158:785–788, 1999.

Gage TW: Drugs in dentistry. In Page CP, Curtis MJ, Sutter MC, et al (eds):Integrated Pharmacology. St. Louis, CV Mosby, 1997, pp 383–398.

Gonzalez del Rey JA, DiGiulo GA: Wound Care and the Pediatric Patient. In Trott AT (ed): Wounds and Lacerations: Emergency Care and Closure, 2nd ed. St. Louis, CV Mosby, 1997, pp 38–52.

Hruza GJ: Dermatologic Surgery: Introduction and Approach. In Fitzpatrick TB, Eisen AZ, Wolff K, et al (eds): Dermatology in General Medicine, 5th ed. New York, McGraw-Hill, 1999, pp 2923–2937.

Page CP, Curtis MJ, Sutter MC, et al: General principles of drug action. In Page CP, Curtis MJ, Sutter MC, et al (eds): Integrated Pharmacology. St. Louis, CV Mosby, 1997, pp 17–52.

Strichartz GR: Drugs affecting peripheral transmission: Local anesthetics. In Brody TM, Larner J, Minneman KP (eds): Human Pharmacology: Molecular to Clinical, 3rd ed. St. Louis, CV Mosby, 1998, pp 151–156.

Trott AT: Infiltration and nerve block anesthesia. In Trott AT (ed): Wounds and Lacerations, 2nd ed. St. Louis, CV Mosby, 1997, pp 53–89.

Usatine RP, Moy RL: Anesthesia. In Skin Surgery: a Practical Guide. Usatine RP, Moy RL, Tobinick EL, et al (eds): St Louis, CV Mosby, 1998, pp 20–30.

Bibliography

• Fine JD, Arndt KA: Medical dermatologic therapy. In Orkin M, Maibach HI, Dahl MV (eds): Dermatology. Norwalk, Conn, Appleton & Lange, 1991, pp 635–656.

• Kechijian P: Nail surgery. In Fitzpatrick TB, Eisen AZ, Wolff K, et al (eds): Dermatology in General Medicine, 5th ed. New York, McGraw-Hill, 1999, pp 2992–3002.

• Kongsiri AS, Ciesielski-Carlucci C, Stiller MJ: Topical nonglucocorticoid therapy. In Fitzpatrick TB, Eisen AZ, Wolff K, et al (eds): Dermatology in General Medicine, 5th ed. New York, McGraw-Hill, 1999, pp 2717–2726.

• Ries CR, Sutter FM, Sutter MC: Drugs used in surgery. In Page CP, Curtis MJ, Sutter MC, et al (eds): Integrated Pharmacology. St. Louis, CV Mosby, 1997, pp 399–410.

• Roenigk HH: Dermatologic surgery in dermatology. In Orkin M, Maibach HI, Dahl MV (eds): Dermatology. Norwalk, Conn, Appleton & Lange, 1991, pp 657–662.

Chapter 23

Wound Closure

▷ Karen A. Newell

Procedure Goals and Objectives

Goal: To reapproximate wound edges with sutures, staples, or skin adhesive successfully in order to facilitate wound healing and reduce the likelihood of infection.

Objectives: The student will be able to . . .

▶ Describe the indications, contraindications, and rationale for performing wound closure.

▶ Identify and describe common complications associated with wound closure.

▶ Describe the essential anatomy and physiology of the skin associated with the performance of wound closure.

▶ Identify the materials and tools necessary for performing wound closure and their proper use.

▶ Identify the important aspects of care after wound closure.

Background and History

Wound closure has been in existence for many years in the practice of medicine. Although wound closure is typically associated with suturing the wound, many materials have been used over time. The word *suture* describes any strand of material used to ligate (tie) blood vessels or approximate (sew) tissues. The first written description of sutures used in operative procedures is recorded in the Edwin Smith Papyrus, the oldest known surgical document. This document has Egyptian origins and dates back to the 16th century BC. As far back as 2000 BC, written references have been found describing the use of strings and animal sinews for suturing.

Rhazes of Arabia was credited in 900 AD with first using kit gut to suture abdominal wounds. The Arabic word *kit* means a dancing master's fiddle. In those days the musical strings of fiddles, called *kit strings,* were made of sheep's intestines. It has been speculated that Rhazes used these to suture. The term *catgut* is thought to have evolved from these origins.

Through the centuries, a wide variety of materials—silk, linen, cotton, horsehair, animal tendons and intestines, and wire made of precious metals—have been used in operative procedures. Some of these are still in use today. The evolution of suturing material has brought us to a point of refinement that includes sutures designed for specific surgical procedures. They not only eliminate some of the difficulties the surgeon may have previously encountered during closure but decrease the potential for infection postoperatively. Despite the sophistication of today's suture materials and surgical techniques, closing a wound still involves the same basic procedure used by physicians to the Roman emperors (Ethicon, 1985).

Indications

Most superficial wounds will heal without intervention. However, a superficial skin laceration extending into the subcutaneous tissues should be considered for closure in order to avoid undesirable outcomes. Suture, staple, or skin adhesive closure of wounds may be warranted for the following:

- To decrease the time required for the wound to heal
- To reduce the likelihood of infection
- To decrease the amount of scar tissue likely to form
- To repair the loss of structure or function, or both, of the tissue
- To improve cosmetic appearance

Contraindications

Before any wound or laceration repair is initiated, a thorough evaluation of the patient must be carried out. Remember that all wounds, no matter how minor they may appear, can be the result of serious injury to underlying structures. The basic history, general physical examination, and wound examination help define the repair strategy and help identify more serious problems necessitating specialized care.

Contraindications to suture closure of wounds relate largely to the risk of infection and disruption of underlying structures such as nerves, arteries, and tendons. Wounds that have the following characteristics should be left unclosed, or at least very careful consideration should be given (weighing the pros and cons of closure) before electing to suture the wound.

- Wounds that have a high likelihood of contamination should not be closed with sutures. Doing so may mask a developing underlying infection, thus delaying appropriate treatment. This delayed treatment may result in spread of infection to underlying and surrounding structures, which has the potential to cause considerable morbidity. Classification of the wound helps the clinician to make an informed decision about the appropriateness of closing the wound (see Review of Essential Anatomy and Physiology).
- Wounds that require suturing to minimize infection and scar potential should be closed within 8 hours of the injury. Some wounds can be closed up to 24 hours after injury if the anatomic location is highly vascular (e.g., face, neck, and scalp) and the cosmetic appearance is an important consideration.
- The presence of foreign bodies in the underlying tissues is a consideration. Foreign bodies will remain a source of repeated infections if not thoroughly removed through irrigation, exploration, and extraction or débridement of devitalized and contaminated tissue.
- Extensive wounds involving tendons, nerves, or arteries should be carefully considered before closure.

Potential Complications

The primary complications associated with wound closure include the following:

- Infection
- Scarring, including keloid formation
- Loss of function and structure (an example might be scarring of an eyelid repair, resulting in incomplete closure of the eyelids)

- Loss of a cosmetically desirable appearance
- Wound dehiscence (wound margins separate and wound reopens)
- Tetanus

Review of Essential Anatomy and Physiology

Anatomy of the Skin and Fascia

The epidermis is a thin layer of skin located on the outermost surface. It is composed completely of squamous epithelial cells. This layer of the skin is void of blood vessels or nerve endings. The epidermis provides an excellent protective barrier when healthy and intact. The stratum germinativum, or basal layer, is the parent layer for new cells. This layer provides the cells for new epidermis formation during wound healing (Fig. 23–1).

The dermis is much thicker than the epidermis. It is composed largely of connective tissue such as fibroblasts; macrophages, lymphocytes, and mast cells are also present. Some small blood vessels and nerve fiber endings are present at this level.

Deep to the dermis is a layer of loose connective tissue that composes the superficial fascia or subcutaneous tissue. Many blood vessels and nerve

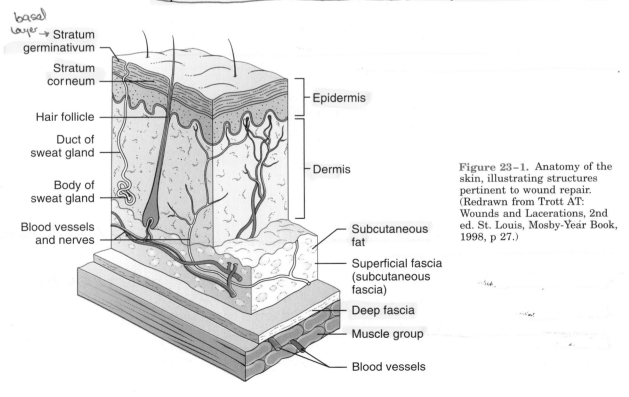

basal
layer → Stratum
germinativum

Stratum
corneum

Hair follicle

Duct of
sweat gland

Body of
sweat gland

Blood vessels
and nerves

Epidermis

Dermis

Subcutaneous
fat

Superficial fascia
(subcutaneous
fascia)

Deep fascia

Muscle group

Blood vessels

Figure 23–1. Anatomy of the skin, illustrating structures pertinent to wound repair. (Redrawn from Trott AT: Wounds and Lacerations, 2nd ed. St. Louis, Mosby-Year Book, 1998, p 27.)

endings are located at this level. Subcutaneous fat is present here, and the quantity varies depending on the region of the body. Sensory nerve branches to the skin travel in the superficial fascia just deep to the dermis, which makes it ideal for injecting local anesthetic, because the anesthetic will spread easily along this plane and abolish sensation in the overlying skin.

The deep fascia is a relatively thick, dense, and discrete fibrous tissue layer. It lies just above muscle, tendon, or bone. If disrupted by the injury, it should be repaired to re-establish the supportive function of this layer. Failure to do so may result in disfiguration of the surrounding area.

Skin Tension Lines (Langer's Lines)

Skin tension lines, also known as Langer's lines or lines of cleavage, are linear clefts in the skin that indicate the direction of orientation of the underlying collagen fibers. If the skin is disrupted parallel to the long axis of the fibers, the wound will tend to reapproximate. However, if the wound crosses the long axis of the fibers perpendicularly, they are disrupted in a manner that causes the wound to "gape" open; therefore, greater tension is required to close it. Lacerations that run parallel to these lines will naturally reapproximate the skin edges. Lacerations that run at right angles to the tension lines will tend to gape apart. Figure 23–2 illustrates the typical orientation of the Langer's lines throughout the body.

Wounds should be classified based on their degree of contamination with bacteria or foreign matter, or both. Timing of the closure is also important to consider. The chance of wound infection developing increases each hour that wound closure is delayed. There is general agreement that wounds less than 6 to 8 hours old that are considered clean are eligible for primary closure with sutures. Highly vascular areas such as the face and scalp can be considered for primary closure with sutures up to 24 hours after the injury. In each case, the clinician must consider the degree of contamination.

Classification of Wounds

- Clean: incisions made during a surgical procedure in which aseptic techniques were followed, without involvement of the gastrointestinal, respiratory, or genitourinary tract; likelihood of infection is less than 2% and warrants routine primary closure
- Clean-contaminated: similar to clean wounds except that the gastrointestinal, respiratory, or genitourinary tract is involved
- Contaminated: similar to clean and clean-contaminated except gross spillage (examples: bile, stool); traumatic wounds fall into this category
- Infected: established infection before wound is made (e.g., incision and drainage of an abscess) or heavily contaminated wounds (e.g., gross spillage of stool)

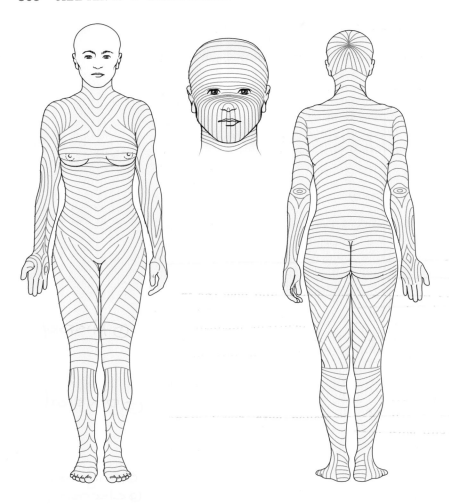

Figure 23–2. Langer's lines. Typical orientation throughout the body. (Redrawn from Trott AT: Wounds and Lacerations, 2nd ed. St. Louis, Mosby-Year Book, 1998, p 31; Adapted from Simon R, Brenner B: Procedures and Techniques in Emergency Medicine. Baltimore, Williams & Wilkins, 1982.

Wound Closure Classification

- Primary intention: All layers are closed.
  - Best chance for minimal scarring
  - Usually performed in clean and clean-contaminated wounds
- Secondary intention: The deep layers are closed, whereas superficial layers are left open to granulate on their own from the inside out.
  - Often leaves a wide scar and requires frequent wound care, consisting of irrigation and assorted types of packing and dressings
  - It is a prolonged process.
  - Reasons for use include excessive tissue loss and infection.
- Third intention or delayed primary intention: The deep layers are closed primarily, whereas the superficial layers are left open until reassessment on the fourth to fifth day after initial closure, at which time the wound is inspected for signs of infection.

[handwritten margin note: 3rd wound class]

- If it looks clean and has begun to granulate, it is irrigated and closed.
- If it looks as if it may be infected, it is left open to heal by secondary intention.
- These wounds often arise initially from contaminated wounds.

Standard Precautions ▷ Every practitioner should use Standard Precautions at all times when interacting with patients, especially when performing procedures. Determining the level of precaution necessary requires the practitioner to exercise clinical judgment based on the patient's history and the potential for exposure to body fluids or aerosol-borne pathogens (for further discussion, see Chapter 2).

Patient Preparation

- Take the patient's history to denote when, where, and how the injury occurred. Other pertinent information in the history may include handedness, tetanus status, other past or concurrent medical problems (e.g., diabetes mellitus, peripheral vascular diseases, immune status), smoking history, occupation, hobbies, family history, medications, and allergies. *(1) History*
- Begin the physical examination with a meticulous inspection detailing the type of wound, anatomic location, extent of injury, and level of contamination. Bleeding can usually be controlled with direct manual pressure applied to the site with a clean bandage. A careful sensory and motor examination should precede any wound exploration or anesthetic infiltration. *(2) physical*
- Prepare the patient for the initial treatment of the wound. This involves irrigation of the wound, which is a major step in reducing the likelihood of infection. The next step is cleansing the wound and then, with the patient properly anesthetized, suturing the wound. *(3) irrigation (4) cleansing (5) anesthesia (6) suture.*
- Immunize the patient against tetanus if necessary. *(7) tetanus. shot*

A discussion regarding tetanus status and potential risk is warranted in any patient with a wound. Tetanus is a preventable endotoxin-mediated disease caused by *Clostridium tetani*. When present, it may cause trismus, neck rigidity, dysphagia, and severe, uncontrolled reflex spasms. Populations at particular risk are the elderly and those who have immigrated to the United States and had inadequate immunization, those who are immunocompromised, and those who inject drugs regularly and have frequent skin abscesses, impaired immune status, and reluctance to seek health care.

It is therefore important to determine when the patient last received a tetanus immunization and to classify the wound as either tetanus prone or non–tetanus prone.

Tetanus-prone wounds are those that are:

- Greater than 6 hours old
- Greater than 1 cm deep
- Stellate or have an avulsion configuration
- Associated with devitalized tissue
- Contaminated with soil, feces, or saliva
- From a missile (e.g., gunshot wound)
- From a puncture or crush
- Associated with a burn or frostbite

All other wounds can be considered non–tetanus prone. To determine the appropriate treatment, see Table 23–1 and the following guidelines:

1. A non–tetanus prone wound in an up-to-date adult patient requires tetanus and diphtheria toxoid (Td) if it has been 10 years since the last immunization.
2. A tetanus-prone wound in a patient with up-to-date immunization requires Td if it has been more than 5 years since the last immunization.
3. A non–tetanus prone wound in an adult patient with inadequate immunization requires Td.
4. Tetanus-prone wounds in adult patients with inadequate immunization require both passive immunity with tetanus immunoglobulin (TIG) and active immunity with Td. Recognize that when both Td and TIG are given, they are placed in different syringes and delivered at separate anatomic locations. Adults with an unknown history should receive the three-dose regimen and therefore will require follow-up. The initial dose of Td toxoid is given at the time of wound closure; 4 to 8 weeks later, a second dose of Td toxoid is administered.

■ Table 23–1

Summary Guide to Tetanus Prophylaxis in Routine Wound Management, 1991

History of Adsorbed Tetanus Toxoid (Doses)	Clean, Minor Wounds		All Other Wounds*	
	Td[†]	TIG (250 U)	Td[†]	TIG (250U)
Unknown or <3	Yes	No	Yes	Yes
≥3[‡]	No[§]	No	No[‖]	No

* Such as, but not limited to, wounds contaminated with dirt, feces, soil, and saliva; puncture wounds; avulsions; and wounds resulting from missiles, crushing, burns, and frostbite.

[†] For children <7 years old; DTP (DT, if pertussis vaccine is contraindicated) is preferred to tetanus toxoid alone. For persons ≥7 years of age, Td is preferred to tetanus toxoid alone.

[‡] If only three doses of *fluid* toxoid have been received, a fourth dose of toxoid, preferably an adsorbed toxoid, should be given.

[§] Yes, if >10 years since last dose.

[‖] Yes, if >5 years since last dose. (More frequent boosters are not needed and can accentuate side effects.)

Adapted from ACIP: Diphtheria, tetanus, and pertussis: Recommendations for vaccine use and other preventative measures. MMWR 1991;40(RR-10):1–50.

(The last dose is given 6 to 12 weeks after the second dose.) Booster doses of Td toxoid should then be given every 10 years to maintain an adequate tetanus status.

5. Diphtheria, tetanus toxoid, and pertussis (DTP) or acellular pertussis (DTaP) is used instead of Td in children.

6. TIG is considered safe in pregnancy, whereas Td toxoid can be safely given in the second trimester and later in those who have high-risk wounds.

Materials Utilized for Performing Irrigation, Cleansing, and Débridement

■ Gloves and goggles

Irrigation
■ 60-mL syringe
■ 21-gauge plastic intravenous catheter or irrigation needle with "blunted" end for fluid irrigation
■ Several liters of saline solution

Cleansing
■ A cleansing agent (Table 23–2)

Table 23–2

Summary of Wound Cleansing Agents

Skin Cleanser	Antibacterial Activity	Tissue Toxicity	Systemic Toxicity	Potential Uses
Povidone-iodine surgical scrub	Strongly bactericidal against gram-positive and gram-negative bacteria	Detergent can be toxic to wound tissues	Painful to open wounds. Other reactions extremely rare	Hand cleanser
Povidone-iodine solution	Same as povidone-iodine scrub	Minimally toxic to wound tissues	Extremely rare	Wound periphery cleanser
Chlorhexidine	Strongly bactericidal against gram-positive organisms, less strong against gram-negative bacteria	Detergent can be toxic to wound tissues	Extremely rare	Hand cleanser. Alternative wound periphery cleanser
Poloxamer 188	No antibacterial activity	None known	None known	Wound cleanser (particularly useful on face)
Hexachlorophene	Bacteriostatic against gram-positive bacteria; poor activity against gram-negative bacteria	Detergent can be toxic to wound tissues	Teratogenic with repeated use	Alternative hand cleanser
Hydrogen peroxide	Very weak antibacterial agent	Toxic to red cells	Extremely rare	Wound cleanser adjunct

Adapted from Trott AT: Wounds and Lacerations, 2nd ed. St. Louis, Mosby-Year Book, 1998, p 91.

- Sterile, fenestrated drape
- Several sterile square or rectangular drapes

Débridement
- Scalpel or sharp tissue scissors

Procedure for Irrigating and Cleansing the Wound

1. Put on gloves and goggles to avoid exposure to blood-borne pathogens.
2. Using a 60-mL syringe and a 21-gauge plastic intravenous catheter or blunt needle designed for irrigation, repeatedly squirt normal saline into the site in short bursts to dislodge remaining particulate matter. Several liters may be necessary for large wounds that are heavily contaminated.
3. Apply a cleansing agent (see Table 23–2) to the wound edges and surrounding skin using a bull's eye or circular motion from the inside moving outward and repeat three times.

Note: One example of a cleansing agent might include three sterile povidone-iodine—soaked 4 x 4 pads.

4. Place a sterile fenestrated drape over the wound site and several sterile square or rectangular drapes around the site to create a sterile field.

Note: If the wound is on a limb, a sterile drape should be placed under the extremity before the other drapes are applied. Drapes are often found in prepackaged suture kits or on a laceration tray and are placed after the clinician dons sterile gloves.

5. If débridement is necessary to remove dead or devitalized tissue, use a scalpel or sharp tissue scissor.

Note: Care should be taken to preserve tissue, yet conversion of a jagged laceration to a surgical one may be required for optimal closure to occur. Sometimes the subcutaneous tissue may need to be undermined to allow for adequate closure of tight wound edges.

Materials Utilized to Perform Suturing

- Sterile gloves

Suture Selection

Note: Once it is determined that a wound should be closed primarily, suture selection begins. The first item to consider is whether to use absorbable or nonabsorbable suture based on anatomic location and healing potential.

- Absorbable suture is used in mucosal areas such as the oral cavity and tongue and disintegrates by one of two methods: enzymatic breakdown of organic material (e.g., surgical gut—plain or chromic) or by hydrolysis of synthetic material (e.g., polyglactin 910 [Vicryl]).

■ Nonabsorbable suture (silk, stainless steel, nylon, polypropylene, polyester fiber) can be further classified into monofilament (single strand) or multifilament (several strands, which are often braided).

Note: One advantage of monofilament is that it passes through tissue more easily than does braided suture. However, a disadvantage is that it has less tensile strength than a multifilament. Advantages of a multifilament suture include better flexibility, whereas a disadvantage would be that it may harbor organisms more easily within the braid. It is also important to recognize that loss of tension strength and absorption are separate processes (i.e., suture may lose tensile strength rapidly but absorb slowly or vice versa).

Note: Suture size is denoted by the number of zeros and increases in number as the diameter of suture decreases, for example, 7–0 is smaller than 1–0. Refer to Table 23–3 as a guide for suggested suture size based on anatomic location.

Table 23–3

Suggested Guidelines for Suture Material and Size for Body Region

Body Region	Percutaneous (Skin)	Deep (Dermal)
Scalp	5–0/4–0 monofilament*	4–0 absorbable[†]
Ear	6–0 monofilament	—
Eyelid	7–0/6–0 monofilament	—
Eyebrow	6–0/5–0 monofilament	5–0 absorbable
Nose	6–0 monofilament	5–0 absorbable
Lip	6–0 monofilament	5–0 absorbable
Oral mucosa	—	5–0 absorbable[‡]
Other parts of face/forehead	6–0 monofilament	5–0 absorbable
Trunk	5–0/4–0 monofilament	3–0 absorbable
Extremities	5–0/4–0 monofilament	4–0 absorbable
Hand	5–0 monofilament	5–0 absorbable
Extensor tendon	4–0 monofilament	—
Foot/sole	4–0/3–0 monofilament	4–0 absorbable
Vagina	—	4–0 absorbable
Scrotum	—	5–0 absorbable
Penis	5–0 monofilament	—

* Nonabsorbable monofilaments include nylon (Ethilon, Dermalon), polypropylene (Prolene), and poly-butester (Novafil).

[†] Absorbable materials for dermal and fascial closures include polyglycolic acid (Dexon, Dexon Plus), polyglactin 910 (Vicryl), polydioxanone (PDS [monofilament absorbable]), and polyglyconate (Maxon [monofilament absorbable]).

[‡] Absorbable materials for mucosal and scrotal closure include chromic gut and polyglactin 910 (Vicryl).

Adapted from Trott AT: Wounds and Lacerations, 2nd ed. St. Louis, Mosby-Year Book, 1998, p 179.

■ Needles

Note: The final consideration for proper suture selection is based on needle characteristics and includes the following:

- ■ The smallest-diameter needle to accomplish the task should be chosen to avoid unnecessary tissue trauma.
- ■ The type of needle should be considered and includes several shapes.
- ■ A conventional cutting needle is often used for skin and has three cutting edges (two lateral and one on the *inner* concave curve).
- ■ A reverse cutting needle is often used for tough tissue such as ligament and also has three cutting edges (two lateral and one on the *outer* concave curve).
- ■ A taper needle is circumferentially rounded with a point and it is useful intraoperatively on delicate tissue such as peritoneum. Figure 23–3 illustrates the various parts of a needle.

Other Instruments

- ■ Needle driver or holder, appropriate for the size of needle and suturing material being used
- ■ Skin forceps
- ■ Suture scissors

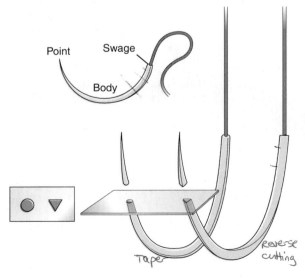

Figure 23–3. The parts of a taper and reverse cutting needle. (Redrawn from Trott AT: Wounds and Lacerations, 2nd ed. St. Louis, Mosby-Year Book, 1998, p 31.)

Procedure for Performing Suture Techniques (General Information)

Caution: **Proper instrument technique is paramount.**

Needle Driver-Holder

1. Using sterile gloves, hold the needle driver with the dominant hand while the nondominant hand holds the forceps.

Note: The tripod grip is an excellent method for use with both the needle driver and scissors as it maximizes hand control (Fig. 23–4). This may include the distal phalanx of the thumb and fourth digit inserted into the rings of the needle driver but never allowing the digits to move into rings more proximal than the distal interphalangeal joint.

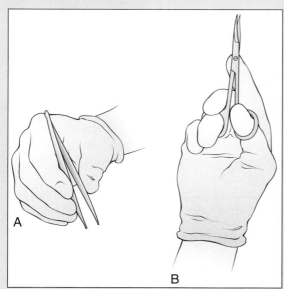

Figure 23–4. *A* Redrawn from Trott AT: Wounds and Lacerations, 2nd ed. St. Louis, Mosby-Year Book, 1998, p 32.

2. Grasp the needle at the tip of the needle driver and load so that it is perpendicular to the needle driver, as shown in Figure 23–5.

Note: The needle concavity will be furthest from the clinician, and the point of the needle will be pointing to the nondominant shoulder as the clinician views the needle.

3. Grasp the needle at the junction of its proximal and middle third so that it can be moved more distal (toward the point) for smaller bites.

Note: The tip of the needle should never be grasped because it can become dull. To minimize needle stick injuries, needles should never be touched with the fingers; they can be loaded easily from the packet they come in or from any flat surface.

Forceps

1. For maximal control, hold the forceps like a pencil, as shown in Figure 23–4.

Note: If the forceps have teeth, avoid a tight tissue grasp to eliminate skin trauma ("teeth marks").

2. One method lifts the tissue rather than grasping it by placing one tooth of the forceps into the wound edge and lifting gently without closing the other toothed face to the skin surface.

Scissors

1. Cut with the tips of the scissors using the tripod grip and with the screw of the scissors facing up and at a 45-degree angle to the suture as in Figure 23–4.

Procedure for Performing Suture Techniques (General Information) – *(continued)*

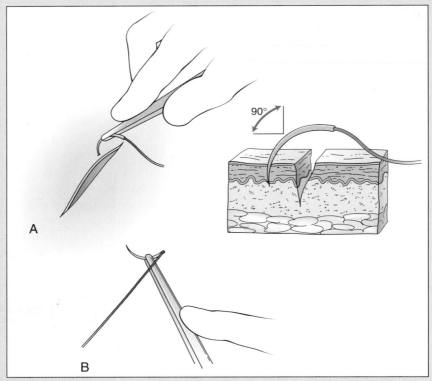

Figure 23–5. *A* Redrawn from Trott AT: Wounds and Lacerations, 2nd ed. St. Louis, Mosby-Year Book, 1998, p 33.

Note: Scissors are manufactured to cut most accurately with the tips.

Note: The technique of cutting at a 45-degree angle helps eliminate the possibility of accidentally cutting out the knots when no tail is left intraoperatively. One should never attempt to cut suture without full visualization of the distal scissor tips to avoid cutting tissue inadvertently.

Procedure for Suture Placement

1. Introduce the suture needle into the tissue at a 90-degree angle or less (toward the wound) (see Fig. 23–5); try to approximate this angle as closely as possible. This can be maximized with full wrist pronation.

   Note: This is to promote skin eversion or a slight tenting of the wound edge at

Procedure for Suture Placement – *(continued)*

closure to minimize the ultimate scar visibility. With time, a normal scar will contract and flatten and appear flush, casting no shadow. Conversely, a wound that initially is closed flush will often later "sink-in" and create a shadow of light that highlights and draws attention to the scar. **Note:** The depth of needle penetration is determined by the wound depth. Sometimes a bite can be completed by one pass through the tissue (skin surface, wound edge, wound edge, skin surface); other times the needle should be reloaded halfway through or after it passes from skin surface through the first wound edge. This allows for specific placement of the wound edge to the adjacent wound edge to ensure a side-to-side match and is necessary for larger bites in a deep wound. Typically, the total stitch length should be as wide as the wound is deep as shown in Figure 23–6. **Note:** If a needle begins to bend, excessive pressure has been placed on it by either poor technique or attempting too large a bite. Taking a bite deeper than the wound may cause important structures to

be traumatized from blind needle placement. Conversely, taking too superficial a bite may leave dead space below the closure, inviting blood accumulation, bacterial growth, and subsequent infection.

2. Place the needle bite just superficial to the wound depth.

Note: This allows complete visualization of structures penetrated and adequately closes the wound.

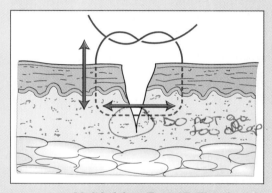

Figure 23–6. Modified from Trott AT: Wounds and Lacerations, 2nd ed. St. Louis, Mosby-Year Book, 113.

Procedure for Performing the Instrument Tie

1. Place the needle driver between the suture ends and, with the nondominant hand, wrap the suture with the needle attached over the instrument twice on the first throw of the first knot only (surgeon's knot, used to prevent slippage) (Fig. 23–7A and B).

2. Grasp the short end of the suture with the needle driver, and the short and long suture ends switch sides (see Fig. 23–7C).

Note: This is considered one throw. Two throws makes one knot. Next, the needle driver is placed between the two suture ends and *one* wrap of the

Procedure for Performing the Instrument Tie – *(continued)*

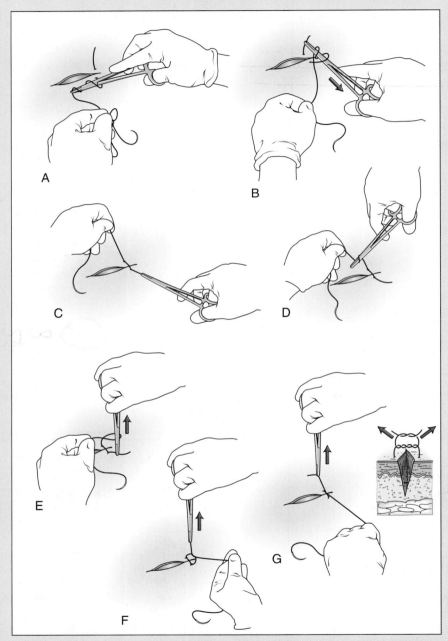

Figure 23–7. Redrawn from Trott AT: Wounds and Lacerations, 2nd ed. St. Louis, Mosby-Year Book, 1998, pp 98–102.

Procedure for Performing the Instrument Tie – *(continued)*

long suture over the instrument is used (Figure 23–7D).

3. Again, grasp the short suture end with the needle driver. The long and short suture ends again switch sides (see Fig. 23–7E).

Note: A circle should be seen as the suture comes down to the skin surface. This suture circle should be placed at 90 degrees to the wound length for simple interrupted and vertical mattress sutures (horizontal mattress sutures will be parallel with the wound) (see Fig. 23–7F).

4. Repeat these steps with only one wrap over the needle driver on every successive throw until the suture is cut.

Note: Remember the only throw that gets two wraps is the first throw of the first knot in a series. Therefore, an even number of throws will ensure completion of all knots. Compare the diagrams of a typical knot (see Fig. 23–6) and a surgeon's knot (see Fig. 23–7G).

Note: The number of knots depends on the anatomic location (below the skin surface requires fewer knots; above the skin surface requires more knots) and suture material (those with "memory" often require more knots). Usually three to four knots on the skin surface will suffice. The needle remains connected throughout these steps and usually poses no problem to the clinician or patient, as it remains stationary lying on the sterile field. There is no need to remember where you are in a sequence, as in the "over-under technique," with this method.

5. After an adequate number of knots are secured, pull the suture knot to one side to avoid knot placement directly over the wound to minimize debris collection and potential infection.

Note: The suture is now ready for cutting. The "suture tail" or "suture tag" will be used during suture removal.

Note: Two helpful rules can be used to estimate this length: (1) The tail length should be equal to the distance from the wound edge to the suture border. (2) The tail length should be slightly less than the distance between adjacent knots. Use the previously described scissor technique to cut the suture.

Procedure for Performing the Simple Interrupted Stitch

Note: It is important to estimate carefully the number and size of sutures necessary to close the wound adequately without placing too many and too small or too few and too large stitches. Most simple interrupted stitches should measure between 3 and 10 mm in length and should be about this same distance apart. The method described in the instrument tie section is consistent with the simple interrupted stitch, which is frequently used to close most lacerations.

1. One method of closure includes closure by halves. Place the first stitch at the halfway point along the length of the wound.

2. Place the next stitches at the halfway point between the first stitch and each end of the wound.

Procedure for Performing the Simple Interrupted Stitch – *(continued)*

3. Place the next stitches between each of the previous stitches until the wound is approximated.

Note: An alternate method involves beginning at one end of the wound and placing evenly spaced sutures along the length until you reach the opposite end of the wound. Be careful to place the sutures evenly on both sides of the wound; failure to do so may result in an asymmetric end to the wound known as a *dog ear,* in which one side of the wound appears to be longer than the other side, creating a redundant "ear" of tissue.

Procedure for Correcting Dog Ear Deformity

If a dog ear develops, the sutures should be removed and the closure reattempted. If it appears that correction cannot be achieved by reapproximation, the following method illustrates an acceptable procedure for correction.

1. Make an incision 45 degrees at the end of the redundant side.

Note: This tissue is undermined to create a small flap, which when gentle traction is applied can be excised as shown.

2. Close the wound in the usual fashion creating a "hockey-stick" appearance (Fig. 23–8, middle).

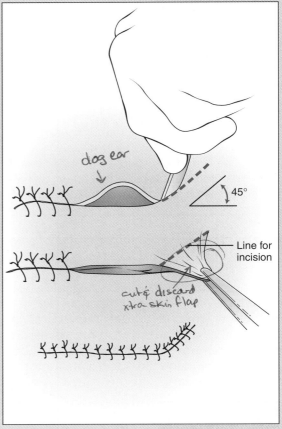

Figure 23–8. Redrawn from Trott AT: Wounds and Lacerations, 2nd ed. St. Louis, Mosby-Year Book, 1998, p 37.

Procedure for Performing the Vertical Mattress ("Far-Far/Near-Near")

The next most commonly performed stitch is the vertical mattress stitch. This stitch is so named because the stitch lies in a plane perpendicular (vertical) to the skin. It is useful for closing deeper wounds (e.g., those of the scalp) in which the closure occurs at two levels (superficial and deep), eliminating dead space.

1. To perform the vertical mattress stitch, introduce the needle "far" and exit "far" from the wound edge, diving deep but just superficial to the wound depth (Fig. 23–9).

Note: Figure 23–9 illustrates a superficial wound with first stitch traversing below the wound margin. Most wounds will have the first stitch traverse within the lower portion of the wound margin, as illustrated in Figure 23–6.

2. Next, starting on the same side as the first exit point, load the needle backhand (needle points to dominant shoulder while all other criteria remain unchanged) and enter "near" the wound edge and exit on the original side "near" the wound edge, both at a level more superficial than the original deep first pass.

3. The remainder of the instrument tying steps is the same (see Fig. 23–7).

Note: Performing the second step first, or a "near-near/far-far" stitch, should be avoided to eliminate "blind" needle placement and creating inadvertent trauma to unseen structures.

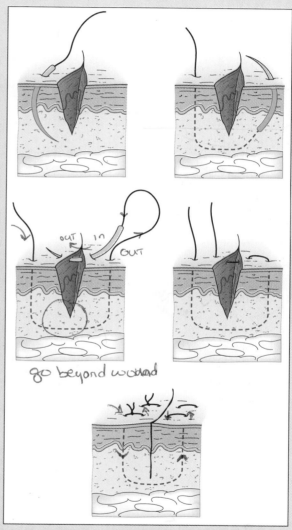

Figure 23–9. Redrawn from Trott AT: Wounds and Lacerations, 2nd ed. St. Louis, Mosby-Year Book, 1998, p 38.

Procedure for Performing the Horizontal Mattress Stitch

The horizontal mattress stitch lies in a plane parallel to the skin. It is useful when there is a flap of tissue or when the tension of the stitch is to be predominantly on one side (the knotted side). For example, this method works well in a wound with a vascular side and a relatively avascular side, as the avascular area is pulled toward the vascular side with most of the tension being on the vascular side. In other stitch types, the tension is shared equally by each side.

1. To perform the horizontal mattress stitch, start on the vascular side and exit on the relatively avascular side.
2. Re-enter backhanded on this avascular side parallel to the wound edge and adjacent to the original exit site; the final exit is on the original vascular side.

Note: The stitch should look like a box. All knot tying steps are performed as previously discussed except that the stitch is brought down parallel (not perpendicular) to the wound line (Fig. 23–10).

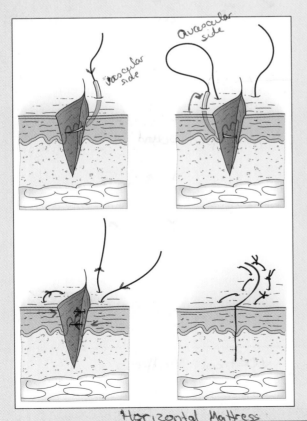

Horizontal Mattress

Figure 23–10. Redrawn from Trott AT: Wounds and Lacerations, 2nd ed. St. Louis, Mosby-Year Book, 1998, p 39.

Procedure for Performing the Continuous-Running-Baseball Stitch

The advantages of the continuous stitch is that it can be performed quickly and can be applied tightly if "locked." The disadvantages are:

■ If <u>one loop is broken, the entire wound may open.</u>

■ It <u>cannot be partially removed</u> as can other stitch types (e.g., every other or a wound segment) to allow for drainage when managing an early wound infection.

■ It may leave a cosmetically suboptimal scar with a "<u>railroad tracks</u>" <u>appearance.</u>

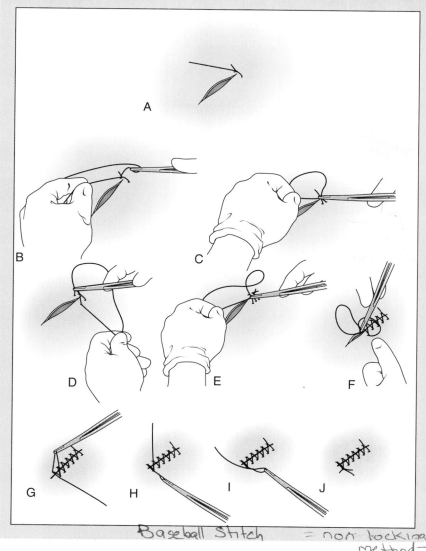

Figure 23–11. Redrawn from Trott AT: Wounds and Lacerations, 2nd ed. St. Louis, Mosby-Year Book, 1998, pp 123–128.

Baseball Stitch = non locking method

Procedure for Performing the Continuous-Running-Baseball Stitch – *(continued)*

The continuous suture is performed as follows:

1. Place a suture at the end of the wound in the same fashion as that outlined for a simple interrupted suture (only cut suture on non-needle side after knot is tied).

2. Using the initial suture as an anchor, additional sutures are placed (throws) in a continuous fashion until the entire wound is reapproximated. Enter next to knot and exit on opposite side skin surface at a 45-degree angle to the wound and reenter through skin surface directly across and repeat. (Fig. 23–11).

3. When the end of the wound is reached, the final suture is tied in the same manner as that outlined for the simple interrupted suture, but the needle side is tied to the last loop before it has been pulled taut. When cut, it will yield three tails.

Note: The method illustrated demonstrates the "non-locking" method. To "lock" the suture, bring the needle up through the previous loop before it has been pulled taut creating a tight seal, which can be particularly useful intraoperatively.

Procedure for Performing the Subcuticular Stitch

The subcuticular stitch is often used to close a surgical incision or a very clean wound. Absorbable suture material must be used if the suture will not be removed at a later time.

1. Create an initial buried knot to anchor the suture (Fig. 23–12).

2. Begin making equal passes through the wound edges in the horizontal plane until you have traversed the length of the wound (entering and exiting the dermal layer from side to side).

Note: It is important to keep the bites equal and approximate the tissue so that it aligns properly.

3. A final buried knot is tied at the opposite wound end to complete and anchor the opposite end of the suture. Leave the needle side of the suture tail uncut (cut the loop side).

Note: The suture is secure because of the final buried anchor knot.

4. Bury the final tail by reentering the closed wound with the needle and attached suture and exiting on the skin surface 1 cm away from the wound edge.

5. Cut it flush with the skin.

6. Apply skin tapes over the wound surface.

Note: No suture will be visible on the skin surface.

Procedure for Performing the Subcuticular Stitch – *(continued)*

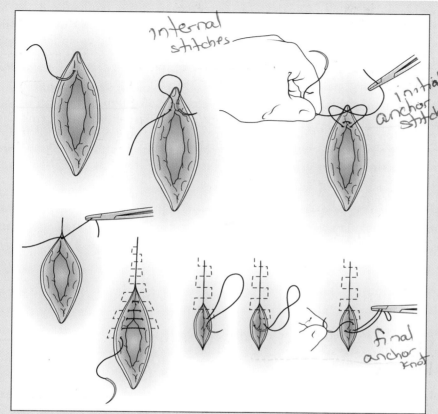

Figure 23–12. Redrawn from Trott AT: Wounds and Lacerations, 2nd ed. St. Louis, Mosby-Year Book, 1998, p 41.

Special Considerations

Several important general concepts exist and are discussed based on anatomic location.

- Hair can be shaved to allow for better wound exploration, irrigation, and closure, but this is *not* mandatory. Often just trimming the surrounding hair is helpful without further traumatizing the skin by creating potential sites of infection from the minute lacerations and skin abrasions that often occur during the shaving process. Cutting the suture tails longer than usual and using an alternate suture color will also facilitate removal in hairy anatomic locations and minimize the need for shaving hair.
- Never shave an eyebrow, as the hair may not grow back at all or will grow back irregularly. It is also critical to line up the hair and skin

borders exactly to avoid misalignment. If an eyebrow has been shaved and the wound is sutured closed, it is difficult to know where these borders exist. Therefore, the possibility of even slight misalignment of the hair to the skin border can occur, and if the hair grows back it will look very disfiguring. Usually these areas can be visualized well enough to suture them adequately without the need for significant hair removal. Infection rates do not seem to be significantly decreased by hair removal and in fact may be elevated because of skin trauma.

- Following this same principle is the concept of aligning the vermilion border of the lips. The best method for doing this begins by placing the first stitch at the border of the skin and mucosal edges (use 6–0 nylon). The remaining wound can be closed using nonabsorbable suture for the skin and absorbable suture for the lip itself. It is critical that this border be aligned exactly.

- If an incision has to be made, it is important to recognize and follow the natural skin tension lines. Scar visibility is minimized when it runs parallel to these lines and is more prominent when placed perpendicular or oblique to them (see Fig. 23–2).

Materials Utilized for Using Skin Staplers

- Stapler with staples—sterile disposable type
- Tissue forceps
- Skin tape

Procedure for Using Skin Staplers

Note: Skin staplers are sterile, disposable, cost-effective, and useful for long, linear lacerations of the scalp, trunk, and extremities because they can be applied quickly with the same ultimate cosmetic result as suture.

1. Place staples over the approximated wound and firmly squeeze the trigger to deliver each staple, everting the tissue edges.

Note: Staplers should not be used to close lacerations of the face or hands or those over a joint. They should also be avoided in areas that might later require computed tomography or magnetic resonance imaging (e.g., head injury).

2. To remove, use a special sterile, disposable device and squeeze this device at each staple. The staple legs are straightened. Then pull the staple from the tissue.

Note: Skin tapes are often placed after removal of the staples.

Materials Utilized for Applying Wound Adhesives

- Ampules of wound adhesive
- Cotton-tipped applicator

Procedure for Applying Wound Adhesives

Note: Wound adhesives are another variation of wound closure that may be used; they can be applied quickly and painlessly for easily approximating skin edges of surgical incisions or lacerations of the face, trunk, and limbs. They are not recommended over skin creases, areas of movement, or long lacerations, or for hand injuries. Other contraindications include wounds with active infection, those that involve mucosal surfaces or occur at mucocutaneous junctions, and areas exposed to body fluids. In addition, some clinicians avoid areas of dense hair such as the scalp. After the usual cleaning, débriding, and care to achieve hemostasis, the area is carefully dried.

1. Crush an ampule and invert it, soaking the cotton-tipped applicator with solution.

2. With the applicator, lightly paint over the approximated wound edge three times in succession with 30 seconds' drying time between.
Caution: It is important to avoid applying the fluid into the wound and to avoid spillage to surrounding areas such as the eye.

3. Because the adhesive is of low viscosity (runny), position the anatomic area in the horizontal plane to avoid runoff or protect surrounding skin with a barrier.

4. After full strength is reached at 2.5 minutes, a protective dressing can be applied at 5 minutes but is not required.

Follow-Up Care and Instructions for Sutured and Stapled Wounds

- Advise the patient to keep the wound site clean and dry. Some clinicians advocate no contact with water at all for 48 hours, whereas others allow gentle bathing with soap and water or a quick shower with careful drying of the site afterward, but all emphasize no prolonged soaking of the site in water.
- If applicable, elevate the area.
- Instruct the patient verbally and in writing regarding the desired frequency of wound checking and dressing changing. It is suggested that the patient remove the dressing twice each day to visualize the site for

signs of infection and to reapply antibiotic ointment.] A clean, dry dressing should then be applied. Some sites may be left open to the air (face, neck, scalp).

- Instruct the patient to apply a cold compress for the first 48 hours after surgery in sites with significant associated soft tissue involvement, such as a contusion (20 minutes each time four to five times per day).]
- Verbalize and write the signs of infection for the patient to watch for and instruct him or her to return if there is an increase in pain, redness beyond the wound margin, or red streaking; if the area becomes warm, swollen, and tender; or if there is discharge or drainage from the wound, tenderness under the arms or groin, fever, or chills.]
- Consider possible activity restriction or immobilization.]
- Consider analgesics] (acetaminophen, nonsteroidal anti-inflammatory drugs [NSAIDs]).
- Advise the patient about when he or she should return for a wound check and suture or staple removal.]
- Educate the patient that scars take 1 year to fully mature and that after initial healing it is best to avoid strong sunlight and to apply sunscreen to the site.]
- Administration of antibiotics is sometimes advised, although small, uncomplicated wounds and lacerations often do not require them. If the particular wound is high risk, a wound check in 24 to 48 hours may be necessary. It is always best to have the original provider assess the wound if possible, because he or she has a baseline for comparison. Antibiotics should be considered in the following high-risk wounds:

Criteria for antibiotic Tx

- Wounds that are more than 12 hours old at initial presentation, especially those of the hands
- Human or animal bites, including those caused by the patient's teeth (intraoral laceration)
- Crush wounds
- Heavily contaminated wounds
- Wounds involving relatively avascular areas, such as the cartilage of the ear
- Wounds involving joint spaces, tendon, or bone
- Severe paronychia and felons
- Wounds in patients with a history of valvular heart disease
- Wounds in patients with immunosuppression (diabetes, chronic steroid use, infection with human immunodeficiency virus [HIV])

Suture Removal

Anatomic location dictates the length of time sutures should be left in place to ensure adequate healing. Table 23–4 may be useful as a general guide. It is important to remember that adults heal more slowly than children do and that other medical conditions may increase healing time.]

Table 23–4
Recommended Intervals for Removal of Percutaneous (Skin) Sutures

Location	Days to Removal
Scalp	6–8
Face	4–5
Ear	4–5
Chest/abdomen	8–10
Back	12–14
Arm/leg*	8–10
Hand*	8–10
Fingertip	10–12
Foot	12–14

* Add 2 to 3 days for joint extensor surfaces.
From Trott AT: Wounds and Lacerations, 2nd ed. St. Louis, Mosby-Year Book, 1998, p 366.

- The wound should be inspected for signs of infection before the sutures are removed, including erythema beyond the wound margin, discharge, swelling, pain, or tenderness.
- Some practitioners advocate the use of povidone-iodine (Betadine) both before and after suture or staple removal.
- Using sterile instruments, cut the suture to minimize dragging contaminated suture through the patient's body.
- If sutures are tight and difficult to cut, use of a No. 11 scalpel blade should be considered. Turn the sharp side away from the patient to sneak under the suture to avoid excessive pulling. Diagrams of correct and incorrect methods of various stitch removals are shown in Figure 23–13.
- It is important to ensure that all the nonabsorbable suture is removed and that none is left inside the body to act as a foreign body.
- Often, minimal erythema surrounding the wound, secondary to local reaction to these materials, is alleviated 24 to 48 hours after the sutures are removed.
- Some practitioners advocate the use of antibacterial ointment.
- Most wounds should be left open to the air at this point and do not require a dressing.

Staple Removal

- Align the staple remover so that it is centered under the staple.
- It is important to recognize that the staple removal device is squeezed and then the staple is lifted in two distinct motions; combining them is painful to the patient and traumatizes tissue.

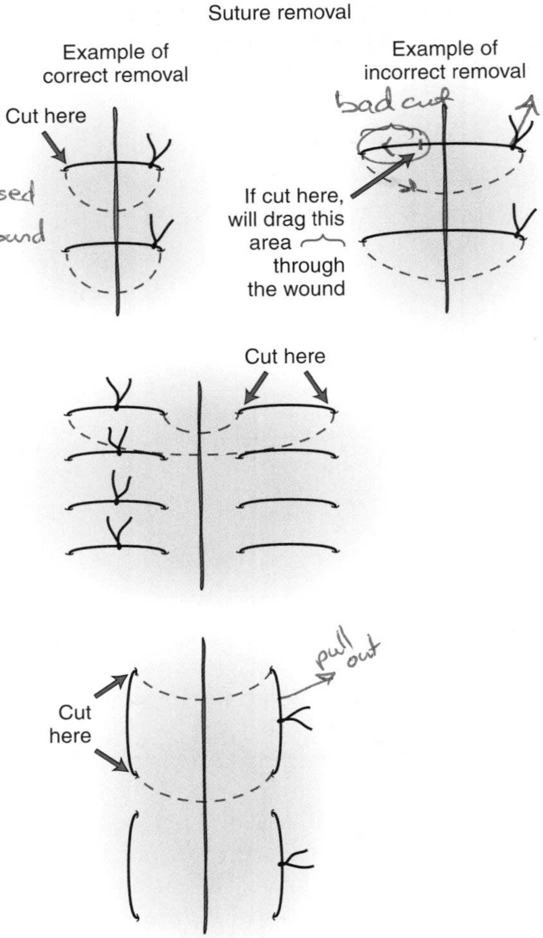

Suture removal

Example of
correct removal

Example of
incorrect removal

bad cut

Cut here

*you want to
avoid dragging exposed
suture material thru wound*

If cut here,
will drag this
area
through
the wound

Cut here

Figure 23–13. Suture removal.

Cut
here

pull out

- Often, minimal erythema surrounding the wound, secondary to local reaction to the staples, is alleviated 24 to 48 hours after the staples are removed.
- Some practitioners advocate the use of antibacterial ointment.
- Most wounds should be left open to the air at this point and do not require a dressing.

Follow-Up Care and Instructions for Adhesive-Closed Wounds

- Notify the patient that the adhesive will naturally start to slough off 5 to 10 days after placement.

- Caution the patient to avoid scratching, rubbing, or picking at the site.
- Instruct the patient that the area should not be scrubbed, soaked, or exposed to prolonged wetness (the area should be kept dry; a quick shower can be taken, if necessary).
- Advise the patient not to apply medication in liquid or ointment form to the site.

The cost of skin adhesives may be comparable when costs for suture kits, suture materials, clinician time, and follow-up visits for suture removal are considered.

Reference

Ethicon: Wound Closure Manual. New Brunswick, NJ, Ethicon, 1985; website available at *http://www.ethiconinc.com/*

Bibliography

- Trott AT: Wounds and Lacerations: Emergency Care and Closure, 2nd ed. St. Louis, CV Mosby, 1998.
- Principles of Primary Wound Management, A Guide to the Fundamentals. Fairfax; Va, Mortiere, 1996.
- Pfenninger JL, Fowler GC, eds: Procedures for Primary Care Physicians, St. Louis, CV Mosby, 1994.

Chapter 24

Dermatologic Procedures

▷ Michelle DiBaise

Procedure Goals and Objectives

Goal: To perform biopsies, electrosurgery, and acne surgery successfully while observing standard precautions and with the minimal degree of risk to the patient.

Objectives: The student will be able to . . .

► Describe the indications, contraindications, and rationale for performing biopsies, electrosurgery, and acne surgery.

► Identify and describe common complications associated with performing biopsies, electrosurgery, and acne surgery.

► Describe the essential anatomy and physiology associated with performing biopsies, electrosurgery, and acne surgery.

► Identify the materials necessary for performing biopsies, electrosurgery, and acne surgery and their proper use.

► Describe the steps in performing biopsies, electrosurgery, and acne surgery.

► Identify the important aspects of care after biopsies, electrosurgery, and acne surgery.

Biopsies

Background and History

Skin biopsies are performed to determine the cause of a lesion or to remove the lesion, or both. The general categories of biopsies include shave, punch, and excision. A shave biopsy removes the epidermis and a portion of the upper dermis and is performed along the horizontal plane. Variations on the shave technique include snip excisions, as performed for skin tag removal, and curettage, as performed for many benign superficial lesions. A punch biopsy can be either incisional or excisional. An incisional biopsy removes only a portion of a lesion, whereas an excisional biopsy removes the entire lesion. Larger excisional biopsies can be completed using a No. 15 blade. Incisional and excisional biopsies extend to the subcutaneous fat. Determining the correct biopsy technique is based on the clinical diagnosis (Fig. 24–1) and the desired cosmetic outcome (Tobinick and Usatine, 1998).

Shave Biopsy

Indications

- Seborrheic keratoses
- Verrucous lesions

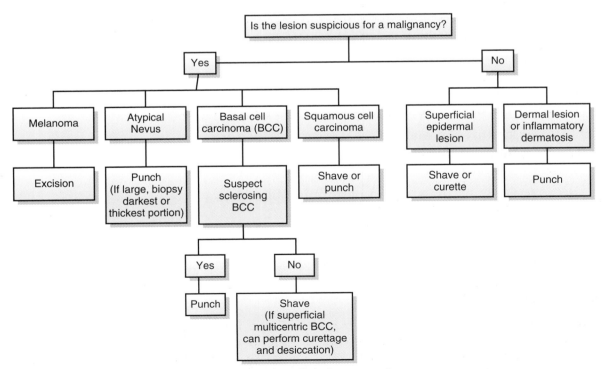

Figure 24–1. Algorithm for biopsy technique based on clinical assessment.

- Molluscum contagiosum
- Superficial basal cell carcinomas

Occasionally, a shave biopsy may be performed on benign nevi, particularly on the face, when a good cosmetic result is essential (Bennett, 1988a; Siegel and Usatine, 1998b; Tobinick and Usatine, 1998).

Snip excisions may be performed for the following (Bennett, 1988a; Siegel and Usatine, 1998b):

- Acrochordons (skin tags)
- Pedunculated nevi

Care must be taken not to perform this technique on dermal nevi without anesthesia, as the patient will experience greater discomfort because of innervation of nevi.

Curettage may be performed on benign superficial lesions such as the following (Ho, 1999):

- Molluscum contagiosum
- Verruca vulgaris
- Seborrheic keratoses, with or without cryotherapy

For superficial multicentric basal cell carcinomas and Bowen's disease, curettage and desiccation are alternatives to excision (Bennett, 1988a; Schwartz and Stoll, 1999; Usatine, 1998a).

When curettage is used, histologic margins are impossible to determine. If tumor margins need to be determined, an alternative biopsy technique should be used.

Contraindications

Contraindications for a shave biopsy include the following (Siegel and Usatine, 1998b):

- Most pigmented lesions, except in the case of benign nevi as stated earlier
- For the diagnosis of infiltrative dermatoses
- In a suspected sclerosing basal cell carcinoma
- Any lesion with a dermal component

Potential Complications

The most common complications seen with shave biopsy include the following (Siegel and Usatine, 1998b):

- Bleeding: Most bleeding is readily stopped with the use of 20% aluminum chloride (Drysol). If bleeding is more brisk, as occurs when patients are taking aspirin or warfarin, or if the shave is too deep into the dermis, hand-held cautery may be used. Monsel's solution (ferric subsulfate) and silver nitrate may be used, but tattooing can occur with its use. It is not recommended that Monsel's solution or silver nitrate be used on the face or highly visible areas (Siegel and Usatine, 1998b; Stasko, 1994; Usatine, 1998b).

- Infection
- Regrowth of the lesion: Lesions such as warts and incompletely removed nevi or seborrheic keratoses can regrow. An estimated 1 in 20 nevi will regenerate (Siegel and Usatine, 1998b).
- Scarring: Scarring, which usually has the appearance of an atrophic, lighter than normal area, may occur even when the procedure is performed correctly. It is more of a risk if the shave is too deep into the dermis.
- Some discomfort may be experienced with the injection of anesthetic.

Review of Essential Anatomy and Physiology

For simplicity, the skin structure consists of the epidermis or topmost layer of the skin, the dermal-epidermal junction, the dermis, and the subcutaneous fat. It is essential that the practitioner have knowledge of the vasculature and nerves of the biopsy site before performing any biopsy of the skin. In addition, adequate knowledge of the lines of skin tension is required to determine the orientation of punch and excisional biopsies. Suture lines will be less likely to develop into a widened scar if placed parallel to the lines of tension (Fig. 24–2) (Moy and Usatine, 1998b; Zalla and Roenigk, 1996). In addition, placing suture lines parallel to wrinkles will improve the cosmetic appearance of the end defect. Caution must be used when performing elliptical excisions on the face—particularly on the forehead or near the eye or lips—so that distortion does not occur. Large excisions in these areas may necessitate a graft or flap closure.

Standard Precautions ▷ Every practitioner should use Standard Precautions at all times when interacting with patients, especially when performing procedures. Determining the level of precaution necessary requires the practitioner to exercise clinical judgment based on the patient's history and the potential for exposure to body fluids or aerosol-borne pathogens (for further discussion, see Chapter 2).

Patient Preparation

- Explain the procedure to the patient or guardian, or both, and be prepared to answer any questions.
- The patient or patient's guardian must give informed consent before the start of the procedure.
- A topical anesthetic can be provided, which must be applied under occlusion approximately 1 hour before the procedure. If the topical anesthesia is used, the occlusive tape is removed and cleaned with gauze.

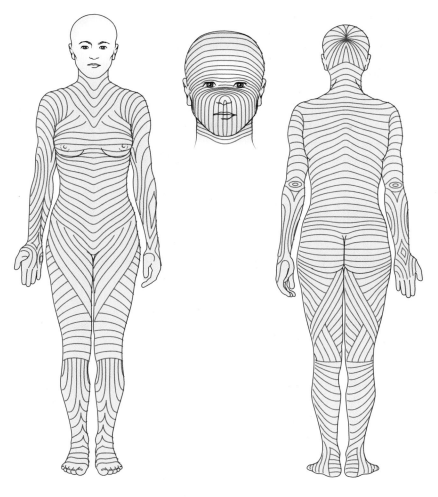

Figure 24–2. Skin tension lines of the body surface. (Adapted from Trott AT: Wounds and Lacerations, 2nd ed. St. Louis, Mosby-Year Book, 1998, p 17.)

Materials Utilized to Perform a Shave, Snip, or Curettage Biopsy

- Topical anesthetic applied under occlusion 1 hour before the procedure
- Sterile gloves
- Sterile towels
- Alcohol pads
- A No. 15 blade or a razor blade
- Lidocaine with or without epinephrine, as indicated
- A 3-mL syringe and a 30-gauge needle for local anesthesia
- 4 × 4 gauze
- Forceps

- Cotton-tipped applicator and 20% aluminum chloride for hemostasis (for more vascular lesions, hand-held cautery may be needed)
- Specimen container

Note: Most biopsy specimens may be sent in formalin containers. The exceptions to this are specimens sent for culture or immunofluorescent studies and specimens in which formalin will break down the tissue, such as in xanthomatous lesions (Fitzpatrick et al, 1999; Schultz, 1996). In these instances, specimens should be sent fresh. This is accomplished by placing the specimen on a sterile 4 × 4 gauze moistened with sterile water or normal saline in a sterile urine cup. All fresh specimens need to be transported immediately to the pathology department for examination.

- Polymyxin B sulfate—bacitracin zinc (Polysporin) and an adhesive bandage

If skin tags (acrochordons) are to be removed, the following equipment is needed:
- Alcohol pads
- Forceps
- Tenometry scissors
- 4 × 4 gauze
- 20% aluminum chloride
- Cotton-tipped applicator
- Polymyxin B sulfate—bacitracin zinc and an adhesive bandage
  For curettage the following equipment is needed:
- Alcohol pads
- 4 × 4 gauze
- 20% aluminum chloride
- Cotton-tipped applicator
- Polymyxin B sulfate—bacitracin zinc and an adhesive bandage
- Optional equipment includes hand-held cautery and cryogun

Procedure for Performing a Shave, Snip, or Curettage Biopsy

1. Place a sterile towel around the biopsy site.
2. Lightly clean the area with an alcohol pad unless cautery use is anticipated.

Note: Because alcohol is flammable, use nonflammable povidone-iodine and water to prepare the skin if cautery may be used.

3. If the lesion has the potential to blanche with an injection of lidocaine with epinephrine, such as in basal cell carcinomas, mark the margins of the lesion with a sterile surgical marker before the anesthetic is injected (Bennett, 1988a; Siegel and Usatine, 1998b).

Procedure for Performing a Shave, Snip, and Curettage Biopsy – *(continued)*

4. Inject the lesion with anesthetic so that a wheal is raised.
5. Hold the No. 15 blade flat and parallel with the skin surface.
6. If a razor blade is used, snap it in half lengthwise and bow the ends so that the middle of the blade is flat and parallel with the skin surface.
7. Use a gentle sawing motion to shave through the lesion (Fig. 24–3).
8. The lesion may be elevated with the use of forceps or by spearing the lesion with a needle.

Note: Care must be taken not to crush the lesion with the forceps, which will distort the histologic specimen, referred to as crush artifact.

9. Attempt to shave the base of the lesion completely by shaving into the uppermost portion of the dermis.

Note: If the specimen is too thin (just epidermis), a good histologic diagnosis may not be made.

10. To complete the shave, it is sometimes useful to stabilize the far end of the lesion with a cotton-tipped applicator to cut against.
11. Once the lesion is removed, most light bleeding can be stopped with direct pressure and 20% aluminum chloride on a cotton-tipped applicator.

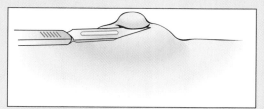

Figure 24–3. Redrawn from Pfenninger JL, Fowler GC: Procedures for Primary Care Physicians. St. Louis, Mosby-Year Book, 1994, p 22.

Note: If bleeding is more brisk or is not stopped with the preceding procedure, hand-held cautery should be used.

12. Place an antibiotic ointment such as mupirocin (Bactroban) or polymyxin B sulfate—bacitracin zinc on an adhesive bandage to dress the wound.

Snip Excision

1. Clean the area lightly with an alcohol pad.

Note: There is usually no need to anesthetize the area. The exception is larger skin tags because they may actually be dermal nevi.

2. Pick up the skin tag with forceps and cut at the base with tenometry scissors.
3. If there is any bleeding, stop with 20% aluminum chloride on a cotton-tipped applicator.
4. Place antibiotic ointment on an adhesive bandage to dress the wound.

Curettage

Note: For seborrheic keratoses, verrucous lesions, or molluscum contagiosum, cryotherapy (see Chapter 27) applied first and followed quickly by curettage will require no local injection because liquid nitrogen acts as a partial anesthetic (Graham, 1999).

1. If the patient is apprehensive, a topical anesthetic can be applied 1 hour before the procedure.
2. For superficial basal cell carcinomas or any other lesion in which the use of cautery is anticipated, the lesion should be injected with anesthetic.

3. Hold the curette like a pencil with the sharp side down.
4. Stabilize the skin and use quick scraping motions.

Note: When the lesion has been removed, the skin feels different under the curette. Differentiating this change develops with the experience of the provider.

5. Once the lesion is completely removed, obtain hemostasis with 20% aluminum chloride on a cotton-tipped applicator or with hand-held cautery.

Note: Curettage and desiccation for basal cell carcinomas and Bowen's disease requires the following procedure: Curette the lesion until all visible signs of tumor are gone (generally 1 to 2 mm onto normal skin), desiccate the whole base of the lesion with hand-held cautery, and then repeat both steps for three full cycles of curettage and desiccation (Schwartz and Stoll, 1999; Usatine, 1998a).

6. Place antibiotic ointment on an adhesive bandage to dress the wound.

Follow-Up Care and Instructions

- Written instructions on wound care can be provided.
- Instruct the patient to keep the area clean and dry for 24 hours (Siegel et al, 1998; Zalla and Roenigk, 1996).
- After that time, instruct the patient to remove the adhesive bandage and to clean the wound site with soap and water as usual.
- Instruct the patient that if an adhesive bandage is applied, more antibiotic ointment should be placed on the biopsy site. For most small shave biopsy sites, however, the adhesive bandage does not need to be reapplied after the first 24 hours.
- Caution the patient that infection is a rare complication, as antibiotic ointment is applied under the dressing after the procedure is complete.
- Instruct the patient to call the office if the following signs appear: erythematous, tender, warm skin with purulent drainage. When this occurs, antibiotic treatment should be initiated. A broad-spectrum oral antibiotic that covers *Staphylococcus* and *Streptococcus* species should be used, such as cephalexin, dicloxacillin, or erythromycin (Moy and Usatine, 1998a).
- Barring infection, it is not necessary to schedule a return appointment, but the patient should be informed of the results of the pathologic examination.

Punch Biopsy

Indications

When there is a lesion or dermatosis that covers a large surface area and diagnosis needs to be confirmed before treatment is started, taking just a portion of the lesion is indicated (Siegel and Usatine, 1998a).

- It is important to take the most representative area of the lesion for the highest diagnostic yield.
- In the case of pruritic dermatoses, it is best to biopsy a lesion that has not been excoriated.
- For vesicular lesions, an intact vesicle or bulla may provide the best diagnostic yield. In suspected melanoma that is too large to excise at that time, the biopsy should be obtained from the darkest or thickest area of the lesion.

Contraindications

Contraindications for an incisional biopsy would be any lesion with highly suspected malignant potential, such as melanoma, that could be easily excised at the initial visit (Siegel and Usatine, 1998a). Any lesion smaller than 8 to 10 mm, regardless of malignant potential, can easily be removed completely with a punch biopsy.

Potential Complications

The risks for a punch biopsy are similar to those of shave biopsies:

- There is discomfort with the injection of anesthetic.
- The risk for bleeding is higher than in shave biopsies because the skin is incised to the subcutaneous fat, increasing the risk of severing small vessels. Hand-held cautery is the method of choice to stop brisk bleeding.
- In any punch biopsy of 8 mm or larger, subcutaneous sutures will also decrease the bleeding and improve wound healing.
- The infection rate is higher because the procedure is slightly more invasive. As with a shave biopsy, secondary infection can be easily treated with a 5- to 7-day course of a broad-spectrum antibiotic.
- Scarring will occur, but the extent is dependent on the patient's ability to heal versus the size of the end defect. In punch biopsies of 1 cm or larger, it is more cosmetically appealing to perform an excision with a No. 15 blade (Moy and Usatine, 1998b; Siegel and Usatine, 1998a). This will avoid the potential problem of dog-eared closures.

Standard Precautions ▷ Every practitioner should use Standard Precautions at all times when interacting with patients, especially when performing procedures. Determining the level of precaution necessary requires the practitioner to exercise clinical judgment based on the patient's history and the potential for exposure to body fluids or aerosol-borne pathogens (for further discussion, see Chapter 2).

Patient Preparation

- Explain the procedure to the patient or guardian, or both, and be prepared to answer any questions.
- The patient or guardian must give informed consent before the start of the procedure.
- A topical anesthetic can be provided to the patient and must be applied under occlusion approximately 1 hour before the procedure. If topical anesthesia is used, the occlusive tape is removed and cleaned with gauze.

Materials Utilized to Perform a Punch Biopsy

- Topical anesthetic applied under occlusion 1 hour before the procedure
- A metric ruler to determine the size of the lesion
- Sterile gloves
- Sterile towels
- Alcohol pads
- Lidocaine with or without epinephrine, as indicated
- A 3-mL syringe and a 30-gauge needle for local anesthesia (for larger lesions use a 27-gauge, 1 1/2-inch needle)
- 4 × 4 gauze
- Forceps
- Curved scissors
- Needle driver
- Appropriate suture to close skin (see Chapter 23)
- Specimen container
- Polymyxin B sulfate—bacitracin zinc and an adhesive bandage
- A punch is selected that is the appropriate size to completely excise the lesion with minimal surrounding normal skin

   Note: Disposable punches are available in the following sizes: 2 mm, 3 mm, 4 mm, 6 mm, and 8 mm. Nondisposable punches are available in 10 mm, 12 mm, and 15 mm sizes. In the case of incisional biopsies, a 3- or 4-mm punch should be sufficient to make the diagnosis. If enough tissue is needed to send a portion for histologic examination and another portion for culture or immunofluorescent studies, two 3- or 4-mm biopsy specimens may be taken. Alternatively, one 6-mm specimen may be sent with a request to the pathology department to split the specimen and explicit directions on what is to be done with each half.

Procedure for Performing a Punch Biopsy

1. With punch biopsy specimens smaller than 1 cm, place a sterile towel around the biopsy site.
2. Use an alcohol pad to lightly clean the area.
3. If the punch biopsy specimen is to be 1 cm or larger, scrub the area first for 3 minutes with chlorhexidine or povidone-iodine (Hruza, 1999; Moy and Usatine, 1998b).
4. Drape the area with sterile towels.
5. If the lesion has the potential to blanche with the injection of lidocaine with epinephrine, such as in basal cell carcinomas, the margins of the lesion should be marked with a sterile surgical marker before the anesthetic is injected.
6. Inject the lesion with the anesthetic so that the area where the punch will be placed and the surrounding tissue will be sutured is anesthetized.

Note: It is also important to ensure that the full depth of where the punch will extend is anesthetized. Local anesthetic works rapidly, within a minute; however, in highly vascular areas such as the scalp it is prudent to wait 10 minutes to allow the epinephrine to work (Siegel and Usatine, 1998a).

7. After selecting the appropriate size punch, hold the skin taut perpendicular to the lines of tension, wrinkle, or skin fold.
8. Hold the punch perpendicular to the skin and place it so that the lesion is centered within the punch area (Fig. 24–4A).
9. Apply downward pressure while rotating the punch.

Note: It is useful to get into the habit of rotating the punch in one direction, as it is necessary for the biopsy of vesicular or bullous lesions. Rotating back and forth in these cases will distort the plane of cleavage (Bennett, 1988c).

10. The punch should extend to the subcutaneous fat.

Note: When performing a punch biopsy over large vessels or nerves and in areas of thin skin, it is sometimes helpful to pinch the skin upward to avoid damaging underlying structures.

11. Once complete, remove the punch, and the specimen will remain attached to the subcutaneous fat by a pedicle (see Fig 24–4B).

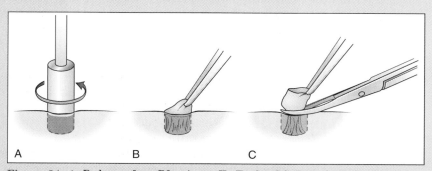

Figure 24–4. Redrawn from Pfenninger JL, Fowler GC: Procedures for Primary Care Physicians. St. Louis, Mosby-Year Book, 1994, p 23.

Procedure for Performing a Punch Biopsy – *(continued)*

12. Gently lift the specimen with a pair of forceps and cut at the base with a pair of scissors (Fig. 24–4C).

Note: Care must be taken not to crush the lesion with the forceps, which could distort the histologic specimen.

Note: If the punch is removed and the pedicle is missing, it may be found in one of two places. Most commonly it is inside the punch. Removal can be accomplished by spearing it with a needle and pulling it out. It may also be under the skin. Gently explore under the skin through the defect to look for the specimen.

13. Once the specimen is removed completely, place it in the specimen container.

14. Suture the wound, placing half as many sutures as the size of the punch (see Chapter 23). For instance, a 6-mm punch would require three evenly spaced sutures.

15. Apply an antibiotic ointment on an adhesive bandage to dress the wound.

Follow-Up Care and Instructions

- Written instructions on wound care can be provided.
- Instruct the patient to keep the area clean and dry for 24 hours. After that time, the adhesive bandage may be removed and the site cleaned with soap and water as usual.
- If a new adhesive bandage is applied, instruct the patient to place more antibiotic ointment on the biopsy site. For most punch biopsy sites, however, the adhesive bandage does not need to be reapplied after the first 24 hours. The exception to this is in areas of friction or if drainage will get on the patient's clothing.
- Schedule a return appointment in 5 to 21 days, depending on the area biopsied. The head tends to heal faster, whereas areas of tension such as the anterior tibia require longer healing times. A basic time schedule for suture removal would be as follows (Hruza, 1999; Moy, 1998):
  - Face and ears: 5 to 7 days
  - Neck: 7 days
  - Scalp: 7 to 10 days
  - Trunk and extremities: 7–14 days
  - Distal lower extremities: 10 to 21 days
- Advise the patient not do any heavy lifting or exercising that might cause the sutures to break or lead to a widened scar.
- The patient should be informed of the results of the pathologic examination, either when the results are provided to the practitioner or when the patient returns for suture removal.

Excisional Biopsy

Indications

Any lesion that is smaller than 8 to 10 mm can be completely excised as stated earlier with a punch biopsy. Most lesions larger than 1 cm will have a better cosmetic appearance if the excision is performed using a No. 15 blade. Lesions that are excised routinely follow (Moy and Usatine, 1998b; Schultz, 1996; Zalla and Roenigk, 1996):

- Suspected melanomas
- Epidermal inclusion cysts
- Lipomas
- Larger basal cell and squamous cell carcinomas
- Dermal lesions larger than 1 cm

Moh's micrographic surgical procedures are beyond the scope of most primary care providers, as they require special training to perform. However, they bear mentioning with respect to removal of malignant lesions. Moh's procedures are preferred in sclerosing and morpheaform basal cell carcinomas, recurrent tumors, and any malignant tumor around the eyes, nose, or lips, and on the ears. They use a special technique of excising and color-coding the specimen before histologic examination. This method has a higher overall cure rate and lower recurrence rate than do standard excisions (Randle and Roenigk, 1996; Russell et al, 1999; Zalla and Roenigk, 1996). Patients who meet the preceding criteria and in whom surgery is being considered should be referred to a dermatologist trained in the Moh's technique.

Potential Complications

The complications are similar to those of punch biopsies.

- There is discomfort with the injection of anesthetic.
- The risk for bleeding is higher because a larger area of skin is incised to the subcutaneous fat, increasing the risk of severing small vessels.
- Hand-held cautery is the method of choice to stop brisk bleeding in addition to subcutaneous sutures.
- The infection rate is also higher because the procedure is more invasive. Secondary infection can be easily treated with a 5- to 7-day course of a broad-spectrum antibiotic covering *Staphylococcus* and *Streptococcus* species.
- Scarring will occur, but the extent is dependent on the patient's ability to heal versus the size and placement of the end defect.
- More than with any other biopsy technique, adequate knowledge of the lines of skin tension is required to determine orientation of excisional biopsies (see Fig. 24–2).

Caution must be used when performing elliptic excisions on the face—particularly on the forehead or near the eyes or lips—so that distortion does not occur (Moy and Usatine, 1998b). Large excisions in these areas may necessitate a graft or flap closure.

Standard Precautions ▷ Every practitioner should use Standard Precautions at all times when interacting with patients, especially when performing procedures. Determining the level of precaution necessary requires the practitioner to exercise clinical judgment based on the patient's history and the potential for exposure to body fluids or aerosol-borne pathogens (for further discussion, see Chapter 2).

Patient Preparation

- Explain the procedure to the patient or the patient's guardian, or both, and be prepared to answer any questions.
- The patient or guardian must give informed consent before the start of the procedure.
- A topical anesthetic can be provided to the patient, which must be applied under occlusion approximately 1 hour before the procedure.
- If topical anesthesia is used, the occlusive tape is removed and cleaned with gauze.

Materials Utilized to Perform an Excisional Biopsy

- Topical anesthesia applied under occlusion 1 hour before the procedure
- Chlorhexidine or povidone-iodine
- A sterile surgical marker
- Sterile gloves
- Sterile towels
- Alcohol pads
- Lidocaine with or without epinephrine, as indicated
- A 3-mL syringe and 27-gauge, $1\frac{1}{2}$-inch needle for local anesthesia
- 4 × 4 gauze
- Forceps
- Curved scissors
- Needle driver
- Appropriate suture to close subcutaneous tissue and skin (see Chapter 23)
- Hand-held cautery
- Specimen container
- Polymyxin B sulfate—bacitracin zinc and a dressing of 4 × 4 gauze and paper tape or a large adhesive bandage
- A metric ruler to determine the size of the end defect

Procedure for Performing an Excisional Biopsy

Note: Proper anesthetic technique is determined by the size of the area being excised and may warrant direct infiltration of the biopsy site, digital block, or a field block (see Chapter 22).

Note: It is also important to ensure that anesthesia is adequate for the full depth and width of the excision and placement of sutures. Local anesthesia works rapidly, within a minute; however, in highly vascular areas such as the scalp it is prudent to wait 10 minutes to allow the epinephrine, when used, to work.

1. Scrub the area for 5 minutes with chlorhexidine or povidone-iodine.
2. Drape the area with sterile towels.
3. If the lesion has the potential to blanche with the injection of lidocaine with epinephrine, such as in basal cell carcinomas, the margins of the lesion should be marked with a sterile surgical marker before the anesthetic is injected.
4. Use a sterile surgical marker to mark the intended incision line, taking into account the lines of tension, wrinkles, or skin folds (see Fig. 24–2).
5. Hold the No. 15 blade like a pencil, perpendicular to the skin.
6. Use the tip of the blade to incise the corner of the ellipse, but the belly is used for the rest of the incision (Moy and Usatine RP, 1998b; Zalla and Roenigk, 1996).
7. Continue the incision through the dermis to the subcutaneous fat (Fig. 24–5).
8. Use the forceps to lift the specimen gently, taking care not to crush it.
9. Use the No. 15 blade to cut the specimen at the base or subcutaneous fat.

Note: In the case of potentially malignant lesions, it is useful to place a tag suture on one corner of the specimen, indicating where the tag was placed on the form

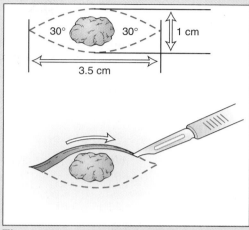

Figure 24–5. Redrawn from Pfenninger JL, Fowler GC: Procedures for Primary Care Physicians. St. Louis, Mosby-Year Book, 1994, p 24.

sent to pathology (e.g., tag is placed on medial corner).

10. Once the specimen is completely removed, place it in the specimen container.
11. In larger excisions, push the skin edges of the defect together or pull them together with skin hooks to see how much tension will be placed on the sutures.

Note: If there is tension, undermining is needed. Undermining is performed by blunt dissection to mobilize adequate tissue for closure.

12. Stop any bleeding with hand-held cautery.
13. Begin wound closure of the excision with the placement of subcutaneous vertical mattress sutures to approximate the wound edges, decrease wound tension, and reduce the risk of wound dehiscence. This is performed with an absorbable suture material.

14. Next, place nonabsorbable sutures to close the skin.
Note: This can be performed with running or simple interrupted sutures for most wounds. In areas of greater tension, mattress sutures may need to be placed for strength.

15. Leave the skin edges everted at the end closure for the best outcome.
16. Apply an antibiotic ointment on a dressing over the wound.

Special Considerations

With any invasive procedure, a good history and review of systems should be taken to determine if there are any contraindications to surgery. In addition, the patient's ability to heal, history of allergies, need for SBE prophylaxis and use of anticoagulants should be assessed. If possible, the patient should discontinue warfarin and nonsteroidal anti-inflammatory agents approximately 2 to 4 days before any invasive procedure, and aspirin should be discontinued for approximately 10 days (Hruza, 1999; Moy and Usatine, 1998a; Stasko, 1996; Zalla and Roenigk, 1996).

It is difficult to perform biopsies on small children, particularly those between the ages of 1 and 5. The provider needs to discuss the absolute need for biopsy with the parents or guardian before deciding to perform the procedure. Once it is determined that the biopsy is necessary, the child may need to be sedated. However, with the use of topical anesthetics, many children experience little discomfort.

Follow-Up Care and Instructions

- Written instructions on wound care can be provided.
- Instruct the patient to keep the area clean and dry for 24 hours.
- After that time, the dressing may be removed and the site cleaned with soap and water as usual.
- If a new dressing is applied, instruct the patient to place more antibiotic ointment on the biopsy site. For most biopsy sites, however, the dressing does not need to be reapplied after the first 24 hours. The exception to this is in areas of friction or if drainage will get on the patient's clothing.
- Schedule a return appointment in 5 to 21 days, depending on the area biopsied. (Refer to the time schedule for suture removal under Punch Biopsy.)
- Care should be taken not to do any heavy lifting or exercising that might cause the sutures to break or lead to a widened scar.
- The patient should be informed of the results of the pathologic examination either when the results are provided to the practitioner or when the patient returns for suture removal.

Electrosurgery

Background and History

Electrosurgery encompasses electrodesiccation, electrocoagulation, electrofulguration, electrosection, electrolysis, and electrocautery. The focus of this section is electrodesiccation. This is a high-voltage, low-amperage damped current, which generates heat in the tissue, causing coagulation and dehydration (Hruza, 1999; Pollack and Kobayashi, 1997). There is no current channeling along blood vessels and nerves with electrodesiccation, so it is relatively safe in patients with cardiac pacemakers. Despite this, it should not be used immediately near the pacemaker (Bennett, 1998b; Hruza, 1999; Pollack and Kobayashi, 1997; Usatine, 1998a). Lesions larger than 3 to 4 mm do better with cryosurgery, whereas smaller, 1- to 2-mm lesions may respond better to electrodesiccation (Graham, 1999).

Indications

Lesions commonly treated with electrodesiccation include the following:

- Acrochordons
- Pyogenic granulomas and other vascular lesions
- Verruca vulgaris
- Condyloma acuminata
- Actinic keratoses
- In combination with curettage for superficial multicentric basal cell carcinomas

Contraindications

- The procedure should not be performed near a pacemaker.
- It should also not be performed if flammable material or gases are present in the immediate surgical field.

Potential Complications

Common complications of electrodesiccation include the following:

- Pain
- Scarring
- Delayed bleeding
- Risk of burns
- Pigment alterations: A crust will form within 24 hours. Within 5 to 7 days, the crust will slough off. Once this occurs, there may be a hypopigmented area remaining, which is generally temporary. Occasionally, an area of hyperpigmentation may develop that could

require further treatment with keratolytic (e.g., topical retinoids) or bleaching agents (e.g., 4% hydroquinone) to lighten the skin (Stasko, 1996). Scarring may be hypertrophic, atrophic, or a keloid on rare occasions.

- The use of alcohol to prepare the skin could lead to fire during electrosurgery. An alternative preparation such as povidone-iodine is preferred and is nonflammable. Care must also be taken when electrosurgery is performed in the perianal area. Bowel gas, which is composed of methane and hydrogen gas, can ignite. This can be prevented with adequate bowel preparation before the procedure or the placement of cotton in the rectum (Bennett, 1998b).

- Viral particles can be aerosolized in cautery and laser smoke, particularly human papillomavirus (HPV) and human immunodeficiency virus (HIV). There are no case reports of HIV transmission through cautery and laser smoke. There are, however, reports of laryngeal papillomatosis in health care providers from cautery and laser ablation of warts (Lowry and Androphy, 1999; Seabury-Stone and Lynch, 1996; Usatine, 1998a).

Standard Precautions ▷ Every practitioner should use Standard Precautions at all times when interacting with patients, especially when performing procedures. Determining the level of precaution necessary requires the practitioner to exercise clinical judgment based on the patient's history and the potential for exposure to body fluids or aerosol-borne pathogens (for further discussion, see Chapter 2).

Patient Preparation

- Explain the procedure to the patient or the patient's guardian, or both, and be prepared to answer any questions.
- The patient or guardian must give informed consent before the start of the procedure.
- A topical anesthetic can be provided to the patient, which must be applied under occlusion approximately 1 hour before the procedure.
- If topical anesthesia is used, the occlusive tape is removed and cleaned with gauze.
- Electrodesiccation does not induce partial anesthesia; therefore, the procedure is better tolerated if a topical anesthetic is applied 1 hour before starting the procedure or local anesthesia infiltration is used. It must be applied under occlusion. After the procedure, most patients rarely need any analgesia, but acetaminophen may be required.

Materials Utilized to Perform Electrosurgery

- Topical anesthetic applied under occlusion 1 hour before the procedure
- Hyfrecator and desiccation electrode needle
- A face mask (for protection from smoke generated during the procedure)
- 4 × 4 gauze
- Antibiotic ointment and an adhesive bandage
- If curettage of a lesion will follow the electrosurgery, a 5- or 7-mm curette and a 4 × 4 gauze are also needed

Performing the Procedure of Electrosurgery

1. Clean the area with povidone-iodine and water only for electrodesiccation. Alcohol is flammable, and therefore should not be used.
2. For electrodesiccation, remove the occlusive tape from the topical anesthetic.
3. Use the hyfrecator with desiccation electrode needle.

Note: Set the hyfrecator at a low setting to begin with and turn it up as needed. Lightly touch the lesion to determine if the power setting is adequate.

4. Once the correct power setting is found, ablate the lesion.

Note: Small lesions are usually ablated immediately, whereas larger lesions require gentle passes with the electrode.

5. Gently wipe the charred lesion with 4 × 4 gauze or curette it off. No bleeding should occur.
6. Apply an antibiotic ointment and an adhesive bandage.

Follow-Up Care and Instructions

- Written instructions on wound care can be provided.
- For areas of electrodesiccation, instruct the patient to keep the area clean and dry for 24 hours.
- After that time, the dressing may be removed and the site cleaned with soap and water as usual.
- If a new dressing is applied, instruct the patient to place more antibiotic ointment on the biopsy site. For most biopsy sites, however, the dressing does not need to be reapplied after the first 24 hours. The exception to this is in areas of friction or if drainage will get on the patient's clothing.
- No return appointment is necessary.

Acne Surgery

Background and History

Acne surgery is performed on comedones and, occasionally, pustules. Open comedones or "blackheads" are removed purely for cosmetic purposes. It will not shorten the resolution of the acne lesions. Removal of closed comedones or "whiteheads" will shorten the resolution time, as acne surgery prevents them from rupturing and becoming larger papules or pustules (Strauss and Thiboutot, 1999).

Indications

Acne surgery may be performed on most patients with comedonal or pustular acne. Pretreatment with a topical retinoid by the patient for approximately 1 month will greatly improve the removal of comedones (Baran et al, 1998; Strauss and Thiboutot, 1999).

Contraindications

Care should be taken with patients who may develop postinflammatory hyperpigmentation, or those who may bruise easily. They should be informed of the possible risks of bruising and hyperpigmentation.

Potential Complications

- Discomfort from the procedure
- Immediate swelling and pinpoint bleeding
- Small amounts of bruising
- Postinflammatory hyperpigmentation
- Rupture of the comedo if improper technique is used (Baran et al, 1998; Strauss and Thiboutot, 1999).

Standard Precautions ▷ Every practitioner should use Standard Precautions at all times when interacting with patients, especially when performing procedures. Determining the level of precaution necessary requires the practitioner to exercise clinical judgment based on the patient's history and the potential for exposure to body fluids or aerosol-borne pathogens (for further discussion, see Chapter 2).

Patient Preparation

- Explain the procedure to the patient or the patient's guardian, or both, and be prepared to answer any questions.
- The patient or guardian must give informed consent before the start of the procedure.

Materials Utilized to Perform Acne Surgery

- Alcohol pads
- A No. 11 blade or a 25-gauge needle
- An Unna-type comedo extractor
- 4 × 4 gauze

Procedure for Performing Acne Surgery

1. Clean the area with an alcohol pad.
2. Use a No. 11 blade or 25-gauge needle to open the pore of the comedo or pustule gently.
3. Place the Unna-type comedo extractor flat against the skin.
4. Apply pressure downward while gently sliding toward the comedo or pustule (Fig. 24–6).

Note: The extractor may need to be moved in all four quadrants to ensure all the comedonal contents are removed.

5. Stop any bleeding with direct pressure with a 4 × 4 gauze.

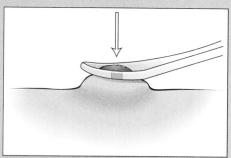

Figure 24–6. Redrawn from Pfenninger JL, Fowler GC: Procedures for Primary Care Physicians. St. Louis, Mosby-Year Book, 1994, p 55.

Note: The patient may want to wash his or her face before leaving the office.

Follow-Up Care and Instructions

- Instruct the patient to wash the area with soap and water as usual.
- Advise the patient that topical retinoids and alpha-hydroxy acids may need to be avoided for 24 hours to prevent irritation of the open areas.
- No return appointment is necessary.

References

Baran R, Chivot M, Shalita AR: Acne. In Baran R, Maibach HI (eds): Textbook of Cosmetic Dermatology, 2nd ed. London, Martin Dunitz, 1998, pp 433–444.

Bennett RG: Curettage. In Fundamentals of Cutaneous Surgery. St. Louis, CV Mosby, 1988a, pp 532–552.

Bennett RG: Electrosurgery. Fundamentals of Cutaneous Surgery. St. Louis, CV Mosby, 1988b, pp 553–590.

Bennett RG: The skin biopsy. In Fundamentals of Cutaneous Surgery. St. Louis, CV Mosby, 1988c, pp 517–531.

Fitzpatrick TB, Bernhard JD, Cropley TG: The structure of skin lesions and fundamentals of diagnosis. In Fitzpatrick TB, Eisen AZ, Wolff K, et al (eds): Dermatology in General Medicine, 5th ed. New York, McGraw-Hill, 1999, pp 13–41.

Graham GF: Cryosurgery. In Fitzpatrick TB, Eisen AZ, Wolff K, et al (eds): Dermatology in General Medicine, 5th ed. New York, McGraw-Hill, 1999, pp 2980–2987.

Ho VCY: Benign epithelial tumors. In Fitzpatrick TB, Eisen AZ, Wolff K, et al (eds): Dermatology in General Medicine, 5th ed. New York, McGraw-Hill, 1999, pp 873–890.

Hruza GJ: Dermatologic surgery: Introduction and approach. In Fitzpatrick TB, Eisen AZ, Wolff K, et al (eds): Dermatology in General Medicine, 5th ed. New York, McGraw-Hill, 1999, pp 2923–2937.

Lowry DR, Androphy EJ: Warts. In Fitzpatrick TB, Eisen AZ, Wolff K, et al (eds): Dermatology in General Medicine, 5th ed. New York, McGraw-Hill, 1999, pp 2484–2497.

Moy RL: Suturing techniques. In Usatine RP, Moy RL, Tobinick EL, et al (eds): Skin Surgery: A Practical Guide. St. Louis, CV Mosby, 1998, pp 88–100.

Moy RL, Usatine RP: Complications and their prevention. In Usatine RP, Moy RL, Tobinick EL, et al (eds): Skin Surgery: A Practical Guide. St. Louis, CV Mosby, 1998a, pp 287–299.

Moy RL, Usatine RP: Elliptical excision. In Usatine RP, Moy RL, Tobinick EL, et al (eds): Skin Surgery: A Practical Guide. St. Louis, CV Mosby, 1998b, pp 120–136.

Pollack SV, Kobayashi T: Cosmetic electrosurgery. In Coleman WP III, Hanke CW, Alt TH, et al (eds): Cosmetic Surgery of the Skin: Principles and Techniques, 2nd ed. St. Louis, CV Mosby, 1997, pp 272–286.

Randle HW, Roenigk RK: Indications for Moh's micrographic surgery. In Roenigk RK, Roenigk HH (eds): Dermatologic Surgery: Principles and Practice, 2nd ed. New York, Marcel Dekker, 1996, pp 703–730.

Russell BA, Amonette RA, Swanson NA: Moh's micrographic surgery. In Fitzpatrick TB, Eisen AZ, Wolff K, et al (eds): Dermatology in General Medicine, 5th ed. New York, McGraw-Hill, 1999, pp. 2988–2991.

Schultz BC: Skin biopsy. In Roenigk RK, Roenigk HH (eds): Dermatologic Surgery: Principles and Practice, 2nd ed. New York, Marcel Dekker, 1996, pp 177–190.

Schwartz RA, Stoll HL Jr: Epithelial precancerous lesions. In Fitzpatrick TB, Eisen AZ, Wolff K, et al (eds): Dermatology in General Medicine, 5th ed. New York, McGraw-Hill, 1999, pp 823–839.

Seabury-Stone M, Lynch PJ: Viral warts. In Sams WM, Lynch PJ (eds): Principles and Practice of Dermatology, 2nd ed. New York, Churchill-Livingstone, 1996, pp 127–133.

Siegel DM, Usatine RP: The punch biopsy. In Usatine RP, Moy RL, Tobinick EL, et al (eds): Skin Surgery: A Practical Guide. St Louis, CV Mosby, 1998a, pp 101–119.

Siegel DM, Usatine RP. The shave biopsy. In Usatine RP, Moy RL, Tobinick EL, et al (eds): Skin Surgery: A Practical Guide. St Louis, CV Mosby, 1998b, pp 55–76.

Siegel DM, Moy RL, Usatine RP: Wound care. In Usatine RP, Moy RL, Tobinick EL, et al (eds): Skin Surgery: A Practical Guide. St Louis, CV Mosby, 1998, pp 278–286.

Stasko T: Complications of cutaneous procedures. In Roenigk RK, Roenigk HH (eds): Dermatologic Surgery: Principles and Practice, 2nd ed. New York, Marcel Dekker, 1996, pp 149–175.

Strauss JS, Thiboutot DM: Diseases of the sebaceous glands. In Fitzpatrick TB, Eisen AZ, Wolff K, et al (eds): Dermatology in General Medicine, 5th ed. New York, McGraw-Hill, 1999, pp 769–784.

Tobinick EL, Usatine RP: Choosing the type of biopsy. In Usatine RP, Moy RL, Tobinick EL, et al (eds): Skin Surgery: A Practical Guide. St Louis, CV Mosby, 1998, pp 40–54.

Usatine RP: Electrosurgery. In Usatine RP, Moy RL, Tobinick EL, et al (eds): Skin Surgery: A Practical Guide. St Louis, CV Mosby, 1998a, pp 165–199.

Usatine RP: Hemostasis. In Usatine RP, Moy RL, Tobinick EL, et al (eds): Skin Surgery: A Practical Guide. St Louis, CV Mosby, 1998b, pp 31–39.

Zalla MJ, Roenigk RK: Excision. In Roenigk RK, Roenigk HH (eds): Dermatologic Surgery: Principles and Practice, 2nd ed. New York, Marcel Dekker, 1996, pp 191–207.

Bibliography

- Pollack SV, Grekin RC: Electrosurgery and electroepilation. In Roenigk RK, Roenigk HH (eds): Dermatologic Surgery: Principles and Practice, 2nd ed. New York, Marcel Dekker, 1996, pp 219–231.
- Sinclair RD, Tzermias C, Dawber R: Cosmetic cryosurgery. In Baran R, Maibach HI (eds): Textbook of Cosmetic Dermatology, 2nd ed. London, Martin Dunitz, 1998, pp 691–700.
- Usatine RP, Moy RL: Anesthesia. In Usatine RP, Moy RL, Tobinick EL, et al (eds): Skin Surgery: A Practical Guide. St. Louis, CV Mosby, 1998, pp 20–30.
- Usatine RP, Tobinick EL: Cryosurgical techniques. In Usatine RP, Moy RL, Tobinick EL, et al (eds): Skin Surgery: A Practical Guide. St. Louis, CV Mosby, 1998, pp 137–164.
- Zacarian SA: Complications, indications and contraindications in cryosurgery. In Roenigk RK, Roenigk HH (eds): Dermatologic Surgery: Principles and Practice, 2nd ed. New York, Marcel Dekker, 1996, pp 259–272.

Chapter 25

Incision and Drainage of an Abscess

▷ Patrick C. Auth

▷ George S. Bottomley

Procedure Goals and Objectives

Goal: To incise and drain an abscess successfully while observing standard precautions and with the minimal degree of risk to the patient.

Objectives: The student will be able to . . .

▶ Describe the indications, contraindications, and rationale for performing incision and drainage of an abscess.

▶ Identify and describe common complications associated with incision and drainage of an abscess.

▶ Describe the essential anatomy and physiology associated with the performance of incision and drainage of an abscess.

▶ Identify the materials necessary for performing incision and drainage of an abscess and their proper use.

▶ Identify the important aspects of care after incision and drainage of an abscess.

Background and History

The world's oldest medical manuscript is a small clay tablet written in Sumerian around 2100 BC. A portion of it translates as, "If a man, his skull contains some fluid, with your thumb press several times at the place where the fluid is found. If the swelling gives way (under your finger) and (pus) is squeezed out of the skull, you shall incise, scrape the bone and (remove) its fluid. . . ." (Manjo, 1977). Advances made over the last 4100 years in the use of minor surgical procedures to treat abscesses are discussed in this chapter.

Indications

- A localized collection of infection that is tender and is not resolving spontaneously. The cardinal signs of infection (pain, fever, redness, swelling, and loss of function) are usually present.

Contraindications

- Facial furuncles should not be incised or drained if they are located within the triangle formed by the bridge of the nose and the corners of the mouth. These infections should be treated with antibiotics and warm compresses, as the risk of septic phlebitis with intracranial extension can follow incision and drainage of a furuncle in this area.
- Abscesses that occur very near the rectum or genitalia must be carefully evaluated, and consideration should be given to referring these patients to a general surgeon for treatment.
- Patients with diabetes, debilitating disease, or compromised immunity should be observed after incision and drainage (incision and drainage) of an abscess.

Potential Complications

- Cellulitis or re-collection of pus. Bacteremia and septicemia are complications of an inadequately treated abscess. In patients with diabetes or disease that interferes with immune function, an abscess on an extremity can be complicated by severe cellulitis or gangrene, with subsequent loss of the affected extremity.
- Perianal abscess incision and drainage frequently results in a chronic anal fistula up to 50% of the time in adults.
- An abscess in the palmar aspect of the hand can extend from superficial to deep tissue via the palmar fascia.
- Deep infection is suspected when the simple incision and drainage fails to reduce the erythema, pain, pus, or swelling. More extensive surgical débridement, hospitalization, and intravenous antibiotics may be necessary in a patient with deep palmar abscess.

Review of Essential Anatomy and Physiology

An abscess is a focal circumscribed accumulation of purulent materials (pus and other inflammatory tissue). An acute or "hot" abscess has all the characteristics of a classic inflammatory episode, producing redness, heat, pain, and swelling. It is a suppurative reaction caused by the invasion of pyogenic (pus-forming) bacteria into a tissue or organ. Grossly (on the skin or surface of an organ), abscesses appear as focal, round or ovoid areas of swelling covered by skin or other tissue. On palpation, there is usually an area where the covering is thin and comes to a head (point), and when palpated that area is more easily compressible or fluctuant due to its liquid or gel-like contents.

A dry abscess is one that resolves without rupture. A sterile abscess is one from which bacteria cannot be cultured. A chronic or cold abscess lacks the redness, heat, pain, and swelling of an acute abscess and is usually associated with liquefactive necrosis of tuberculous lesions.

Clinical Evaluation

The patient usually complains of pain and swelling. Abscesses commonly occur in the perianal region. A subcutaneous abscess is often seen. Evaluation includes a search for the underlying cause of the abscess, that is, infection secondary to puncture wound or foreign body, exposure to unusually pathogenic organisms, a faulty or overwhelmed immune system, the presence of hyperglycemia, bacteremic spread from another focus, and development of a deep abscess in badly contused muscle tissue in which there was no preceding penetration of skin. When a sweat gland or hair follicle forms an abscess, it is called a furuncle or boil. When the furuncle extends into the subcutaneous tissue, it is referred to as a carbuncle. Paronychia is an abscess that involves the nail. Perifollicular abscesses are commonly found on the extremities, buttocks, breasts, or in hair follicles. A subcutaneous abscess is often seen. When signs and symptoms of localized infection or an abscess are present, incision and drainage should be considered.

Therapy

A small abscess may respond to warm compresses or antibiotics and may drain spontaneously.

As the abscess enlarges, the inflammation, collection of pus, and walling off of the abscess cavity renders such conservative treatments ineffectual. If done properly, such treatment renders antibiotics unnecessary.

In nonlactating women, a breast abscess that is not subareolar is rare and should prompt a biopsy in addition to incision and drainage of the abscess. Indications include a localized collection of pus that is tender and is not resolving spontaneously.

A culture should be obtained by aspiration or swabbing of the abscess cavity, because unusual organisms may have caused the abscess. The infection may also warrant the administration of antibiotics.

Etiology

Healthy skin and its protective mechanisms are usually successful at fending off potentially pathogenic microorganisms. If, however, this barrier is interrupted through trauma (mechanical, chemical, or thermal) to the stratum corneum, inflammation, or through the often more ingenious mechanisms of infectious agents themselves, skin infections and abscesses develop. Most often, *Staphylococcus aureus* is the causative agent in abscesses, but some abscesses are due to *Streptococcus* species or a combination of microorganisms, including gram-negative and anaerobic bacteria. The flora found in the affected area usually causes the abscess. Puncture wounds or the presence of foreign bodies are common underlying causes of abscess formation. The skin of the debilitated, elderly, diabetic (hyperglycemic state), or otherwise immunocompromised patient may also offer a damaging agent easier access.

Histologically, an abscess is a central area of pus composed of dead white blood cells, bacteria, degenerating tissue debris, and proteins from the immune response to the bacteria. Surrounding this is a zone of healthy neutrophils. Depending on the age of the abscess, peripheral to this is a circumferential area of vascular dilatation, macrophages, fibroblasts, and fibrocytes in varying stages of development and collagen. Ultimately, a connective tissue capsule surrounds the area, which inhibits the penetration of anti-infective agents. A diffuse abscess is a localized accumulation of pus that is not well encapsulated.

Abscesses can interfere with normal function of nearby tissue, either by expansion and subsequent pressure on adjacent structures (such as an abscess adjacent to the trachea) or through expulsion of its contents and seeding of bacteria into surrounding areas or the vascular system, with resultant septicemia.

In the treatment of abscesses, the important anatomic structures underlying the abscess must be appreciated and anticipated before an incision is performed. The location of the abscess is critical to the direction of the incision. the abscess locations listed here are in close proximity to major vessels and should be aspirated with an 18-gauge needle attached to a 10-mL syringe before drainage to avoid inadvertent incision into an artery.

- Peritonsillar and retropharyngeal regions
- The anterior triangle of the neck

- The supraclavicular fossa
- Deep in the axilla
- The antecubital space
- The groin
- The popliteal space

Standard Precautions ▷ Every practitioner should use Standard Precautions at all times when interacting with patients, especially when performing procedures. Determining the level of precaution necessary requires the practitioner to exercise clinical judgment based on the patient's history and the potential for exposure to body fluids or aerosol-borne pathogens (for further discussion, see Chapter 2).

Patient Preparation

- Advise the patient regarding the potential benefits and risks associated with the procedure.
- Be sure to describe the care required to pack the wound after the procedure.
- Provide an opportunity for the patient to ask questions and receive answers.
- Assist the patient into a comfortable supine position that affords complete access to the abscess site.

Materials Utilized for Performing Incision and Drainage of Abscesses

- Alcohol or povidone-iodine (Betadine) wipe
- 1% to 2% lidocaine (Xylocaine) without epinephrine
- 19- to 22-gauge needle
- Three to four towels for drapes
- No. 11 or No. 15 scalpel blade
- Scalpel handle
- Kelly's clamps
- Adson's forceps
- Curved hemostats
- 4 × 4 inch gauze pads
- Sterile gloves
- 500 mL of normal saline solution
- ¼- to ½-inch Nu-Gauze strip for packing the wound
- Bandage scissors
- Dressing of choice to cover wound

Procedure for Performing Incision and Drainage of Abscesses

Skin Preparation

1. Apply a single layer of povidone-iodine to the abscess and allow to air-dry before performing the incision.

Anesthesia

1. Use a regional field block anesthetic technique to anesthetize the abscess by injecting a ring of anesthetic agent approximately 1 cm away from the erythematous border of the abscess around its perimeter.

Note: This will allow the lesion to be anesthetized circumferentially. The onset of action of the anesthetic is approximately 5 to 10 minutes. Complete anesthesia is difficult to provide, especially when breaking the septum within the cavity of the abscess with a hemostat.

2. After alcohol preparation of the skin, superficially infiltrate the skin in a linear course across the abscess and then traverse the second linear course directly perpendicular to the first. Be careful to remain superficial to the abscess cavity.

Drapes

1. Place drapes to ensure isolation of the abscess and the prepared surrounding skin.

Incising and Drainage

1. Make the incision along the relaxed skin tension lines (Langer's lines) to reduce scarring (Fig. 25–1).

2. Open the abscess widely by extending the incision across its full dimension. If more drainage is desired, make a second incision perpendicular to the first, forming a cruciate pattern (Fig. 25–2).

Note: This technique typically results in a less aesthetically pleasing scar when fully healed.

3. Obtain a specimen for culture as soon as the purulent material is expressed from the abscess cavity.

Note: If a culture is obtained, it should be from the abscess cavity and not from the superficial skin over the abscess. Alternatively, the abscess cavity can be aspirated with a large-bore (18-gauge) needle before the incision is made. The aspirated contents can then be sent for the appropriate cultures in more complicated cases. Rarely is it helpful in routine cases.

4. Explore the abscess cavity thoroughly. This can be accomplished with a sterile cotton-tipped applicator or with hemostats. Insert the blunt end of the hemostat into the abscess cavity and spread the hemostat to break up the septum and loculations within the abscess, thus releasing any further pockets of purulent material (Fig. 25–3).

5. Thoroughly irrigate the cavity with normal saline before any gauze is inserted to pack the cavity (Fig. 25–4).

6. After complete drainage of the cavity, insert iodoform gauze into the abscess cavity, with 1 cm of gauze exiting from the cavity (Fig. 25–5) and then pack the cavity with packing material, such as iodoform gauze. The length and width of the gauze are dependent on the abscess size.

Note: The iodoform gauze serves two purposes: it prevents the incision from sealing

Procedure for Performing Incision and Drainage of Abscesses – *(continued)*

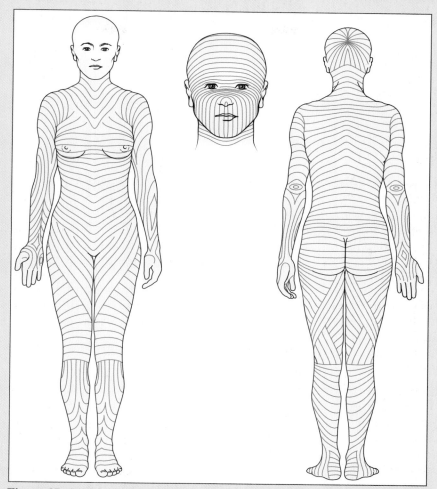

Figure 25–1. Redrawn from Trott TA: Wounds and Lacerations: Emergency Care and Closure, 2nd ed. St. Louis, Mosby-Year Book, 1998, pp 16–17; adapted from Simon R, Brenner B: Procedures and Techniques in Emergency Medicine. Baltimore, Williams & Wilkins; 1982.

over and provides for adequate drainage of the abscess cavity. The iodoform gauze is removed and reinserted every 12 to 24 hours by either the patient or a caregiver. **Note**: Healing should progress from the inside out, that is, epithelialization of the abscess cavity should occur before healing of the incision site to minimize the chance of recurrence.

7. Apply a sterile dressing over the abscess site to absorb drainage and prevent foreign materials from entering the wound.
8. Instruct the patient or caregiver on the procedure for packing the wound and twice daily changes at home until healthy closure of the wound occurs.

Procedure for Performing Incision and Drainage of Abscesses – *(continued)*

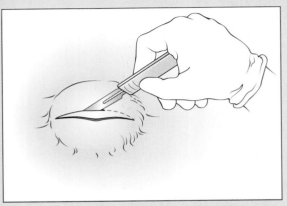

Figure 25–2. Redrawn from Rosen P, Barkin R, Sternback G: Essentials of Emergency Medicine. St. Louis, Mosby-Year Book, 1991, p 645.

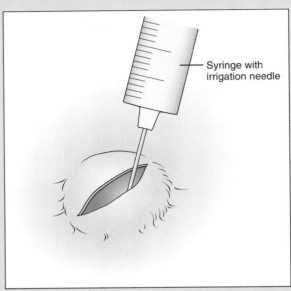

Syringe with irrigation needle

Figure 25–4

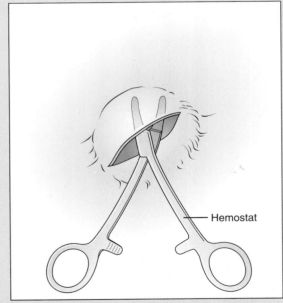

Hemostat

Figure 25–3

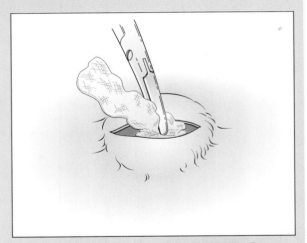

Figure 25–5. Redrawn from Rosen P, Barkin R, Sternback G: Essentials of Emergency Medicine. St. Louis, Mosby-Year Book, 1991, p 645.

Special Considerations

Primary management of abscesses should be incision and drainage and routine culture. Usually incision and drainage is sufficient treatment to cure an abscess. Antibiotic therapy is not indicated for the typical abscess in patients with normal defenses. However, for patients fitting into the following situations, additional treatment may be necessary:

- Abscesses to be treated with oral antibiotic therapy are those that are surrounded with lymphangitis or a large area of cellulitis. The cellulitis is determined by tenderness peripheral to the area of the abscess as well as increased warmth and redness, as opposed to the nontender induration palpated around an abscess that is well localized and that would not benefit from the addition of oral antibiotics. When surrounding cellulitis is present or when the patient has risk factors mentioned previously, dicloxacillin (250 to 500 mg every 6 hours) may be used. Alternative antibiotics can be used, but they must cover *Staphylococcus* organisms until the culture results have been returned and a more specific antibiotic treatment is determined.
- Purulent material from immunosuppressed patients (including diabetic patients) should be cultured, with the patient placed on oral antibiotics pending the culture results. Antibiotics may be used in conjunction with surgical incision and drainage in patients who are immunocompromised, that is, those who have diabetes, leukemia, or acquired immune deficiency syndrome or those who are undergoing chemotherapy. This purulent material should be examined by Gram stain, and the specimen should be sent for culturing (both aerobic and anaerobic) and sensitivity testing before any antibiotic treatment is started.
- Aspiration is used for diagnostic confirmation. The rationale to drain the abscess is to avoid incision of a mycotic aneurysm and imminent exsanguination. The aspiration confirms that the material within the cavity is purulent and not serosanguineous or pure blood.
- In nonlactating women, a breast abscess that is not subareolar is rare and should prompt the consideration of a biopsy in addition to incision and drainage of the abscess. A culture should be obtained by aspiration or swab of the abscess cavity, because unusual organisms may have caused the abscess. The infection may also warrant the administration of antibiotics.

Pain Relief

If the packing is tight in the abscess cavity, the pain can be sufficient to warrant the use of acetaminophen or nonsteroidal anti-inflammatory drugs. Rarely are narcotics needed beyond the initial incision and drainage procedure. The procedure alone may provide sufficient pain relief from a tense abscess so that no pain medication is needed.

Follow-Up Care and Instructions

Advise the patient that following removal of the iodoform pack, the patient is to apply warm wet soaks to the areas four to six times a day for 5 to 7 days.

- A nonadherent dressing (Adaptic, Telfa) should be applied over the wound and covered with sterile gauze.

Immobilization

- Advise the patient that in some areas of the body (particularly hand and foot injuries involving joints), motion may interfere with healing.
- Instruct the patient to elevate an injured extremity to help improve venous and lymphatic drainage and control swelling and pain and focal edema control.

Analgesics

- Usually a nonsteroidal analgesic provides sufficient pain relief.

General Follow-Up Care

- Advise the patient to keep the wound clean and dry.
- Instruct the patient about how to remove the dressing 2 days after the procedure, replace with a dry, sterile dressing, and change the dressing daily.
- Some patients can be taught to change their own packing, replace the dressings, and advance the drain.
- Instruct the patient to watch for signs of recurrence of the abscess or for evidence of further infection such as cellulitis.
- Instruct the patient to notify the clinician immediately if any of the following occur: recollection of pus in the abscess, fever and chills, increased pain or redness, red streaks near the abscess, or increased swelling in the area.

References

Manjo, G: The Healing Hand: Men and Women in the Ancient World. Cambridge, MA, Harvard University Press, 1977, pp 58–59.

Bibliography

- Goroll, AH, May LA, Mulley AG: Primary Care Medicine, 3rd ed. Philadelphia, Lippincott-Raven, 1995, pp 951–952.
- Kelly WN: Essentials of Internal Medicine. Philadelphia, JB Lippincott, 1994, p 482.
- Lawrence PF: Essentials of General Surgery, 3rd ed. Philadelphia, Lippincott Williams & Wilkins, 2000, pp 129, 288–289.
- Simmon RR, Barry BE: Emergency Procedures and Techniques, 3rd ed., Baltimore, Williams & Wilkins, 1994, pp 357–360.

Chapter 26

Wound Dressing Techniques

▷ Paul F. Jacques

Procedure Goals and Objectives

Goal: To apply wound dressings correctly, which will optimize conditions for healing.

Objectives: The student will be able to . . .

▶ Describe the indications and contraindications for applying a dressing over a wound.

▶ Identify the common complications associated with wound dressings.

▶ Describe the types of wounds.

▶ Describe the three biologic phases of wound healing.

▶ Identify the appropriate types of dressings and the rationale for their use.

Background and History

There are several types of skin lesions that require or benefit from the application of dressings: wounds from trauma or surgical intervention, ulcers from an arterial, venous, diabetic or pressure-type cause, or burn injury. This chapter presents some of the basic principles of dressing techniques for wounds. The sources in the bibliography are provided for more in-depth information for the clinician who works in a setting where wound management is an ongoing responsibility.

Research and technology have significantly enhanced the medical community's ability to optimize healing and thus better treat wounds. Many new dressing materials are available, and much more is known and understood about the body's mechanisms of wound healing. When trauma occurs, either by accident or surgical intervention, the goal of managing the wound is to optimize the healing potential while preventing possible complications such as infection or deformity.

During the Middle Ages, Henri de Mondeville (1260–1320) made a major stand on the principle of cleanliness to avoid suppuration, a popular belief that remained in effect for centuries. In 1460, Heinrich von Pfolspeund wrote a book regarding trauma titled *Bundth-Ertznel,* which means "bandage treatment." Von Pfolspeund had considerable war experience, where he developed a breadth of knowledge about war-related traumatic wounds. He subscribed to the belief that only certain types of wounds should be closed and that for most war wounds, oil of turpentine should be poured into the wound, with the resulting suppuration being a sign of healing. Von Pfolspeund wrote that wounds should be bound with clean white cloths, for if not clean, harm would result. He also advocated that physicians wash their hands before tending to individual patients.

In 1545, Ambroise Paré, a military surgeon, was accustomed to treating wounds with boiling oil. The custom was to pour boiling oil into the wound to stop suppuration. When Paré's supply of boiling oil ran out he simply dressed the wounds with clean cloths and minimal medication. He was dumbfounded to find on the following morning that the soldiers treated without the boiling oil were relatively free of pain, afebrile, and resting comfortably. Paré spent the rest of his life advocating keeping medications out of wounds and letting nature work. His expression, "I dressed him, and God healed him," made medical history.

It was during the 19th century that a better understanding of wound healing emerged, and antiseptic surgery was introduced in 1867. With the development of general anesthesia in 1847, surgeons were better able to carry out more deliberate surgical procedures. However, at that time, pus was still believed to be necessary to the healing of wounds. The brilliant work of Louis Pasteur in France and the discovery of bacteria as the source of infection changed the management of surgical cases. A British surgeon, Joseph Lister, concluded that microorganisms were the cause of the high mortality rate and implemented the use of carbolic acid (a powerful antiseptic). With the advent of spraying carbolic acid into the wound and around the surgical operative site, Lister's patient mortality rate dropped precipitously. The theory of asepsis was developed and is the standard of care today.

Today, there are more than 2000 brands of wound dressings. The clinician should be aware of the major types and categories of dressings and the indications for each.

Indications

A wound dressing decreases the risk of infection, and the correct material covering the wound optimizes the healing process. The ideal dressing accomplishes the following:

- Maintains a high degree of humidity between the wound and the dressing
- Provides a thermal insulation for the wound, which provides a better environment for cellular growth (Fig. 26–1)
- Removes excess exudate and toxic substances from the wound
- Allows gas exchange
- Is impermeable to bacteria to prevent infection
- Does not leave particular material or contaminants within the wound

Dressings are also indicated for the following:

- To apply the aesthetic principle of hiding the injury
- To protect the wound from accidental trauma, abrasions, self-inflicted "picking," or other irritations
- To provide support, immobilization, and compression

There is no single ideal product available that provides all these functions at once, but the clinician should consider carefully which characteristics of the dressing are the most important for your patient's wound. The wound treatment plan should consider factors such as the cause, severity, environment, size and depth, anatomic location, volume of exudate, and the risk or presence of infection. Patient considerations such as medical status, preferences, level of comfort, and cost-benefit analysis must also be taken under advisement. The final factors to consider are the availability, durability, adaptability, cost, and uses of the wound care products.

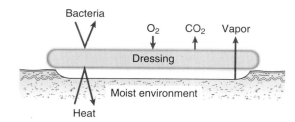

Figure 26–1. The ideal dressing.

Contraindications

Ultimately, the dressing should not cause pain or traumatize the wound with removal. It is essential to avoid applying a dressing that may compromise the blood supply to the tissue within and surrounding the wound. There are no other significant contraindications to dressing a wound. Relative contraindications include the following:

- Skin sensitivity to the dressing and related products (i.e., allergies to tape, adhesives, latex, iodoform gauze, povidone, neomycin or bacitracin): These should be discussed with the patient before application of the dressing of choice.
- Persistent povidone application to a wound causes damage to the normal tissue and inhibits healing, and thus should be avoided.
- Decreased circulation in affected area: Dressings can interfere with circulation in a digit or extremity if applied too tightly. Therefore, only material that stretches should be applied when the dressing will encircle the extremity.
- Application of gauze dressings, such as gauze squares (2-inch × 2-inch or 4-inch × 4-inch), directly on a wound; the gauze can adhere to the wound as the epithelial cells intertwine within the gauze. Removal of the dressing can cause removal of the eschar (scab) and new epithelial cells from the wound as well as cause the patient some significant discomfort. If a dressing has become adherent to a wound, it should be soaked in normal saline for approximately 10 minutes before removal is attempted. Some dressing materials have been designed to adhere less to wounds than traditional gauze does, and these should be considered when the potential for wound adherence is high.
- When dealing with the elderly, carefully consider the texture and integrity of the skin before applying an adhesive tape directly to the skin. With the aging process, there is a loss of collagen within the dermis and an increased friability of the skin. Therefore, adhesives can readily tear the "normal" aged skin when removal of the adhesive tape is warranted to change the dressing. The way to keep a dressing in place is to use a gauze roll or elastic roll over the dressing and around the body part affected and apply tape only to the gauze or elastic roll ends or edges.
- When treating infants and children, be sure to reinforce the wound dressing with additional gauze covering the wound, thereby making it more difficult for the child to remove the dressing.

Review of Essential Anatomy and Physiology

Wound Types

The material used for a dressing is dependent on the type, size, and location of the wound. The wound types include closed, open (full- or partial-thickness), necrotic, infected, granulating, and epithelializing.

Closed and Open Wounds

For a closed wound, in which the skin integrity is intact, there is no evidence that a dressing decreases the risk of infection. Applying nonadherent gauze dressing will absorb exudate and prevent irritation. For an open wound, the objective is to encourage clean granulation by creating a moist environment without slough.

Necrotic Wounds

Necrotic wounds must be surgically débrided, if possible, to remove nonviable tissue, because necrotic tissue impedes the healing process. If the patient is not a surgical candidate, the use of hydrocolloids or hydrogels can facilitate débridement. Contact with the exudate causes the hydrophilic particles of the hydrocolloids to swell and form an impermeable gel. Rehydrating necrotic tissue separates from the normal tissues and sloughs off. Separation may take a few weeks depending on the size of the lesion. Hydrocolloids (DuoDerm) absorb exudate and produce a moist environment without maceration of the surrounding tissues.

Infected Wounds

Infected wounds should be treated with normal saline irrigation. Minor infections are adequately treated with saline bathing. Alginates are used for more extensive infected wounds. This product contains calcium and sodium alginic acid prepared in a fiber form. Moisture causes the calcium alginate to convert to a soluble sodium salt and produces a hydrophilic gel. The gel is easily removed with saline irrigation or by bathing. This dressing removal is comfortable for the patient.

Granulating Wounds

Granulating wounds require a moist environment, and removal of the dressing should not damage the tissue. Impregnated gauze [Xeroform] works well as long as the dressing is not allowed to dry out, in which case it will then débride the wound of new granulation tissue when the dressing is pulled off. Hydrocolloids or hydrogels with a transparent film covering are good alternatives to impregnated gauze.

Epithelializing Wounds

Epithelializing wounds (abrasions) should be treated in the same manner as granulating wounds, being careful not to remove the new epithelial layer when changing the dressing. Therefore, they should be covered with a nonadherent dressing (Telfa), a biosynthetic sheet, or a transparent film.

Wound Healing

There are three stages in the healing process of a wound, regardless of whether the wound is surgical or traumatic in nature.

Inflammatory (0 to 6 Days)

Edema, erythema, heat, and pain characterize the inflammatory phase, which begins at the time of injury and lasts 4 to 6 days. Hemostasis controls bleeding, and polymorphonuclear leukocytes control bacterial growth. After about 4 days, macrophages migrate into the wound area and produce chemoattractants and growth factors, which facilitate wound healing.

Proliferative (4 to 24 Days)

In an open wound, granulation tissue is generated, which produces red, beefy, shiny tissue with a granular appearance. This tissue consists of macrophages, fibroblasts, immature collagen, blood vessels, and ground substance. As the granulation tissue proliferates, fibroblasts stimulate the production of collagen, which gives tissue its tensile strength and structure.

As the wound fills with granulation tissue, its margins contract, decreasing the wound's surface area. During epithelialization, cells migrate from the wound margins, ultimately sealing it. Epithelization can occur only in the presence of viable, vascular tissue. When this phase is complete, a scar forms.

Maturation (21 Days to 24 Months)

During the maturation phase, the collagen fibers reorganize, remodel, and mature, gaining tensile strength. The maximal tensile strength that is regained is approximately 80%.

Poor Wound Healing

Advanced age, diabetes mellitus, immunosuppression, radiation therapy, vitamin deficiency, malnutrition, cancer, vascular insufficiencies, or wound infection are some of the more common causes of poor wound healing. If a wound is not healing readily, the clinician should undertake a comprehensive evaluation of the patient, looking for systemic inhibitors of wound healing.

Environmental factors can impede the healing of a wound, such as recurrent trauma or pressure on the site of the wound (which may occur with bending the affected area), edema that impedes oxygen flow to and from the wound, necrotic tissue within the wound, and patient incontinence, which can expose the wound to urine or feces. Poorly healing wounds are at increased risk for infection, hemorrhage, dehiscence, evisceration, and fistula formation.

Prevention of Infection in Wounds

Clinicians must wash their hands before and after dressing a wound. A study conducted in April 2000 demonstrated a 16% compliance with hand washing before patient interaction and a 25% hand-washing rate after patient contact. Nosocomial infections can be prevented only by increased compliance with effective hand washing.

The skin is the barrier against infection. When the skin is compromised, through trauma or surgical intervention, the patient is at risk for bacterial growth within the wound. The longer the wound is exposed to air particles, dirt, water, and so forth, the risk of infection increases exponentially. The appropriate surgical management, such as débridement, irrigation, or suturing, should be undertaken before wound dressings are applied. Débridement refers to the removal of tissue that is likely to impede the healing process, such as necrotic and unnecessary fibrinous tissue or damaged tissue that is unlikely to survive. This is typically performed as a surgical procedure and its description is beyond the scope of this chapter. Irrigation involves cleaning the wound to minimize contamination by infectious and foreign materials. Typically, large quantities of normal saline solutions are used, and large-capacity syringes can be used to spray the solution with sufficient pressure to irrigate structures that may be difficult to reach. Wound closure and wound contamination classification are covered in depth in Chapter 23.

There are four steps in the prevention of wound infection in the trauma patient. First and foremost is adequate and timely resuscitation of the patient. Hypoxia or hypovolemia, or both, increase the risk of infection. Second is early wound care, which includes débridement, irrigation, hemostasis, and primary wound closure. Third is the application of antibiotics. Although most wounds do not require antibiotic therapy, if antibiotics are indicated, they should be administered early using an agent that provides appropriate coverage of the most likely infecting microbes. In addition, achieving adequate concentrations of the antibiotic for bactericidal effects is essential. The fourth stage is tetanus immune prophylaxis when indicated (see Chapter 23). These basic infection prevention principles are also applicable for nontraumatic wounds.

Standard Precautions ▷ Every practitioner should use Standard Precautions at all times when interacting with patients, especially when performing procedures. Determining the level of precaution necessary requires the practitioner to exercise clinical judgment based on the patient's history and the potential for exposure to body fluids or aerosol-borne pathogens (for further discussion, see Chapter 2).

Patient Preparation

- Inform the patient about the procedure of wound dressing.
- Explain to the patient exactly what is being done and why, and answer any questions that he or she might have.

Materials Utilized for Performing Wound Dressing

Note: Dressings should have the following characteristics: softness, permeability, sterility, and elasticity.

Primary Dressings

■ Alginates

Note: These products are derived from brown seaweed. Alginates (AlgiDerm, AlgiSite, Dermastat) are absorbent and conform to the shape of a wound because they are provided in the shape of a rope (twisted fibers) or pads. An alginate interacts with wound exudate to form a soft gel that maintains a moist healing environment. Alginates can absorb up to 20 times their weight. These products absorb heavy exudate from a deep, draining wound, regardless of whether or not it is infected (Fig. 26–2).

■ Biosynthetic Dressings

Note: Biosynthetic dressings (E-Z DERM, GLUCAN II) were developed as temporary coverings for burns. A biosynthetic dressing may be a gel or a semiocclusive sheet that can be left in place for 1 to 10 days, depending on the clinical situation. Biosynthetic dressings facilitate wound healing by re-epithelialization. These dressings may be used to treat partial-thickness wounds, such as tears, burns, abrasions, and some pressure ulcers (Fig. 26–3).

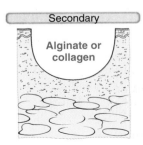

Use alginate in presence of heavy exudate with or without the presence of infection.

Use collagen with or without the presence of infection.

Collagen particles or gel

Figure 26–2. Alginate is used in the presence or absence of infection.

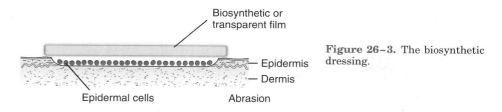

Figure 26-3. The biosynthetic dressing.

■ Collagens

Note: Collagen dressings may be used as primary dressing for partial- and full-thickness wounds, whether they are infected or not (see Fig. 26–2). During wound healing, collagen encourages the deposition and organization of newly formed collagen fibers and granulation tissue in the wound bed. It stimulates new tissue development and wound débridement. With the use of collagen, a secondary dressing needs to be applied to absorb exudate. Collagen dressing products are available as sheets, pads, particles, and gels (FIBRACOL PLUS, Kollagen Medifil, hyCURE).

■ Foams

Note: Foam dressings (CURAFOAM PLUS, SOF-FOAM Dressing, 3M Reston Self-Adhering Foam, Tielle hydropolymer dressing) are absorbent, nonadhering, and lint free. Foams may be either hydrophilic or hydrophobic and are nonocclusive unless they have a film coating. They are used as either a primary dressing, directly on the wound to provide absorption and insulation, or as a secondary dressing overlying a wound packing. Foams may require a secondary dressing to hold them in place if they do not have an adhesive border or film coating as an additional bacterial barrier. (Fig. 26–4).

■ Hydrocolloids

Note: Hydrocolloids (DuoDerm, Exuderm, OriDerm hydrocolloid, 3M Tegasorb hydrocolloid dressings) are occlusive or semi-occlusive dressings that can be composed of gelatin, pectin, or carboxymethylcellulose (see Fig. 26–4). These types of dressings provide a moist healing environment that allows clean wounds to granulate or necrotic lesions to débride autolytically. These types of products are manufactured in various shapes, sizes, and forms, such as wafers, pastes, and powders. Hydrocolloid dressings are self-adhesive, provide light to moderate absorption capacity, minimize skin trauma, and may be used underneath a compression product such as Unna boots. However, they are not recommended for infected wounds or wounds with

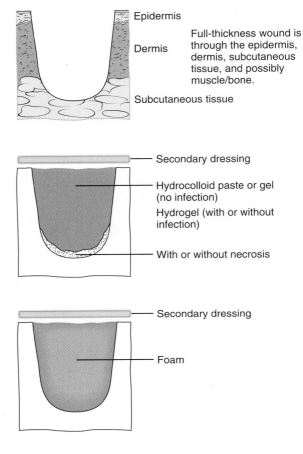

Epidermis

Dermis

Full-thickness wound is through the epidermis, dermis, subcutaneous tissue, and possibly muscle/bone.

Subcutaneous tissue

Secondary dressing

Hydrocolloid paste or gel (no infection)

Hydrogel (with or without infection)

With or without necrosis

Secondary dressing

Foam

Figure 26–4. The foam dressing.

heavy exudate or exposed tendons or bones. Another benefit of this type of dressing is that it protects the lesion from contamination and can be left in place 1 to 10 days, depending on the type of lesion and placement.

■ Hydrogels

Note: Hydrogels are water or glycerin-based amorphous gels (CURASOL, SK Integrity amorphous hydrogel, 3M Tegagel hydrogel wound filler products). The gels can be applied to wounds directly, or there are gauze or sheets impregnated with the hydrogel. They do not absorb exudate because of their high water content. These dressings maintain a moist wound environment, thereby promoting granulation and epithelialization or autolytic débridement of necrotic lesions. They are indicated for the management of partial- and full-thickness wounds, deep wounds,

wounds with necrosis, slough, minor burns, and tissue damaged by radiation (Fig. 26–5). These dressings are applied and removed easily and can be used when infection is present.

Secondary Dressings
■ Transparent films

Note: Transparent films (OpSite, Bioclusive transparent dressing, Polyskin II, 3M Tegaderm transparent dressing) are adhesive, semipermeable, polyurethane membrane dressings that vary in thickness and size. These films are waterproof and impermeable to bacteria, yet they permit water vapor to cross the barrier. Transparent films allow direct observation of the wound and do not require a secondary dressing.

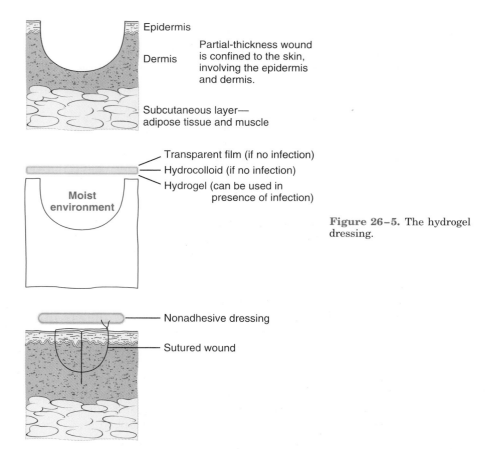

Epidermis

Dermis — Partial-thickness wound is confined to the skin, involving the epidermis and dermis.

Subcutaneous layer— adipose tissue and muscle

Transparent film (if no infection)
Hydrocolloid (if no infection)
Hydrogel (can be used in presence of infection)

Moist environment

Figure 26–5. The hydrogel dressing.

Nonadhesive dressing

Sutured wound

The limitations are that they should not be used on fragile skin or with infected wounds.
- Dressing gauze
  - **Note:** Gauze dressings are manufactured in many forms. They can be used as primary, secondary, or securing dressings. The various categories of gauze are: (1) Gauze for cleaning, débriding, packing, and covering. These types are usually in the form of packets containing sterile 4-inch × 4-inch or 2-inch × 2-inch squares. (2) Nonadherent and impregnated gauze. Nonadherent gauze [Telfa pads] are an important improvement in gauze dressings because they do not stick to wounds and facilitate exudate transmittal away from the wound. Gauze comes impregnated with many different substances, such as oil emulsions, petrolatum, saline, scarlet red, sodium chloride, water, Xeroform or zinc-saline solution. Some impregnated gauze dressings serve as occlusive dressings and prevent drainage from the wound.
- Flexible collodion
  - **Note:** Flexible collodion is a preparation of nitrocellulose dissolved in alcohol and ether. It is a plastic-like substance that is applied aseptically to a wound and forms a thin, clear sealant layer of plastic over the wound. This product is a good choice for scalp lacerations, where gauze dressing is difficult to apply.
- Dressing stabilizer (wrapping or rolling gauze)
  - **Note:** Rolls of dressing material are used to hold other materials against a wound. The ideal roll gauze will have some elastic properties; they are used to add bulk and cushion to the dressing (Kling, Kerlex). Another type of wrapping gauze that is categorized as a dressing stabilizer is tubular gauze used to stabilize a dressing circumferentially (Tube-gauze). These types of dressings are applied using a stainless steel metal-cage applicator and are useful for dressing digits.
- Tape
- Ace bandage
- Tube gauze
- Cleansing materials
  - Irrigation set
  - Normal saline

- Povidone-iodine
  - **Note:** Antiseptic agents such as povidone-iodine can injure skin, delaying healing; therefore, they should be used only when necessary and used sparingly on damaged skin.
- Hydrogen peroxide

Procedure for Performing Wound Dressing

1. Wash hands and put on clean sterile gloves.
2. Clean the wound.

Note: Clean wounds with dirt or grease contamination with mild soap and irrigate with water to remove the detergent. Irrigate deep wounds to remove excessive exudate, slough, or loose necrotic tissue (see Chapter 23). Closed wounds should be cleansed gently with normal saline or hydrogen peroxide to remove clotted blood from the wound edge, which can contribute to scarring or infection, or both. Excessive exposure to hydrogen peroxide can injure damaged skin, so an effort should be made to limit exposure to intact, dry skin surfaces only.

3. Determine the appropriate primary dressing based on the factors described previously. Maintain aseptic technique when applying dressings (see Chapter 3).
4. Apply the secondary dressing to absorb excessive exudate as well as to provide a cushion (Figs. 26–6 and 26–7).
5. Secure the dressing in a fashion that will provide flexibility and not restrict the movement of the patient, unless such restriction is warranted by the nature of the wound (Fig. 26–8).
6. Make sure that the tape is wide enough and long enough to adhere the gauze to the skin.
7. Wounds overlying flexor surfaces on the extremities or digits will be unduly stressed with flexion of the joint; therefore, range of motion should be

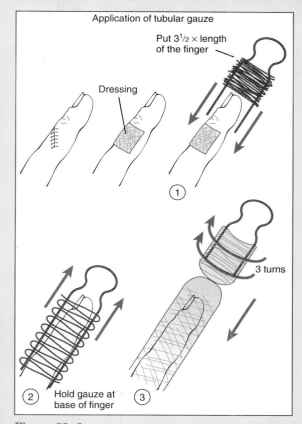

Figure 26–6

somewhat restricted to prevent dehiscence (Fig. 26–9). Splints or bulky dressings should be considered to reduce the range of motion of the affected joint.

8. Apply dressings to cover sutured wounds.

Procedure for Performing Wound Dressing – *(continued)*

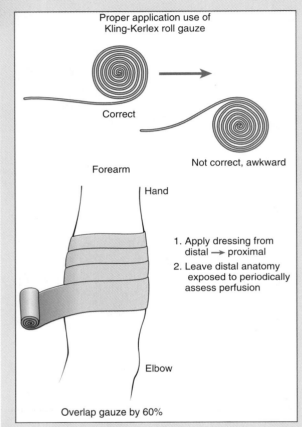

Proper application use of Kling-Kerlex roll gauze

Correct

Not correct, awkward

Forearm

Hand

1. Apply dressing from distal → proximal
2. Leave distal anatomy exposed to periodically assess perfusion

Elbow

Overlap gauze by 60%

Figure 26–7

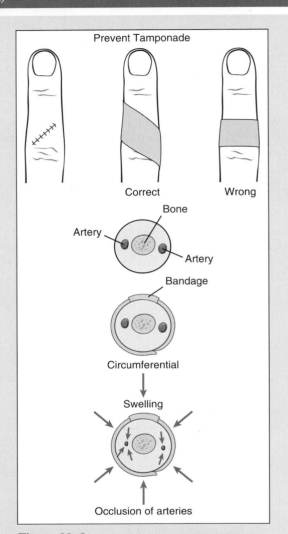

Prevent Tamponade

Correct   Wrong

Bone

Artery

Artery

Bandage

Circumferential

Swelling

Occlusion of arteries

Figure 26–8

Procedure for Performing Wound Dressing – *(continued)*

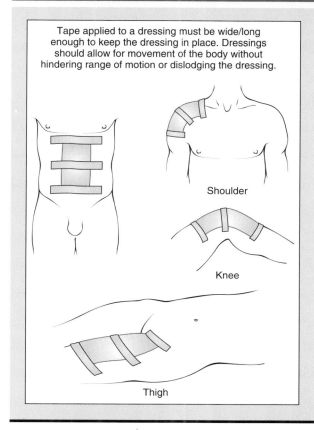

Tape applied to a dressing must be wide/long enough to keep the dressing in place. Dressings should allow for movement of the body without hindering range of motion or dislodging the dressing.

Shoulder

Knee

Thigh

Figure 26–9

Follow-Up Care and Instructions

- When indicated, the patient or caregiver should undertake dressing changes. Carefully explaining the procedure will help facilitate timely, appropriate, and effective wound management. Noncompliance or the inadequate communication of information can result in poor healing, infection, pain, and disfiguring scars.
- Instruct the patient to change the dressing after cleansing the wound, if the dressing becomes wet or dirty, or after a certain amount of time has passed, typically 2 to 3 days.
- Instruct the patient to clean the wound gently with some hydrogen peroxide on cotton swabs or gauze and then gently blot the wound dry approximately three times a day. Dried blood or superficial coagulum should be removed from the wound edges to prevent widening of the final scar.

- Reassure the patient that body hygiene can be maintained by showering but that the shower spray should not spray directly on the wound of the patient. Advise against bathing in a tub because of the possibility of an infection developing in the wound.
- Instruct the patient to observe the wound edges for increased redness or increased tenderness and to contact the office for assessment.
- Make the patient aware of what to expect concerning the progress of the wound over time. Normal wound healing often exhibits characteristics that can be confused with wound infections; therefore, describe in detail what the wound should look like and feel like in the course of the normal healing process. The normal healing process often involves a limited inflammatory response that produces erythema and tenderness for a few days.
- Additionally, make the patient aware of the signs and symptoms of a wound infection, which include erythema, pain, warmth, edema, discharge, throbbing, fever, regional adenopathy, and spreading erythema.
- Patients not able to perform dressing changes or evaluate the progress of their wounds may be candidates for visiting nursing services.
- Wound infections may require interventions that vary by factors such as severity and the proximity to other organ systems. Infections in closed wounds may require that sutures be removed or incision and drainage be performed. Some infections may require aggressive systemic antibiotic therapy, especially those that are spreading by vascular or lymphatic systems or are following tissue lines such as fascia or muscle.
- Infected wounds should be cleaned with normal saline solution at least four times a day and the dressing changed.
- Instruct the patient to wash his or her hands with soap and water before and after tending to the wound.
- Instruct the patient to use the same primary and secondary dressing materials as used by the primary provider.
- When a wound is free of infection, sutures have been removed, all skin surfaces are dry, and the wound is no longer draining, the use of dressings can be discontinued. At this point, dressings may be still be used when indicated as padding to protect the fragile, newly healed tissues from damage due to physical trauma. However, in most cases, dressings can be discontinued when the indications for them, primarily protection of the wound, are no longer present.

Bibliography

- Bischoff WE, Reynolds TM, Sessler CN, et al: Handwashing compliance by health care workers: The impact of introducing an accessible, alcohol-based hand antiseptic. Arch Intern Med 2000;160:1017–1021.
- Felciano DV, Moore EE, Mattox KL: Trauma. Norwalk, Conn, Appleton & Lange, 1996.

- Grossman JA: Minor Injuries and Disorders: Surgical and Medical Care. Philadelphia, JB Lippincott, 1984.
- Hess CT, Salcido R: Wound Care, 3rd ed. Springhouse, Pa, Springhouse, 2000.
- Schwartz SI: Principles of Surgery, 7th ed. New York, McGraw-Hill, 1999.
- Trott AT: Wounds and Lacerations: Emergency Care and Closure. St. Louis, Mosby-Year Book, 1997.
- Wardrope J, Edhouse J: The Management of Wounds and Burns, 2nd ed. Oxford, England, Oxford University Press, 1999.
- Westaby S: Wound Care. St. Louis, CV Mosby, 1998.
- World Wide Wounds: The Electronic Journal of Wound Management Practice. Available at *http://www.smtl.co.uk/world-wide-wounds*

Chapter 27

Cryosurgery

▷ P. Eugene Jones

Procedure Goals and Objectives

Goal: To perform cryosurgery on a lesion successfully, using technique that will facilitate wound healing and reduce the likelihood of infection while observing standard precautions and with a minimal degree of risk to the patient.

Objectives: The student will be able to . . .

▶ Describe the indications, contraindications, and rationale for performing cryosurgery.

▶ Identify and describe common complications associated with the use of cryosurgery on small skin lesions.

▶ Describe the essential anatomy and physiology of the skin associated with the performance of cryosurgery on small lesions.

▶ Identify the materials and tools necessary for performing cryosurgery on skin lesions and their proper use.

▶ Identify the important aspects of care after cryosurgery on small skin lesions.

Background and History

The therapeutic use of cold for treatment of injuries and inflammation dates back to as early as 2500 BC, when Egyptians appreciated its adjunctive value. Over the centuries, famous physicians such as Hippocrates and Baron Dominique Jean Lorie used cold for analgesia and hemorrhage control (Graham, 1999). The modern era of cryosurgery began when James Arnott developed the application of cold for a variety of conditions. He achieved a temperature of −24°C with a salt and crushed ice brine to treat neuralgia and for palliative care in terminally ill cancer patients. The first dermatologic application of cryosurgery was in New York in 1899 when the dermatologist A. C. White applied liquefied air via cotton-tipped applicators to warts, nevi, and premalignant and malignant skin lesions (Graham, 1998). Liquid nitrogen was introduced as a cryogen about 1948. By 1962, Irving Cooper developed a more modern apparatus that facilitated cryosurgical spray application techniques (Grekin, 1990).

Biologic effects on the skin and subcutaneous tissue are achieved by selective destruction of tissue as heat is transferred from the skin to a heat sink (typically liquid nitrogen). The subzero temperatures achieved results in intra- and extracellular ice crystal formation, disruption of cell membrane integrity, pH changes, and thermal shock (Kuplik, 1997). To achieve maximal tissue destruction effect, a series of freeze-thaw cycles can be used (Gage, 1978).

Indications

Cryosurgery has several indications and advantages over other surgical modalities in selected patients with appropriate lesions. Specific lesions that may be treated with cryosurgery are listed in Table 27–1.

In addition to the rapid healing and technical ease of cryogen application, lesions with more sharply demarcated borders are more responsive to cryosurgery, and the portability of cryosurgical application renders it advantageous for most body areas.

Because of the ease of application and relatively minimal associated risks, cryosurgery is especially useful to treat the following patients:

- Elderly, high-risk surgical patients
- Patients allergic to local anesthetics
- Patients with coagulopathies and pacemakers (Drake et al, 1994)

Contraindications

Cryosurgery is contraindicated in patients with the following:

- Cryoglobulinemia
- Cold intolerance, such as Raynaud's disease or cold urticaria

Table 27-1

Lesions Treatable with Cryosurgery

Benign Lesions	Precancerous Lesions or Tumors of Uncertain Behavior	Malignant Lesions
Acne vulgaris	Actinic cheilitis	Basal cell carcinoma
Angiolymphoid hyperplasia	Actinic keratosis	Bowen's disease
Angiokeratoma	Keratoacanthoma	Kaposi's sarcoma
Angioma, cherry and spider	Lentigo maligna	Squamous cell carcinoma
Chondrodermatitis nodularis chronica helicis	Bowenoid papulosis	Actinic keratosis with squamous cell
Dermatofibroma	Leukoplakia	carcinoma
Disseminated superficial actinic porokeratosis		
Granuloma faciale		
Granuloma fissuratum		
Hemangioma		
Hidradenitis suppurativa		
Keloid		
Leishmaniasis		
Lentigines, lentigo simplex, solar lentigo		
Lichen planus		
Lichen sclerosis et atrophicus		
Lichen simplex chronicus		
Lymphocytoma cutis		
Molluscum contagiosum		
Mucocele		
Myxoid cyst		
Nevi		
Porokeratosis of Mibelli		
Prurigo nodularis		
Psoriatic plaques		
Pyogenic granuloma		
Rosacea		
Sebaceous hyperplasia		
Seborrheic keratosis		
Syringoma		
Venous lake		
Verrucae		
Other		

From Drake LA, Ceilley RI, Cornelison RL, et al: Guidelines of care for cryosurgery. J Am Acad Dermatol 31:648–653, 1994.

- Lesions overlying nerves (Arndt et al, 1997)
- Lesions of dark-skinned individuals; treatment in these individuals may leave hypopigmented scars

Potential Complications

- Immediate complications can include dizziness and vasovagal syncopal episodes during cryosurgery procedures, particularly on the fingers or plantar surfaces. Unless contraindicated because of lesion location or other reasons, place the patient in a supine position before initiating the procedure.
- Soft tissue erythema, edema, and pain are not uncommon, and occasional large, bloody postprocedural bullae are seen when treating lesions of the dorsal hand surface. Facial lesions typically crust over without vesicle or bulla formation.
- Occasional localized hemorrhage and vascular headache are noted immediately after cryosurgery.
- Because of melanocyte sensitivity to cold, the potential for postinflammatory pigmentation changes must be considered in all patients. More typical is hypopigmentation in darker skinned patients and hyperpigmentation in others.
- Delayed complications can include infection, hemorrhage, and excessive formation of granulation tissue (Young and Sinclair, 1997). It is not uncommon for verruca vulgaris lesions to recur as a larger lesion circumferentially after cryosurgery. Patients should be cautioned about the possible appearance of these "ring warts" of recurrent hyperkeratotic verruca at previously treated sites.
- Prolonged complications can include postprocedure hypo- and hyperpigmentation, altered sensation, alopecia in hair-bearing areas, and atrophy. Prolonged postprocedure pain can usually be alleviated with nonsteroidal anti-inflammatory drugs (NSAIDs).
- When freezing over bones and tendons, one should continually move the skin back and forth while performing cryosurgery in order to avoid freezing the skin to the bone or tendon surface.
- Treating lesions of the scalp, forehead, or temple may produce a transient headache (Arndt et al, 1997).
- Avoidance of overfreezing will reduce instances of prolonged residual hypopigmentation, atrophy, and cartilage necrosis.

Review of Essential Anatomy and Physiology

Knowledge of local neurovascular anatomy is imperative before performing cryosurgery. Areas of concern include the skin near the medial epicondyle of the elbow and the lateral aspects of the digits and the angle of the mandible, as nerves are more superficial in these areas and are prone to freeze injury (Habif, 1996). For example, a lesion on the pinna of the ear may respond well to cryosurgery, whereas a lower extremity lesion in a patient with peripheral vascular disease may not. Patient selection criteria include lesion location, skin color and type, size and number of lesions, response to previous therapy, and condition of the skin and subcutaneous tissue. Because melanocytes are more sensitive to cold injury, postinflammatory hypopigmentation is more common in darker skin. Cryogens and their Celsius temperature are noted in Table 27–2.

Standard Precautions ▷ Every practitioner should use Standard Precautions at all times when interacting with patients, especially when performing procedures. Determining the level of precaution necessary requires the practitioner to exercise clinical judgment based on the patient's history and the potential for exposure to body fluids or aerosol-borne pathogens (for further discussion, see Chapter 2).

Patient Preparation

- Have the patient sign a consent form after the procedure and its risks have been explained.
- Ensure patient comfort in a seated or supine position, if not contraindicated.
- The application of liquid nitrogen can be painful, particularly for children; therefore, additional efforts may be necessary to prepare children psychologically before the procedure is performed.
- Consideration for precryosurgery anesthesia with topical agents such as lidocaine-prilocaine (EMLA) or lidocaine (ELA-Max) cream is worth considering before the procedure, unless contraindicated.
- Outlining the lesion with a surgical marking pen may be helpful, as freezing may temporarily obliterate visual lesion margins.

Table 27–2

Cryogens and Their Effective Celsius Temperature

Cryogen	Temperature (°C)
Ice	0
Salt ice	−20
CO_2 slush	−20
CO_2 snow	−70
CO_2 solid	−78.5
Liquid nitrous oxide	−89.5
Liquid nitrogen	−20 (swab)
Liquid nitrogen	−195.8 (spray/probe)

Materials Utilized for Performing Cryosurgery

Sterile Cotton-Tipped Applicator/Swab Method
- Liquid nitrogen
- Styrofoam cup
- Cotton-tipped applicator
- Gloves

Spray Method
- Liquid nitrogen spray gun
- Gloves
- Spray extension (necessary to treat difficult to reach lesions) (Fig. 27–1)

Cryoprobe Method
- Liquid nitrogen spray gun
- Probes (see Fig. 27–1)
- Gloves
- Probe extension (necessary to treat difficult to reach lesions; see Fig. 27–1)

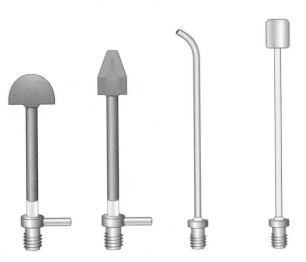

Figure 27–1. Materials used to perform cryosurgery.

Procedure for Performing Cryosurgery

Note: Because longer time and depth of freeze destroys more tissue, care must be exercised to not overtreat. It is better to treat conservatively and re-treat a lesion at a later date than to overtreat once and risk permanent hypopigmentation.
Note: The depth of freeze achieved typically approximates 1.5 times the lateral

spread of the visible cutaneous ice ball (Torre, 1979).

Note: Lesion thickness typically dictates length and depth of freeze. For example, a large, flat, thin seborrheic keratosis should be frozen in sections and not from the center out, as this will result in too deep a freeze. Thicker lesions, such as a hyperkeratotic verruca, require more prolonged freezing that typically results in hemorrhagic bulla formation beneath the lesion (Habif, 1996).

Cotton-Tipped Applicator/Swab Method

Note: The cotton-tipped applicator/swab method is useful on smaller lesions and around the eye or ear canal where unconcentrated spray may be deleterious, as spray is less concentrated.

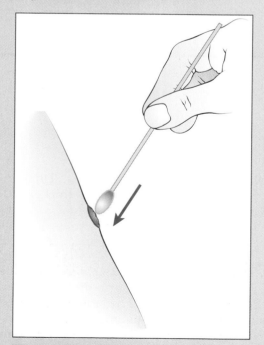

Figure 27–2

1. Pour enough liquid nitrogen from holding tank into a disposable polystyrene (Styrofoam) cup to cover cotton tip of applicator when dipping applicator into cup.
2. With gloved fingertips, loosen tight weave of swab while maintaining pointed tip to allow absorption of more liquid nitrogen.
3. Dip swab in liquid nitrogen, and apply swab tip to lesion (Fig. 27–2).
4. Repeat dipping and application procedure until an ice ball extends 1 to 2 mm beyond the clinical lesion, lasting from 10 to 20 seconds.

Note: Treating twice with a slow thaw between cycles is more destructive to cells than a single treatment with a rapid thaw.

Note: Lesion size, thickness, and location determine the duration of freeze required.

Note: A disposable ear speculum can be used as a focal cone to concentrate spray to a specific circumferential area.

Spray Method

Note: This method is more useful for larger or multiple lesions.

1. Hold the spray tip 1 to 2 cm from the lesion surface and gently squeeze the trigger mechanism (Fig. 27–3).

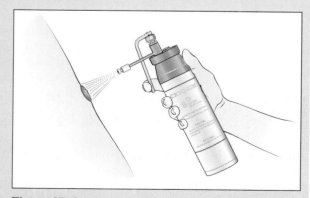

Figure 27–3

Procedure for Performing Cryosurgery – *(continued)*

2. Apply spray in a pulsatile, rotary, spiral, or paintbrush fashion.
3. For better control, maintain an intermittent, pulsatile spray rather than a continuous spray. Cones can be used to confine spray to a specific focal point.

Note: Freeze and thaw cycles are similar to swab application technique.

Note: Consideration should be given to all lesions regarding freeze time. Premalignant lesions such as actinic keratoses require a freeze time of approximately 8 to 12 seconds. Hypertrophic lesions may require 20 to 30 seconds of freeze or longer, and debulking before the procedure may be indicated to reduce excess keratinous tissue.

Cryoprobe Method

Note: More commonly used for malignant lesions such as superficial or nodular basal cell carcinoma, the cryoprobe technique requires additional training and experience before it can be used clinically.

1. Select the appropriate probe based on the size and shape of the lesion (see Fig. 27–1).
2. Precool the tip to prevent skin adhesion.
3. Apply the tip to the lesion with direct pressure for the specified period (Fig. 27–4) (Arndt et al, 1997).

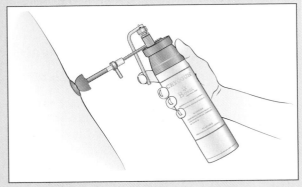

Figure 27–4

Special Considerations

Tissue damage increases with longer freeze-thaw cycles. Thinner lesion depth (e.g., lentigines) requires less freezing, and thicker lesion depth (e.g., dermatofibromas) requires more. Severe residual pain is not uncommon after cryosurgery to thicker tissue areas such as the palms, soles, and anatomically confined areas such as periungual tissue (Habif, 1996).

Cryosurgery of malignant lesions requires additional expertise and training acquired under the tutelage of an experienced cryosurgeon. A thermocoupled temperature probe needle device positioned under the base of the lesion facilitates appropriate length and depth of tissue freeze until sufficient experience is acquired. Table 27–3 compares typical freeze times for benign and malignant lesions.

Table 27-3

Comparison of Freeze Times for Benign and Malignant Lesions and Range of Expected Cosmetic Results Using Intermittent Spray

Lesion	Freeze Time (sec)	Range of Expected Cosmetic Results
Acne scarring	10	Good to fair
Actinic keratoses	5-10	Excellent to good
Chondrodermatitis	30	Good to fair
Granuloma faciale	30	Good to fair
Hemangioma	60+	Good to fair
Hypertrophic scarring	20	Good to fair
Keratoacanthoma	30	Excellent to good
Lentigines	10	Excellent to good
Lentigo maligna	60-120	Excellent to good
Morphea-type BCC	90-120	Good to fair
Nevi	10	Good to fair
Nodular BCC	60-90	Excellent to good
Sebaceous hyperplasia	5-10	Excellent to good
Seborrheic keratoses	10	Good to fair
Superficial BCC	60	Excellent to good

BCC, Basal cell carcinoma.
From Freedberg IM, Eisen AZ, Wolff K, et al (eds): Fitzpatrick's Dermatology in General Medicine, Vol II, 5th ed. New York, McGraw-Hill, 1999.

Follow-Up Care and Instructions

Lesion care after cryosurgery should include the following:

- Instruct the patient to wash the area with soap and water gently twice daily.
- Advise the patient not to use gauze or an occlusive dressing because of the possibility of prematurely removing the eschar.
- Prescribe polymyxin B sulfate/bacitracin zinc (Polysporin) topical ointment to soften hardened eschar (Graham, 1998).
- Inform the patient that, after cryosurgery, it is common for a blister to form. This blister may be hemorrhagic at the treated site and dries, crusts, and peels along with the lesion.
- Reassure the patient that erythema and edema are common immediately after cryosurgery.
- Tell the patient to expect crusting to separate in approximately 10 days.

References

Arndt KA, Wintroub BU, Robinson JK, LeBoit PE. (Eds.) Primary Care Dermatology. Philadelphia, WB Saunders, 1997.

Drake LA, Ceilley RI, Cornelison RL, et al: Guidelines of care for cryosurgery. J Am Acad Dermatol. 31:648–653, 1994.

Gage AA: Experimental cryogenic injury of the palate: Observations pertinent to cryosurgical destruction of tumors. Cryobiology 21:157–69;1978.

Graham GF: Cryosurgery. In Freeberg IM, Eisen AZ, Wolff K, et al: (Eds.). Fitzpatrick's Dermatology in General Medicine. 5th ed. New York, McGraw-Hill, 1999.

Graham GF: Cryosurgery. In Ratz JL (ed): Textbook of Dermatologic Surgery. Philadelphia, Lippincott-Raven, 1998.

Grekin RC: Physical modalities of dermatologic therapy. In Arnold HL, Odom RB, James WD (eds): Andrews' Diseases of the Skin: Clinical Dermatology. 8th ed; Philadelphia, WB Saunders, 1990.

Habif TP: Clinical Dermatology: A Color Guide to Diagnosis and Therapy, 3rd ed. St. Louis, Mosby-Year Book, 1996.

Jones SK, Darville JM: Transmission of virus by cryotherapy and multi-use caustic pencils: A problem to dermatologists? Br Dermatol 121:481, 1989.

Kuplik EG: Cryosurgery for cutaneous malignancy. Dermatol Surg 3: 1081–1087, 1997.

Torre D: Understanding the relationship between lateral spread of freeze and depth of freeze. J Dermatol Surg Oncol. 5:51–53, 1979.

Young R, Sinclair S: Practical cryosurgery. Aust Fam Phys 26:1045–1047, 1997.

Chapter 28

Treating Ingrown Toenails

▷ Sue M. Enns

Procedure Goals and Objectives

Goal: To treat problems associated with an ingrown toenail by removing all or part of the affected nail.

Objectives: The student will be able to . . .

- ▶ Describe the indications, contraindications, and rationale for removing an ingrown toenail.

- ▶ Identify and describe common complications associated with removing an ingrown toenail.

- ▶ Describe the decision process used to determine when to remove an ingrown toenail.

- ▶ Describe the essential anatomy and physiology associated with removal of an ingrown toenail.

- ▶ Identify the materials necessary for performing removal of an ingrown toenail and their proper use.

- ▶ Identify the important aspects of care after removal of an ingrown toenail.

Background and History

The management of an ingrown toenail is one of the most common procedures that the primary care practitioner will be asked to perform. The ingrown toenail can be painful, causing limitation in function and mobility in many patients. Typically, only the great toe is affected, and either the medial or lateral border may be involved. In their protective role, nails bear the brunt of daily activities. Walking, running, wearing shoes, or participating in sports are just a few of the stresses that feet must endure. The most frequent underlying cause of an ingrown toenail is improper trimming of the nail, resulting in impingement, inflammation, and even infection in the surrounding and overlying skin of the nail fold. Improperly fitted shoes (i.e., high-heeled, narrow toe) that compress the toes together are also a significant contributing factor to the development of ingrown toenails. Other injuries to the nail bed that change the shape of the nail or a congenitally increased curvature of the lateral edges of the nail plate may also result in an ingrown nail.

Patients present with pain along the margin of the toenail that is aggravated by any type of pressure, especially when wearing shoes. Erythema and swelling are usually present and if infection has occurred, pustular drainage may be noted. Conservative measures such as elevation of the nail plate with a small cotton wick, frequent soaking, wearing loose-fitting shoes, and selective trimming of the nail may be attempted; however, either partial or total removal of the nail remains the definitive treatment (Peggs, 1994).

Indications

The most common indication for the removal of a nail is onychocryptosis (ingrown nail).

Other indications include the following:

- Onychomycosis (fungal infection of the nail)
- Chronic, recurrent paronychia (inflammation of the nail fold)
- Onychogryposis (deformed, curved nail) (Peggs, 1994)

Contraindications

Relatively few contraindications to the procedure exist but include a bleeding diathesis or an allergy to local anesthesia (Peggs, 1994). In these rare situations, conservative measures should be attempted first, with consideration of referral to a specialist if operative treatment is still indicated.

Potential Complications

Infection is a possible complication; however, it should be easily treatable with appropriate antibiotics and frequent soaks. If the nail bed is not cauterized (ablated), the nail will regrow and symptoms may return. If the nail bed is cauterized (ablated), there is still a potential for regrowth and return of symptoms (approximately 10% with phenol ablation).

Review of Essential Anatomy and Physiology

Nails are derived by keratinization of cells from the nail matrix, which is located at the proximal end of the nail plate (Fig. 28–1). The nail plate consists of the nail root embedded in the posterior nail fold, a fixed middle portion, and a distal free edge. The whitish nail matrix of proliferating epithelial cells grows in a semilunar pattern. It extends outward past the posterior nail fold and is called the *lunula* (Swartz, 1998). Sensory supply to the great toe is through the digital nerves that have an extensor and plantar branch on both the medial and lateral aspects of the toe.

Standard Precautions ▷ Every practitioner should use Standard Precautions at all times when interacting with patients, especially when performing procedures. Determining the level of precaution necessary requires the practitioner to exercise clinical judgment based on the patient's history and the potential for exposure to body fluids or aerosol-borne pathogens (for further discussion, see Chapter 2).

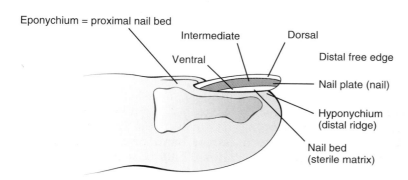

Figure 28–1. Anatomy of a nail. (Redrawn from Pfenninger JF, Fowler GC: Procedures for Primary Care Physicians. St. Louis, Mosby-Year Book, 1994, p 40.)

Patient Preparation

- Explain the procedure to the patient to help alleviate as much anxiety as possible.
- Reassure the patient that the procedure is not painful except for the initial injection.
- Indicate the need for the patient's cooperation in keeping the foot still.

Materials Utilized to Remove an Ingrown Toenail

- Local anesthetic without epinephrine (vasoconstricting agents should never be used in anesthetizing a digit)
- 5-mL syringe with a 1- to 1½-inch, 25- to 27-gauge needle
- Povidone-iodine (Betadine) swabs
- Sterile drape
- Rubber band or small Penrose drain
- Straight hemostats
- Sterile straight scissors
- Sterile periosteal elevator
- Sterile gauze pads
- Sterile cotton-tipped applicators
- Phenol solution (88%) if permanent ablation of nail bed is desired
- Antibiotic ointment
- Rolled or tubular gauze dressing

Procedure for Removing an Ingrown Toenail

1. Place the patient in a supine position.
2. Scrub the digit with povidone-iodine and drape the toe in a sterile fashion.

Anesthesia (see Chapter 22)

3. Withdraw approximately 5 mL of local anesthetic (without epinephrine) into syringe.
4. Inject the anesthetic in a ring fashion around the toe. The initial injection should be proximal to the edges of the medial nail fold on the dorsal surface of the toe. There are four digital nerves that should be anesthetized: both extensor and plantar branches of the medial and lateral nerves.
5. Inject approximately 1 mL of anesthetic around each nerve site, starting dorsally and directing the needle gently in a plantar direction, injecting around the plantar digital nerve.
6. Repeat the procedure on the lateral side of the toe.
7. After the toe is anesthetized (approximately 5 to 10 minutes), apply a tourniquet to the base of the toe (either a rubber band or small Penrose drain clamped with a hemostat).

Procedure for Removing an Ingrown Toenail – *(continued)*

Toenail Removal

8. For partial nail removal, first cut the nail lengthwise with sterile scissors or nail cutters, 4 to 5 mm from the affected nail fold (Fig. 28–2).

Note: If the entire nail is to be removed, cutting the nail in half in a lengthwise manner will facilitate easier removal.

9. Loosen and lift the nail with a narrow periosteal elevator, flat edge of the scissors, or any similar instrument. If the entire nail is to be removed, the nail can first be cut in half with sterile scissors or nail cutters.

10. Gradually separate the nail from the underlying nail bed by applying gentle, upward pressure, taking care to minimize trauma to the underlying nail bed. It is important to ensure that the proximal nail underneath the cuticle is fully loosened.

Ablation of the Nail Matrix

11. If permanent removal of the nail is desired to prevent recurrent problems, the matrix of the nail bed must be ablated.

12. Dry the nail bed with sterile gauze and apply an 88% phenol solution to the nail matrix with a sterile cotton-tipped applicator for approximately 3 minutes.

Note: Care must be taken not to expose surrounding tissue to the phenol solution.

13. Neutralize the area with isopropyl alcohol.

14. Remove the tourniquet.

Care after the Procedure

15. Apply antibiotic ointment to the nail bed and apply a sterile gauze pad to the site.

16. Wrap the toe with rolled or tubular gauze dressing.

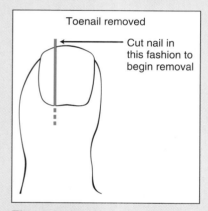

Toenail removed

Cut nail in this fashion to begin removal

Figure 28–2

Follow-Up Care and Instructions

- Instruct the patient to keep the foot elevated for 24 to 36 hours, with gradual return to ambulation.
- Over-the-counter analgesics are generally sufficient for pain relief.
- Advise the patient to change the dressing in approximately 24 hours and to soak the toe in warm water twice a day for several days.
- Instruct the patient to report back to the office with any signs of infection (fever, increasing swelling or erythema, pustular drainage).

- To prevent recurrence of the ingrown nail, advise the patient to wear low-heeled shoes with adequate room for the forefoot and toes.
- Instruct the patient not to trim the nails too short and to trim in a flat, straight-across fashion.

References

Peggs JF: Treatment of ingrown toenails. In Pfenninger JL, Fowler GC (eds): Procedures for Primary Care Physicians. St. Louis: Mosby-Year Book, 1994, p 38–43.
Swartz MH: Textbook of Physical Diagnosis: History and Examination, 3rd ed. Philadelphia, WB Saunders, 1998, p 94.

Bibliography

- Nail Disorders and Treatments: American College of Foot and Ankle Surgeons [cited May 2, 2000]. Available from *http://www.acfas.org/brnailds.html*

Chapter 29

Draining Subungual Hematomas

▷ Darwin Brown

Procedure Goals and Objectives

Goal: To drain a subungual hematoma successfully with a minimal degree of risk and discomfort to the patient.

Objectives: The student will be able to . . .

▶ Describe the indications, contraindications, and rationale for draining a subungual hematoma.

▶ Identify and describe common complications associated with draining a subungual hematoma.

▶ Describe the essential anatomy and physiology associated with draining a subungual hematoma.

▶ Identify the materials necessary for draining a subungual hematoma and their proper use.

▶ Identify the important aspects of care after draining a subungual hematoma.

Background and History

Subungual hematoma is an injury that is common to the nail bed of both fingers and toes. The vast majority are caused by simple trauma, which can result in bleeding into the space between the nail bed and fingernail. The subungual hematoma may also occur as a result of repetitive, indirect trauma to the distal end of the nail plate, typically in a tight-fitting shoe.

The patient often presents with intense pain secondary to the pressure produced by the hematoma. The primary goal of treatment is to relieve the pressure created by the hematoma. Drainage of the hematoma provides dramatic pain relief for the patient and decreases the secondary pressure effects to the digit. If the pressure is not relieved, damage to the nail matrix and the germinal layer may occur, causing delayed regrowth or dystrophy of the nail plate (Donnelly, 1992). The procedure itself is simple and can be performed safely in the practitioner's office.

Clinicians who perform this procedure should familiarize themselves with the anatomy of the nail bed and surrounding structures. The procedure is easy to perform with basic training and can be one of the more rewarding clinical treatments encountered in primary care or urgent care settings.

Indications

This procedure is indicated for relief from the acute pain associated with visible, painful subungual hematomas.

Contraindications

All patients presenting with nail trauma must be carefully assessed by history, physical examination and, when indicated, laboratory studies such as radiographs. Based on the clinical impression from these data, a decision can be made about the appropriateness of proceeding with the draining of the hematoma. Potential contraindications include the following:

- Crushed or fractured nails
- Fracture of the distal phalanx, which can inadvertently be converted to an open fracture by draining the hematoma
- Suspected subungual melanoma
- Hematomas involving 50% or more of the nail may indicate laceration of the underlying nail bed (Zook and Brown, 1999; Van Beek et al, 1990). It has been generally recommended that these patients be referred for nail removal and repair of the laceration (Simon and Wolgin,

1987; Melone and Grad, 1985). Others, however, recommend leaving the nail in place (Meek and White, 1998).

Potential Complications

Significant complications associated with this procedure are rare. Patients should be informed that there is potential for nail bed deformities to persist even after healing of the injury has occurred.

* The most likely complication resulting from a subungual hematoma is permanent nail deformity, especially if a nail bed injury is missed. Meek and White (1998) noted that from the perspective of many patients, nail deformity resulting from a subungual hematoma is considered minimally important.
* Infection of any remaining hematoma is uncommon but can occur. Using sterile technique and covering the site with a dressing after the procedure is completed can minimize the risk of this complication.
* Use of a cautery may result in an inadvertent burn to the nail bed after penetrating the nail, causing permanent damage.
* Functional deficits (numbness) are also a rare complication.

The procedure itself has no significant complications.

Review of Essential Anatomy and Physiology

The nail anatomy is shown in Figure 29–1. The nail plate is produced by the underlying matrix or nail bed. The nail plate and the underlying nail bed are supported by the distal phalanx. The nail plate is not directly innervated; however, the nail bed is richly innervated. The nail bed consists of all the tissue directly beneath the nail that functions in nail generation and migration. The arterial blood supply to the nail bed comes from two terminal branches of the volar digital artery (Zook and Brown, 1999).

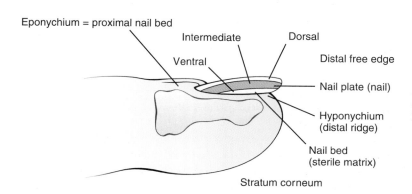

Eponychium = proximal nail bed
Intermediate   Dorsal
Ventral   Distal free edge
Nail plate (nail)
Hyponychium (distal ridge)
Nail bed (sterile matrix)
Stratum corneum

Figure 29–1. Anatomy of the nail bed. (Redrawn from Pfenninger JF, Fowler GC: Procedures for Primary Care Physicians. St. Louis, Mosby-Year Book, 1994, p 40.)

Standard Precautions ▷ Every practitioner should use Standard Precautions at all times when interacting with patients, especially when performing procedures. Determining the level of precaution necessary requires the practitioner to exercise clinical judgment based on the patient's history and the potential for exposure to body fluids or aerosol-borne pathogens (for further discussion, see Chapter 2).

Patient Preparation

- Describe the procedure to the patient and reassure him or her that there is rarely any more pain than what is already being experienced.
- Anesthesia usually is not needed and is often more painful than the procedure.
- If the hematoma is to be evacuated using a large-bore needle or scalpel blade, a digital block may be useful (see Chapter 22), as this method is more painful than cautery because of the pressure applied to the nail (Concannon, 1999).
- Inform the patient that, depending on the selected technique, an irritating odor may occur.
- The patient should be instructed to hold the digit very still during the procedure.

Materials Utilized for Draining a Subungual Hematoma

- Gloves
- Face shield
- Povidone-iodine (Betadine) or other antiseptic-germicidal solution
- Alcohol wipes
- Cautery (battery-operated or electrocautery unit), No. 11 scalpel, 18-gauge needle, or a paper clip
- Lighter to heat paper clip
- Sterile gauze
- Antibiotic ointment
- Bandage

Procedure for Draining a Subungual Hematoma

1. Place the patient in a sitting or supine position in which he or she can rest comfortably during the procedure without risk of further injury should lightheadedness occur. Examine the injured digit to determine the extent of injury.
2. Note the size of the hematoma.

Procedure for Draining a Subungual Hematoma – *(continued)*

3. Assess for fractures of the digit, especially the distal phalanx.
4. If a nondisplaced fracture is suspected, splint in an anatomic position until swelling improves.

Note: Radiographs should be obtained whenever you suspect a fracture.

5. Allow the affected digit to soak in an antiseptic solution such as povidone-iodine.

Note: Care must be taken to use aseptic technique in preparation for evacuation.

6. Clean the nail with alcohol.

Caution: Alcohol is a highly flammable material. Wash off alcohol with sterile water or allow the alcohol to dry before placing hot cautery or flame near the nail.

7. Burn a small hole in the nail using a conventional hand-held cautery or the straightened end of a paper clip (Fig. 29–2).
8. If using a paper clip, hold it with a hemostat.

9. Heat the straightened portion of the paper clip with a lighter until the tip is red hot.
10. Apply the hot tip with gentle pressure to the nail over the site of the hematoma (Fig. 29–3).

Note: It may take two or three attempts to burn through the nail with the heated paper clip.

11. Make a 1- to 2-mm hole, which is large enough to allow for long-term drainage.

Note: A sudden burst of blood may occur if the pressure beneath the nail is great enough.

12. Alternatively, with an 18-gauge needle or a No. 11 scalpel blade, using a rotary motion bore a hole through the nail to the hematoma. Consider using a digital block for this method (see Chapter 22).

Note: After the blood has drained, the associated pain should improve significantly. If pain does not subside significantly, underlying fractures should be reconsidered.

13. Clean the area with alcohol wipes.
14. Apply antibiotic ointment and a light dressing to the nail.

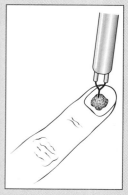

Figure 29–2. Redrawn from Pfenninger JF, Fowler GC: Procedures for Primary Care Physicians. St. Louis, Mosby-Year Book, 1994, p 48.

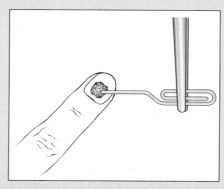

Figure 29–3. Redrawn from Pfenninger JF, Fowler GC: Procedures for Primary Care Physicians. St. Louis, Mosby-Year Book, 1994, p 48.

Special Considerations

For young children, providing guardians more information on the procedure can be helpful. Also, secure immobilization may be needed when performing this procedure in this population.

Follow-Up Care and Instructions

Advise the patient of the proper follow-up care after this procedure.

- The affected digit should be soaked in warm, soapy water two to three times a day.
- A light dressing should be kept over the area until the evacuation site closes completely.
- The patient should notify the practitioner if pain persists. The practitioner should also be notified if there is a change in sensation, purulent or foul-smelling drainage, fever, or erythema of the skin surrounding the area.
- The patient should understand that the nail and discomfort should improve progressively over the following few days.
- If any change occurs or the injury is not improving as expected, the patient should call or return to the office.

References

Concannon MJ: Common Hand Problems in Primary Care. Philadelphia, Hanley & Belfus, 1999, p 119.

Donnelly RE: Step-by-step procedures for treating common nail problems. Part I: Paronychia and subungual hematoma. J Am Acad Phys Assist 5:145–150, 1992.

Meek S, White M: Subungual haematomas: Is simple trephining enough? J Accid Emerg Med 15:269–271, 1998.

Melone CP, Grad JB: Primary care of fingernail injuries. Emerg Med Clin North Am 3:255–261, 1985.

Simon R, Wolgin M: Subungual haematoma: Association with occult laceration requiring repair. Am J Emerg Med 5:302–304, 1987.

Van Beek AL, Kassan MA, Adson MH, et al: Management of acute fingernail injuries. Hand Clin 6:23–35, 1990.

Zook EG, Brown RE: The perionychium. In Green DP, Hotchkiss RN, Pederson WC (eds): Green's Operative Hand Surgery, 4th ed, vol II. Philadelphia, Churchill Livingstone, 1999 pp 1354, 1356.

Bibliography

- Chang P: Nail bed repair. In Blair WF (ed): Techniques in Hand Surgery. Baltimore, Williams & Wilkins, 1996.

Chapter 30

Anoscopy

▷ Sue M. Enns

Procedure Goals and Objectives

Goal: To examine the anus and rectum thoroughly, with minimal discomfort to the patient, and obtain accurate information while maintaining patient modesty.

Objectives: The student will be able to . . .

▶ Describe the indications, contraindications, and rationale for performing anoscopy.

▶ Identify and describe potential complications associated with performing anoscopy.

▶ Describe the essential anatomy and physiology associated with the performance of anoscopy.

▶ Describe how to perform a digital rectal examination.

▶ Identify the materials necessary for performing anoscopy and their proper use.

▶ Properly perform the actions necessary to perform anoscopy.

Background and History

Anorectal disorders are a common source of discomfort for many patients, and adequate visualization of the anorectal canal is important for appropriate diagnosis and treatment of these conditions. Anoscopy is a relatively simple procedure to perform, but adequate patient education and clinical skill is required to reduce the patient's anxiety and embarrassment about the procedure. This procedure is performed in ambulatory, emergency, and inpatient settings and is commonly carried out before colonoscopy.

Indications

Indications for performing anoscopy include, but are not limited to, the evaluation of the following:

- Rectal bleeding
- Anorectal pain
- Pruritus
- Anal discharge
- Prolapse of the rectum
- A mass detected in the rectal vault on digital examination

Therapeutic procedures may be performed along with routine anoscopy and include biopsy of suspicious lesions, removal of foreign bodies, and collection of a specimen for culture.

Contraindications

Relatively few contraindications to the procedure exist. In the following situations, further patient education or referral to a specialist may be necessary if the examination is indicated:

- The presence of severe rectal pain
- Anoscopic examination in patients with perirectal abscess, acutely thrombosed hemorrhoid, or acute anal fissure, as severe discomfort may result as well as, in the case of anal fissure, possible bleeding
- A patient unwilling to have the procedure performed
- A patient not able to cooperate appropriately so that an adequate examination can be performed
- The presence of severe anal stricture

Potential Complications

- Anal or perianal tears (Fry and Kodner, 1985): Tears may occur but are usually mild and respond to conservative measures.
- Bleeding: This is rare but may occur with an anal tear or in the presence of internal hemorrhoids and will usually respond to conservative measures unless a coagulation defect is present.

Review of Essential Anatomy and Physiology

Understanding the anatomy of the anus and surrounding tissues facilitates accurate diagnosis and treatment of anorectal disorders. Careful visual inspection of the perianal region may reveal evidence of hemorrhoids, skin tags, fissures, dermatitis, abscesses, fistulous openings, or lesions. A thorough digital examination before anoscopy should evaluate the competency of the external anal sphincter and assess for palpable lesions.

The rectum is the distal 10- to 12-cm portion of the alimentary tract continuous proximally with the sigmoid colon and distally with the anal canal (Fig. 30–1). The rectum ends anteroinferior to the tip of the coccyx by turning sharply posteroinferiorly (the anorectal flexure) as it perforates the pelvic diaphragm (levator ani) to become the anal canal. The most distal point of the anal canal is the anal verge. The anal verge, the dentate line, and the anorectal ring are the three main anatomic points of reference.

- The anal verge, the external boundary of the anal canal, is the junction between the anal and perianal skin.
- The dentate line, the cephalad border of the anatomic anal canal, is a true mucocutaneous junction. Squamous epithelium is located distal to the dentate line, and columnar epithelium is located proximal to the

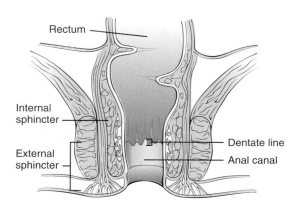

Figure 30–1. Anatomy of the rectum.

dentate line in the rectum. At this junction is a circular ring of glands that secrete mucus to lubricate the anal canal. The dentate line lies approximately 1 to 2 cm above the anal verge.

- The anorectal ring, 1 to 2 cm above the dentate line, is the upper border of the anal sphincteric complex and is easily palpable during digital examination.

The superior rectal artery, the continuation of the inferior mesenteric artery, supplies the proximal portion of the rectum. The two middle rectal arteries, usually arising from the inferior iliac arteries, supply the middle and inferior portions of the rectum, and the inferior rectal arteries, arising from the internal pudendal arteries, supply the anorectal sphincter muscles and anal canal. It is important to remember that the internal hemorrhoidal plexus arises above the dentate line, and the external hemorrhoidal plexus arises below the dentate line.

Both sympathetic and parasympathetic nerves innervate the rectum. The external sphincter (a voluntary skeletal muscle) and the levator ani muscles are innervated by the inferior rectal branch of the internal pudendal nerve (S2, S3, S4) as well as by fibers from the fourth sacral nerve. The internal sphincter (an involuntary muscle approximately 2.5 cm in length) is innervated by both sympathetic and parasympathetic nerves. It is generally accepted that either an intact functional external sphincter or anorectal ring (puborectalis muscle that encircles the very distal rectum) can provide nearly perfect anal continence. The internal sphincter plays little part in maintaining voluntary anal continence. This is important when counseling patients who are considering surgical treatment of anal fissures (Surrell, 1994).

Standard Precautions ▷ Every practitioner should use Standard Precautions at all times when interacting with patients, especially when performing procedures. Determining the level of precaution necessary requires the practitioner to exercise clinical judgment based on the patient's history and the potential for exposure to body fluids or aerosol-borne pathogens (for further discussion, see Chapter 2).

Patient Preparation

The only patient preparation needed is adequate education about the purpose of the examination and the technique used. Many patients have a degree of embarrassment about undergoing the examination and should be reassured that they will be appropriately draped. Although the procedure may be slightly uncomfortable and may cause an urge to defecate, it should not be painful (unless predisposing conditions are present). No bowel preparation is usually necessary.

Materials Utilized for Anoscopy

- Anoscope: The anoscope is a cylindrical instrument with a removable obturator, made of clear polyethylene or reusable metal (Fig. 30–2). Some anoscopes have their own attached light source; if not, another external light source must be used.
- Water-soluble lubricant
- Latex gloves
- Light source (directed or a light worn on the head)
- Appropriate culture swabs (when indicated)
- Monsel's solution
- Large-tipped cotton swabs

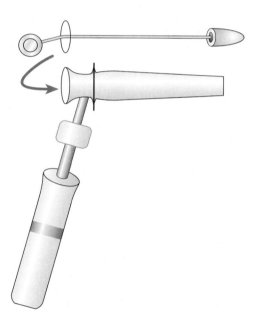

Figure 30–2. An anoscope.

Procedure for Anoscopy

Position

1. The patient should be placed in a lateral decubitus or dorsal lithotomy position with appropriate draping.

Inspection

1. Understanding the anatomy of the anus and surrounding tissues facilitates

Procedure for Anoscopy – *(continued)*

accurate diagnosis and treatment of anorectal disorders.

2. Careful visual inspection of the perianal region may reveal evidence of fissures, dermatitis, abscesses, fistulous openings, or lesions.

3. Asking the patient to bear down while inspecting may reveal prolapsing hemorrhoids.

Digital Rectal Examination

A thorough digital examination should be performed before anoscopy.

1. With a gloved, lubricated finger, gently press on the anal verge and ask the patient to relax. This should allow the finger to enter the anal canal.

2. The examiner should then evaluate the competency of the external anal sphincter by asking the patient to simulate interrupting a bowel movement.

3. After the patient relaxes, the examiner should also assess the rectal canal for any palpable lesions or masses. Finally, the prostate gland should be assessed in the male patient. The examiner should rotate the finger a full 360 degrees to ensure that all rectal structures are fully evaluated.

4. Generally, internal hemorrhoids and the dentate line are not palpable.

5. Any stool present on the examining finger should be examined for occult blood (Fry and Kodner, 1985).

Anoscopy

1. After lubricating the anoscope, gently spread the patient's buttocks and gently insert the anoscope into the anal canal and slowly advance until the flange at the base of the anoscope rests on the perianal skin.

2. Remove the obturator and inspect the mucosa of the perianal canal thoroughly for suspected pathology (Fig. 30–3).

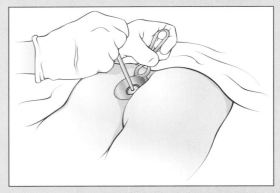

Figure 30–3. From Wigton RS: Gastrointestinal procedures. In Mosby's Primary Care Procedures, CD-ROM series. St. Louis, CV Mosby, 1999.

3. The procedure may need to be repeated in order to ensure adequate inspection of the entire canal (Fry and Kodner, 1985).

4. If a biopsy is necessary, a variety of long-handled biopsy instruments may be used.

5. Control any bleeding with Monsel's solution and pressure (Moesinger, 2000).

Follow-Up Care and Instructions

Examination findings should be discussed thoroughly with the patient. Complications are rare with this procedure, and follow-up care should be based on the treatment of any condition found during the examination.

The patient should be instructed to notify the provider if significant, unexpected bleeding or pain occurs after the procedure.

References

Fry RD, Kodner IJ: Anorectal disorders. Clin Symp 37:2–5, 1985.
Moesinger RC: Gastrointestinal Procedures. In Chen H, Sonnenday CJ (eds): Manual of Common Bedside Surgical Procedures. Philadelphia, Lippincott Williams & Wilkins, 2000, pp 159–160.
Surrell JA: Clinical anorectal anatomy and examination. In Pfenninger JL, Fowler GC (eds): Procedures for Primary Care Physicians. St. Louis, Mosby-Year Book, 1994, pp 898–901.

Bibliography

• Moore KL, Dalley AF: Clinically Oriented Anatomy, 4th ed. Philadelphia, Lippincott Williams & Wilkins, 1999.
• Varma JR: Clinical anorectal anatomy and examination. In Pfenninger JL, Fowler GC (eds): Procedures for Primary Care Physicians. Philadelphia, Mosby-Year Book, 1994, pp 902–905.

Chapter 31

Flexible Sigmoidoscopy

▷ Dawn Morton-Rias

Procedure Goals and Objectives

Goal: To perform flexible sigmoidoscopy on a patient safely and accurately.

Objectives: The student will be able to . . .

► Describe the indications, contraindications, and rationale for performing flexible sigmoidoscopy.

► Identify and describe common complications associated with performing flexible sigmoidoscopy.

► Describe the essential anatomy and physiology associated with the performance of flexible sigmoidoscopy.

► Identify the materials necessary for performing flexible sigmoidoscopy and their proper use.

► Describe the steps associated with safely performing a flexible sigmoidoscopy examination.

Background and History

The need to examine and evaluate the rectum and colon has existed for centuries. Hippocrates mentions the use of a rectal speculum for the diagnosis and treatment of anal disorders. Early instrumentation of the lower bowel was hampered by the lack of light. Several inventors experimented with endoscopic illumination, but Max Nitze of Germany (1879) and Howard Kelly of the United States (1895) are credited with the development of modern rigid proctosigmoidoscopy. Early proctosigmoidoscopy involved visual inspection of the lower bowel through a rigid scope inserted into the patient's anus and advanced to the rectum and sigmoid colon. Later, distal illumination, proximal illumination, and air insufflation expanded the visualization capabilities. Overholt of the United States reported the first experiences with fiberoptic flexible sigmoidoscopy by successfully examining the colon beyond the 25-cm limit of rigid sigmoidoscopy.

Modern flexible sigmoidoscopy involves the visual inspection and evaluation of the anal canal, rectum, and variable portions of the sigmoid colon. The procedure facilitates evaluation of lower bowel pathology, such as rectal bleeding, pain, constipation or diarrhea, and pathologic findings identified on digital or radiologic examination of the colon. Rigid sigmoidoscopy, considered optimal for visualization, biopsy, or culture of large surfaces, was not a welcome clinical intervention. Patient comfort was secondary to the evaluative and diagnostic benefits obtained from the procedure. Screening and the diagnostic benefits of rigid sigmoidoscopy were minimal because of a lack of public awareness of the value of the test, limited clinical training of physicians to perform sigmoidoscopy properly, a high cost-benefit ratio in asymptomatic patients and, perhaps most importantly, poor patient perception and dissatisfaction with rigid sigmoidoscopy. Consequently, rigid sigmoidoscopy was not well utilized. This remains so even today.

According to the American Society for Gastrointestinal Endoscopy, Standards for Training and Practice Committee, flexible sigmoidoscopy, which also involves direct visualization and evaluation of the lower colon, enables detection of three to four times as many precancerous polyps and is more widely accepted by patients. Both flexible and rigid sigmoidoscopy are appropriate for evaluation of colonic symptoms, and yet neither substitute for full colonoscopy when the latter is indicated. Modern biotechnology has facilitated the integration of instrument flexibility, illumination, and therapeutic as well as photographic capabilities into the modern flexible sigmoidoscopy.

Colorectal cancer represents the fourth most common cancer and the second most common cause of cancer death in the United States. Screening and surveillance guidelines endorsed by federal agencies and professional medical societies call for enhanced use of flexible sigmoidoscopy in conjunction with a complete history and physical examination, digital examination, and fecal occult blood assessment in the early detection and treatment of colon cancer. Evidence exists that a reduction in mortality from colorectal carcinoma is feasible through early detection and removal of polyps. Flexible sigmoidoscopy is a valuable screening tool in the early detection of changes in colonic mucosa, even before symptoms become evident. It allows direct visualization of changes, polyps, and other lesions and allows direct sampling. Flexible sigmoidoscopy is a reliable and cost-effective procedure that yields accurate findings when proper techniques are used.

Flexible sigmoidoscopy is safely and effectively performed by gastroenterology nurses, physician assistants, and physicians. All health care providers are strongly encouraged to acquire proper training and supervision in performing this procedure. It is recommended that providers perform at least 20 flexible sigmoidoscopies under direct supervision by a physician trained in the technique before attempting to perform the procedure independently. Flexible sigmoidoscopy is a therapeutic and diagnostic procedure that is best used in conjunction with other screening and diagnostic practices. The screening protocol includes assessment of risk, a digital examination, assessment of occult blood, and sigmoidoscopy. Full colonoscopy and barium radiography of the colon may be indicated. Flexible sigmoidoscopy is not simply a one-time test. Continuity of care and follow-up are key to realization of the benefit of this diagnostic procedure.

Indications

Specific indications for flexible sigmoidoscopy include evaluation and the diagnosis of:

* Frank rectal bleeding
* Occult blood
* Hemorrhoidal inflammation
* Anal fissures
* Polyps
* Inflammatory conditions of the colon

In addition, flexible sigmoidoscopy is indicated for the following:

* To monitor inflammatory bowel disease
* For follow-up and further evaluation of findings identified through barium enema radiography
* Current cancer screening guidelines outlined by the American Cancer Society recommend baseline flexible sigmoidoscopy for all adults by age 50.
* The American Society for Gastrointestinal Endoscopy recommends baseline and annual flexible sigmoidoscopy for individuals with a positive family history of familial polyposis, for individuals who have a

first-degree relative with a history of colonic neoplasia, and for those with a positive family history of hereditary nonpolyposis or colon cancer.

- Some surgeons recommend flexible sigmoidoscopy before hernia repair to rule out a colonic tumor.

Contraindications

Flexible sigmoidoscopy is a relatively safe procedure with few contraindications. Some sources suggest that polypectomy is not recommended using flexible sigmoidoscopy because of possible hemorrhage and risk of electrocautery-induced explosion. Others suggest that removal of polyps that are smaller than 0.5 cm during flexible sigmoidoscopy is safe and acceptable.

Contraindications to flexible sigmoidoscopy include:

- Fulminant colitis
- Severe or acute diverticulitis
- Toxic megacolon
- Acute peritonitis
- Poor bowel preparation
- Poor patient cooperation
- Severe cardiopulmonary disease

As with any diagnostic or therapeutic procedure, one must always weigh the importance of the information to be obtained against the risks associated with the procedure.

Potential Complications

Complications are rare but they can occur.

- Minor complications from flexible sigmoidoscopy include spotting and minor bleeding from the site.
- The most serious complication of flexible sigmoidoscopy is perforation of the bowel. This may occur by pushing the instrument directly through the mucosa, usually in an area of sharp flexion or through a diverticulum, which has been mistaken for bowel lumen.
- Tears at the site of an anastomosis in patients who have undergone rectal surgery is also a possible complication.
- A perforation or tear of the lumen requires surgical repair.

These complications may be avoided by taking a complete history, using proper technique, obtaining supervision and training, and using a reduced pace and rate of examination.

Review of Essential Anatomy and Physiology

The anal canal is the terminal end of the gastrointestinal tract (Fig. 31–1). It is a tubular structure of approximately 3 to 4 cm in length. The anorectal junction is an important landmark, characterized by a change in the pinkish mucosa to pale squamous epithelium. This landmark will not be observed if the instrument is advanced too rapidly. The rectum is the fixed terminal portion of the large intestines. The rectum is generally 15 cm long, and its inferior portion is continuous with the anal canal. The rectal mucosa is generally pink, moist, and glistening. The lumen of the rectum has three shelflike projections called the superior, middle, and inferior valves of Houston. These values are composed of mucous membranes, circular muscle, and fibrous tissue. The entrance to the sigmoid colon is marked by the presence of haustrations that are seen as small mucosal projections into the lumen. These haustrations appear to divide the sigmoid lumen into compartments. Branches of the inferior mesenteric artery and sigmoid arteries provide the arterial blood supply of the sigmoid colon. Venous drainage is achieved via the inferior mesenteric vein. Lymphatic drainage is achieved via the intermediate colic lymph nodes on the branches of the left colic arteries and left inferior mesenteric lymph nodes around the inferior mesenteric artery.

Standard Precautions ▷ Every practitioner should use Standard Precautions at all times when interacting with patients, especially when performing procedures. Determining the level of precaution necessary requires the practitioner to exercise clinical judgment based on the patient's history and the potential for exposure to body fluids or aerosol-borne pathogens (for further discussion, see Chapter 2).

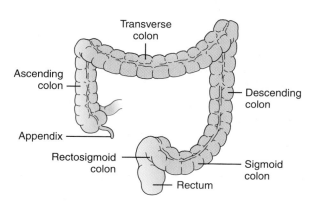

Figure 31–1. Anatomy of the large intestine and rectum.

Patient Preparation

- Explain the procedure to the patient, allowing an opportunity for the patient to ask questions and for them to be answered satisfactorily.
- Obtain informed consent for the procedure.
- Preparation before the procedure may include:
  - A liquid diet for 24 hours before the procedure
  - One to two bowel-cleansing enemas before the procedure. Patients are encouraged to use a commercially prepared enema product. Harsh laxatives may irritate the mucosa and cause retention of soft or watery stool, which may interfere with the quality of the examination. Complete and meticulous bowel preparation must be achieved to avoid explosion of combustible gases.
- Patients are to continue taking their prescribed medications.
- Patients are generally advised to discontinue use of aspirin, non-steroidal anti-inflammatory agents, and blood thinners before the procedure because these agents generally interfere with coagulation.
- Prophylactic antibiotic therapy may be prescribed for patients with cardiac valvular disease.
- The patient must be aware of the indications and expected outcomes as well as the logistics of the examination before positioning and draping.

Materials Utilized to Perform a Flexible Sigmoidoscopy

- A standard, small-caliber, flexible fiberoptic sigmoidoscope, either 35 or 60 cm in length (Fig. 31–2), and an appropriate light source
  Note: The basic unit consists of a control head, flexible insertion tube, and maneuverable tip. The most important features of the scope are flexibility, optics, and a small outside diameter with the largest internal biopsy channel possible. Durability as well as cleaning and ease of maintenance are essential.

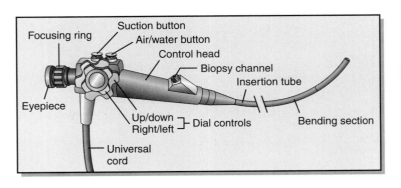

Figure 31–2. Schematic diagram of a fiberoptic sigmoidoscope. (Redrawn from Pfenninger JL, Fowler GC: Procedures for Primary Care Physicians. St. Louis, Mosby-Year Book, 1994, p 916.)

The coated glass fibers allow transmission of images longitudinally and transmit light to the distal end of the scope as well as to the proximal end. Smaller channels within the scope allow for the insufflation of air that is necessary for distention of the lumen, water infiltration, and fulguration apparatus. These are useful for aspiration of retained liquid stool, mucus, or enema water. The water, suction, and air controls are located on the control head and the scope. The exterior of the scope is housed in a plastic sleeve.

- Large, cotton-tipped swabs may be used to push aside stool or to assess mucosal integrity.
- Culture and biopsy materials must be available so that lesions and suspicious mucosa may be adequately sampled.
- Appropriate draping materials to protect patient modesty
- Nonsterile gloves
- Water-soluble lubricant
- Suction machine
- Containers with and without water
- Forceps

Procedure for Performing a Flexible Sigmoidoscopy

Note: Flexible sigmoidoscopy is an outpatient procedure. The success of the examination relies on provider technique and rapport with the patient, as well as patient comfort, preparation, and cooperation.

Note: Sedation is rarely necessary. Low-dose intravenous diazepam may be indicated for patients with significant apprehension or anal disease or for children.

1. Place the patient in any one of three positions: knee chest position, an inverted position or left Sims' position. Some prefer the left Sims' position in that it is perceived to be a less embarrassing position. The knee-chest position as well as the inverted position allows for greater access, as the bowel tends to move away from the pelvis. Encourage the patient in the knee-chest position or inverted position to remain still and to keep the hips straight.

2. Dim the room lighting; an assistant should be available in the examination room.

3. Begin the procedure with a well-lubricated digital examination of the anus.
Note: This examination also serves to ensure proper rectal clearance as well as to relax the rectal sphincter and lubricate the anal canal.

4. Palpate the anal region for abnormalities, fissures, and inflammation of internal or external hemorrhoid tissue. Palpate the ischional fossae and perineum between the thumb and forefinger.

Procedure for Performing a Flexible Sigmoidoscopy – *(continued)*

5. Insert the examining finger farther to palpate the anterior wall and then sweep down to the posterior wall.

Note: This step in effect becomes a bidigital examination because while the index finger is within the anus, the thumb is palpating the tissue of the perineum, ischioanal, fossae and coccygeal areas. In addition, this step allows the provider to assess the anal diameter to determine if the selected caliber scope is appropriate.

6. The distal 10 to 15 cm of the scope may be lubricated, but care should be used to avoid lubrication of the tip, as this will cloud the lens.

7. To minimize patient discomfort, a common approach for insertion of the scope involves gradual replacement of the examining digit during withdrawal with the insertion of the scope (Fig. 31–3).

8. While advancing the scope, you will feel a slight "give" as the scope passes the anal canal and enters the rectum.

9. Advancement, as well as deflection, of the scope via the hand-held control knobs must be slow and gradual.

10. Small turns of the control knobs result in significant movement of the scope. You may observe a "red out" during advancement of the scope. This finding suggests that the lens of the scope is pressed against the lumen, and the instrument must be retracted slightly.

11. Avoid excessive suctioning during the procedure, as the mucosal wall may be suctioned directly to the scope and may become dry and erythematous as well.

12. Use the least amount of air insuffla-

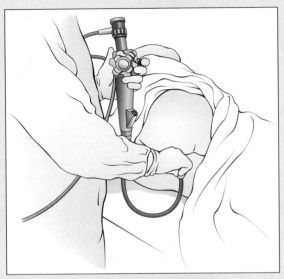

Figure 31–3. Redrawn from Wigton RS: Gastrointestinal procedures. In: Mosby's Primary Care Procedures, CD-ROM series. St. Louis, CV Mosby, 1999, graphic fldo0002.jpg.

tion as possible for visualization to minimize distention and avoid patient discomfort.

Note: Overinsufflation may cause the mucosa to become less flexible and may cause perforation or serosal lacerations.

Note: The normal healthy mucosa is pink and glistening. Plaques, lesions, masses, and polyps must be noted.

Note: Transition to the rectum is generally evident by recognition of three prominent haustral folds called the valves of Houston. These angulations must be successfully negotiated, and this component of the examination is considered most technically challenging.

Note: Dutta and Kowalewski (1987) suggest the following general rules for insertion of the flexible fiberoptic sigmoidoscope.

Procedure for Performing a Flexible Sigmoidoscopy – *(continued)*

- Clockwise torque decreases bowel angulation; counterclockwise torque does the reverse.
- Slight suction may aid in negotiation of sharp angulation in the bowel.
- If spasms occurs, pause and then resume.
- If you reach sharp curves, it is best to withdraw a bit before advancing the scope.

13. Throughout the procedure, sampling, culture, and biopsy specimens may be obtained. Use the largest forceps available that will fit through the scope. Survey samples should be obtained from fold edges because they yield the greatest results.
14. Under rare circumstances and with specialized and specific training and certification, small polyps may be removed via electrosurgery under endoscopic conditions.
15. Small sessile polyps (5 mm or less) may be removed with hot biopsy forceps.

Note: Some providers attempt polypectomy of larger lesions through mechanical debulking.

Note: Dutta and Kowaleswski's 10 overall golden rules for flexible sigmoidoscopy are listed below:

- Never attempt the procedure on an uncooperative or unwilling patient.
- Always obtain written consent.
- Talk with your patient before, during, and after the procedure.
- Allow yourself enough time.

- Do not spend 20 minutes inserting the scope. The best visualization of colonic mucosa may be on the way out.
- Proper bowel preparation is essential. Postpone the test if necessary.
- Do not insist on inserting the instrument the full 60 cm. Thirty to 40 cm may be all that is possible.
- Never advance the scope blindly.
- The 90- to 180-degree deflection available on most scopes is very helpful. Use it.
- Use less air; suction as necessary.

16. Withdraw the scope gradually, and carefully inspect the colon during this process.

Note: Withdrawal of the scope is a crucial part of the examination. The examiner must ensure that the steering knob is not locked, and he or she must use torque combined with in-and-out movements to deflect and observe while exiting.

17. When the tip of the sigmoidoscope is withdrawn from the anus, be careful that it does not strike anything, as the anus can be easily damaged.
18. Reinsert the scope 5 to 6 cm to remove the remaining air. Take care not to suck the mucosa into the scope. The patient can be instructed to tell the examiner when all the air has been removed.
19. Inspect the anal canal thoroughly using either an anoscope or the sigmoidoscope. This can also be performed at the beginning of the procedure.

Special Considerations

Flexible sigmoidoscopy of infants, children, teenagers, and elders requires attention to positioning, preparation, and communication. Infants and children may be understandably apprehensive and may require mild sedation. Special attention to concerns and an explanation of details may be necessary in preparing teenagers and young adults. Teenagers and young adults may be particularly sensitive to traffic within the examination suite. Hence, attention should be paid to limiting exposure. Elders, patients with limited mobility, and those with circulatory compromise may prefer or require left lateral (Sims') positioning for enhanced patient comfort. Full disclosure, communication, and rapport remain key in attending the needs of special populations.

Follow-Up Care and Instructions

Flexible sigmoidoscopy is a relatively safe and benign procedure. Postprocedural complications are rare but may include the following:

- Patients may complain of mild cramping and bloating from distention of the colon. Patients may also notice spotting after biopsy. These reactions are normal.
- Instruct the patient to seek immediate medical attention if he or she experiences severe abdominal pain, significant abdominal distention, nausea, vomiting, fever, chills, or a rectal bleed of greater than 1/2 cup after the procedure.

Reference

Dutta S, Kowalewski E: Flexible Sigmoidoscopy for Primary Care Physicians. New York, Alan R. Liss, 1987.

Bibliography

- American Society for Gastrointestinal Endoscopy: ASGE Publication No 1011. Available at *http://www.asge.org/resources/manual/lge_flex.html*
- Clinical Abstracts—Guidelines for Colorectal Cancer Screening. Available at *http://www.medscape.com*
- Fincher RK, Osgard EM, Jackson JL, et al: A comparison of bowel preparations for flexible sigmoidoscopy: Oral magnesium citrate combined with oral bisacodyl, one hypertonic phosphate enema, or two hypertonic phosphate enemas. Am J Gastroenterol 94:2122–2127, 1999.
- Gitnick G: Gastroenterology: Medical Outline Series. New York, Medical Examination, 1985.

- Hellinger M: Screening and detection of colorectal cancer. Cancer Control 5:17–18, 1998.
- Jednak MA, Nostrant TT: Screening for colorectal cancer. Prim Care 25:293–308, 1998.
- Johnson BA: Flexible sigmoidoscopy: Screening for colorectal cancer. Am Fam Phys 59:313–324, 327–328, 1999.
- Katon K, Keeffe E, Melnyk C: Flexible Sigmoidoscopy. New York, Grune & Stratton, 1985.
- Lewis JD, Asch DA, Ginsberg GG, et al: Primary care physicians' decisions to perform flexible sigmoidoscopy. J Gen Intern Med 14:297–302, 1999.
- Lichtenstein P, Holm NV, Verkasalo PK, et al: Environmental and heritable factors in the causation of cancer. N Engl J Med 343:78–85, 2000.
- Manoucheri M, Nakamura DY, Lukman RL: Bowel preparation for flexible sigmoidoscopy: Which method yields the best results? J Fam Pract 49:273, 2000.
- Moore K: Clinically Oriented Anatomy. Baltimore, Williams & Wilkins, 1985.
- National Digestive Diseases Information Clearinghouse, Bethesda Md. Email address: *nddic@aerie.com*
- National Institute of Diabetes and Digestive and Kidney Diseases: NIH Publication No. 95–1133, December, Bethesda, Md, 1992.
- Painter J, Saunders DB, Bell GD, et al: Depth of insertion at flexible sigmoidoscopy: Implications for colorectal cancer screening and instrument design. Endoscopy 31:227–231, 1999.
- Rex D: Colonic disease: Advances in screening, management and perspectives on health care utilization. Paper presented at the annual meeting of the American College of Gastroenterology, October 15, 1999. Available at *http://www.Medscape.com/medscape/CNO/1999/ACG-09.html*
- Ruffin M, Gorenflo D, Woodman B: Predictors of screening for breast, cervical, colorectal and prostatic cancer among community-based primary care practices. J Am Board Fam Pract 13:1–10, 2000.
- Schoen RE, Weissfeld JL, Bowen NJ, et al: Patient satisfaction with screening flexible sigmoidoscopy. Arch Intern Med 160:1790–1796, 2000.
- Schoenfeld P, Piorkowski M, Allaire J, et al: Flexible sigmoidoscopy by nurses: State of the art 1999. Gastroenterol Nurs 22:254–261, 1999.
- Shaukat MS, Ramirez FC: The utilization of flexible sigmoidoscopy by family practitioners after residency training. Gastrointest Endosc 52:45–47, 2000.
- Society of American Gastrointestinal Endoscopic Surgeons (SAGES) Patient Information—Flexible Sigmoidoscopy. Available at *http://www.medscape.com*
- Stewart BT, Keck JO, Duncan AV, et al: Difficult or incomplete flexible sigmoidoscopy: Implications for a screening programme. Aust N Z J Surg 69:2–3, 1999.
- Taylor T, Williamson S, Wardle J, et al: Acceptability of flexible sigmoidoscopy screening in older adults in the United Kingdom. J Med Screen; 7:38–45, 2000.
- Tuggy M: Virtual reality flexible sigmoidoscopy simulator training: Impact on resident performance. J Am Board Fam Pract 11:426–433, 1998.
- Wallace MB, Kemp JA, Meyer F, et al: Screening for colorectal cancer with flexible sigmoidoscopy by nonphysician endoscopists. Am J Med 107:286–287, 1999.
- Zubarik R, Eisen G, Zubarik J, et al: Education improves colorectal cancer screening by flexible sigmoidoscopy in an inner city population. Am J Gastroenterol 95:509–512, 2000.

Chapter 32

Patient Education Concepts*

▷ Richard D. Muma

Procedure Goals and Objectives

Goal: To perform effective patient education.

Objectives: The student will be able to . . .

► Describe the reasons why patient education is a worthwhile effort.

► Identify and describe Cole's suggestions for enhancing the patient education process.

► Identify and describe the proposed factors that influence patient education.

► Identify several sources for patient education materials.

---

* This chapter was adapted from Muma R, Lyons BA, Newman TA, Carnes BA (eds): Patient Education: A Practical Approach. New York, McGraw-Hill, 1996.

Background and History

This chapter summarizes recommendations as originally proposed by Collier and colleagues in *Patient Education: A Practical Approach* (Cole, 1996; Muma, 1996). Cole points out that there have been dramatic changes in the number of providers, advances in medical technology, and the understanding of disease, as well as striking developments in various methods to treat these problems. The goal of these advancements in health care delivery is to be able to provide better patient treatment, working toward the goal of affecting a healthy outcome. The chief means to accomplish this goal is through an interactive educational process. Whether it involves asking an individual to take medication or to make substantial lifestyle changes to promote better health, providers must be able to communicate, educate, and motivate the patient effectively.

Various approaches to patient education have been outlined over the years and are currently used in the training of physician assistants. All emphasize the importance of providing accurate information and encouraging patients to assume more responsibility for their own treatment. Many of the techniques used to accomplish such education share common characteristics. For example, explanations need to be given in simple terms, avoiding jargon that might be confusing. Also, the health care provider must assess the patient's understanding of the information in case further explanation is necessary to clarify questions or reduce confusion. Careful attention must also be given to patients' emotional responses to a particular diagnosis or treatment method, as these reactions can have a significant impact on outcome.

Effective patient education should be duly recognized as an integral building block in the entire health delivery process, of equal importance to clinical and technologic advancements in the field. Good patient education provides the following benefits (Greenberg, 1989):

- Enables patients to assume greater responsibility for their own health care
- Improves patients' ability to manage acute as well as chronic illness
- Provides patients with opportunities to choose healthier lifestyles and practice preventive medicine
- Improves compliance with medication and treatment regimens
- Increases patients' satisfaction with their medical care and thus reduces the risk of liability
- Attracts patients to your practice
- Leads to a more efficient, cost-effective health care system

Cole's Suggestions for Enhancing the Patient Education Process

Pay Attention to Using Good Interviewing Techniques. Helping patients deal successfully with medical problems involves being able to both educate and motivate for change. This requires the use of skillful interpersonal techniques. One needs to be attuned to both verbal and nonverbal aspects of the interaction. With time and practice, one develops a sense of when it is best to be silent and listen to a patient and when to provide specific educational information or support. Being prepared and organized beforehand (e.g., having laboratory work on the chart, pulling together handouts, having a treatment plan written out specifically for the patient) facilitates the entire process and will likely improve understanding and compliance.

Present Information through Several Channels. Do not rely solely on direct verbal communication to ensure a patient's understanding. For some individuals, verbal learning is not as successful as visual learning. Some individuals may understand and retain information better if they are able to view a handout or chart or follow an explanation concerning a radiograph. Also, some patients may benefit from the opportunity to meet and talk with others who have dealt with a certain problem or are currently undergoing treatment for a particular medical condition. Such peer support can be an effective tool in motivating an individual to comply with treatment.

Always Supplement the Educational Process with Patient Education Resources. The patient education process can be overwhelming because so much information may need to be covered. It is therefore recommended that patients be provided with brochures, handouts, medication inserts, an outline of the treatment plan, or other materials that will permit later perusal to reinforce what was covered during the actual interview.

Involve Families or Significant Others When Possible. Remember that patients are part of a larger family system. Most often, these family members are concerned about the health of their loved one, and involving them in the treatment process can be useful. Indeed, such involvement may in some cases ensure compliance with a treatment plan. Ask how the patient is going to explain a particular health problem to his or her family. Invite family members to attend a follow-up appointment so that they, too, can hear about the situation and learn how they can help.

Be Sure to Raise the Sensitive Issues. There are certain subjects that tend to be highly sensitive, and some patients may have underlying concerns or fears that they may not openly voice. Topics such as sexuality or death and dying often fall into this category. Because these topics may produce embarrassment or feelings of despondency, a patient may be reluctant to inquire about them. Therefore, it is critical for the health care professional to initiate such discussion when it is clearly pertinent to the treatment plan (e.g., medications that might interfere with sexual functioning, the need for a patient to recognize that the treatment options for a particular condition may be only palliative). Raising these issues signals that it is all right to talk about more sensitive matters and allows the patient to express his or her underlying fears and concerns openly.

Be Attuned to Emotional Reactions. As already noted, patients experience emotional reactions to learning of a particular illness and the need to follow a course of treatment. Providing comprehensive health care requires exploring these emotional topics. Whether the patient is expressing fear, anger, anxiety, or depression, unless the health care professional inquires about such reactions and takes steps to address them, treatment outcome may be in jeopardy. Allowing the patient to express feelings and offering him or her support are viewed as an integral part of the patient education process.

Do Not Feel That Once the Topic Is Covered It Is Completely Resolved for the Patient. For some individuals, providing education about a disease or treatment plan will be enough to motivate them to go forward and carry out the prescribed treatment. For others, however, there may be lingering confusion or questions after the interview that will need to be addressed at a later time. In addition, certain aspects of the treatment plan that are more difficult for a patient to deal with (e.g., making lifestyle changes such as smoking cessation or weight reduction) will need to be reviewed and re-encouraged at a later appointment. It is always prudent to review a patient's treatment plan at each subsequent follow-up visit, offering praise for the accomplishments and noting areas that need additional attention.

Proposed Factors That Influence Patient Education

There are many parts to the concept of health, including how one thinks about disease and its cures. Health care in the United States is based primarily on treating acute, well-advanced disease processes, using an infectious disease paradigm. However, the causes of poor health and serious disease processes are linked to multiple factors, particularly behavioral and cognitive habits, along with specific social and physical environments. Patients often react to illness and its management in ways learned from others, according to their cultural norms, and according to their own perception of the severity of the illness. Before engaging in a patient education session, one must realize that every patient responds differently, and several variables or factors play a role in that response. Some of those factors identified for discussion in this chapter include age, ethnicity, family issues, socioeconomic status, and the chronicity of illness.

Age

Although an obvious consideration, age is not always reflected in patient education materials and is often overlooked in the patient education counseling session. One must remember that the range of care starts with infants and ends with the elderly. Let us start with children. They are not small adults, and their wants, needs, thinking process, and emotional and physical status differ from those of an adult. For example, small children often view hospitalization as a punishment, not as a means of getting well (Anderson, 1990). This belief is further reinforced when parental figures make statements such as, "If you go outside without a coat you may get sick and have to go see the doctor." This type of belief often leads to false perceptions about clinicians and to a child's difficulty in accepting medical advice or treatment. Infants, although not directly involved in patient counseling sessions, have special needs and respond to touch and nonverbal communication (Anderson, 1990). As children grow older, however, one must keep in mind the current fads, language, and norms that exist. For example, teenagers often believe themselves to be experts in every area and in some cases, do not heed advice. Furthermore, certain instructions given to teenagers regarding prevention of illness may not be "cool" or in line with the thinking of their peer group.

Adults are more mature and have concerns that are different from those of adolescents. For instance, young adults (ages 20 to 40) are at a point in life in which multiple activities (e.g., college, relationships, children) keep them busy (Anderson, 1990). These patients need practical approaches to education; approaches that are not time-consuming and unrealistic in relation to their lives. As adults grow older (ages 41 to 60), they become more conscious of the possibility of health problems and in most cases are willing to follow a patient education prescription. However, some may lack self-confidence, which can cause avoidance of the risk of failure in learning anything new (Anderson, 1990). Adults older than age 65 are similar to middle-aged adults in their willingness to learn new ideas, but the provider must be aware of the individuals' past experiences, involve them in the learning process, and motivate them to learn (Anderson, 1990). Elderly patients may feel that it is hardly worth the effort to learn new information and skills because they think their life is nearing an end (Anderson, 1990).

Ethnicity

Before we discuss ethnicity, it is important to define the adjective, *ethnic*. Ethnic is defined in the 1982 edition of the *American Heritage Dictionary of the English Language* as follows: . . . "of or pertaining to a social group that claims or is accorded special status on the basis of complex, often variable traits including religious, linguistic, ancestral, or physical characteristics." Ethnicity is defined as the condition of belonging to a particular ethnic group. Examples of ethnic groups in the United States include African American, Asian, white, Hispanic, and Native American. There are at least 106 ethnic groups, including more than 170 Native American groups in the United States (Thernstrom, 1980). Ethnic groups should not be confused with minority groups, as the latter are seen as different from the majority group of which they are part. However, some ethnic groups are also classified as minorities, for example,

African Americans in the United States. One can see that the phenomenon of ethnicity is complex, ambivalent, paradoxical, and elusive (Senior, 1965). As clinicians, it is important to be aware of the ethnic backgrounds of patients. The differences in language and culture each group exhibits will certainly influence the way patient education is communicated. For example, some think that human immunodeficiency virus (HIV) infection prevention literature is not communicated effectively to African American populations. HIV prevention programs are hampered because of the presence of culturally specific attitudes and beliefs, including those pertaining to the roles of males and females (Lyons, 1994).

Family

Although consideration of the individual is important in patient education, the patient's family is also of central importance if teaching is to be effective (Falvo, 1985). How a family functions influences the health of its members as well as how an individual reacts to illness. Including the family members and significant others in patient education sessions facilitates adherence, understanding of the disease process, and the confidence needed to perform specific skills. Hence, the health care professional should capitalize on what family members can do for the patient and work with them in encouraging the patient in tasks that may be difficult. For example, when educating a patient with diabetes mellitus who requires insulin injections, involvement of the family in teaching sessions that demonstrate insulin injections most likely will improve compliance. Family members can also serve as troubleshooters when the patient has difficulty performing complex tasks. However, not all patients have family or significant others available for support. This is frequently seen in cases of HIV infection. Patients are often isolated from others after their diagnosis is made known. These patients are often on complex medical regimens involving the use of intravenous catheters. Lack of support sometimes leads to poor care, missed doses, and increased morbidity and mortality.

The health care professional can do much to facilitate the effectiveness of patient teaching by fostering discussion among significant others. A professional who has continued contact with the patient and his or her significant others may check on the progress of the patient when necessary and identify any new problems that may interfere with optimal care.

Socioeconomic Status

The socioeconomic status of the patient should be carefully considered when initiating education sessions. Individuals in lower socioeconomic groups are less likely to seek treatment; if they seek treatment they tend to access health care later in the course of their illness, and they die sooner than do individuals in higher socioeconomic classes. Hence, the clinician should be aware of the patient's personal income, living arrangements, and employment status but should also have an increased awareness of the patient's health. Lower socioeconomic status has been linked to the development of disease states, the most noted being coronary artery disease (Marmot et al, 1978; Morgenstern, 1980). For example, the provider clearly cannot erase poverty and improve access to health care for all; however, he or she can exert a positive impact on lower socioeconomic groups by working with their members to promote healthier lifestyles (Lyons, 1994). Some individuals often do not know what resources are available. The provider should point individuals to local resources that provide services and, if that is not possible, attempt to arrange for those services for the patient.

Chronicity of Disease

Finally, acute illnesses present differently from chronic ones and cause a variety of reactions among patients. Health care providers must be aware of the illnesses that require extra emotional support and possible psychiatric intervention when preparing for patient education sessions. Furthermore, it is not enough to simply inform a patient of his or her medical condition without time for an initial reaction. Patients require time to react to a new diagnosis. The perceived seriousness and natural course of a disease will help determine how a patient will respond. For instance, the patient diagnosed with acute pharyngitis may feel really terrible during the illness but knows that it is a curable disease and usually self-limiting. Hence, this patient may have fewer emotional problems and require less counseling. Conversely, the patient diagnosed with stage IV breast cancer, in which the long-term prognosis is known to be poor, will have an emotional response that may need further intervention involving a psychiatrist, social worker, or nursing care.

Sources of Patient Education

Finally, as pointed out by many (Lyons, 1996), patient education draws on a broad-based set of materials that can help explain a spectrum of topics. Traditionally, patient education has been accomplished with fact sheets; pamphlets; disease picture books; magazines; anatomic pictures; audiovisual materials such as videotapes, interactive video, computer-assisted instruction, laser disk technology, and the Internet; and verbal instructions or materials of a practitioner's own creation (Graber et al, 1999; Lyons, 1996). The Internet, particularly the World Wide Web, has become a ready source of educational materials, but clinicians should be cautious because much of the material on the Web is not written at a level that is comprehensible to many of our patients (Graber et al, 1999). Further investigation of Web resources is necessary by the clinician or others knowledgeable about patient education materials before referring patients to the Web. Particular attention should be paid to readability and accuracy of the information. Many of the chapters in this text refer to appropriate sites for patient education, and the reader should refer to those chapters for specific Web addresses.

References

Anderson C: Patient Teaching and Communication in an Information Age. Albany, NY, Delmars, 1990, pp 76–102.

Cole CM: An approach to patient education. In Muma RD, Lyons BA, Newman TA, Carnes BA (eds): Patient Education: A Practical Approach. New York, McGraw-Hill, 1996, pp 3–9.

Falvo DR: Effective Patient Education. Rockville, Md, Aspen, 1985, pp 99–109.

Graber MA, Roller CM, Kaeble B: Readability levels of patient education material on the World Wide Web. J Fam Pract 48:58–61, 1999.

Greenberg L: Build your practice with patient education. Contemp Pediatr September, 85–106, 1989.

Lyons BA, Valentine P: Prevention. In Muma RD, Lyons BA, Borucki MJ, et al, (eds): HIV Manual for Health Care Professionals. Norwalk, Conn, Appleton & Lange, 1994, p 257.

Lyons BA: Selecting and evaluating sources of patient education materials. In Muma RD, Lyons BA, Newman TA, Carnes BA (eds): Patient Education: A Practical Approach. New York, McGraw-Hill, 1996, pp 15–21.

Marmot MG, Adelstein AM, Robinson N, et al: Changing social-class distribution of heart disease. Br Med J 2:1109–1112, 1978.

Morgenstern H: The changing association between social status and coronary heart disease in a rural population. Soc Sci Med 14A:191–201, 1980.

Muma RD: Factors influencing patient education. In Muma RD, Lyons BA, Newman TA, Carnes BA (eds): Patient Education: A Practical Approach. New York, McGraw-Hill, 1996, pp 11–12.

Senior C: The Puerto Ricans: Strangers Then Neighbors. Chicago, Quadrangle Books, 1965, p 21.

The American Heritage Dictionary of the English Language. New York, Dell, 1982, p 247.

Thernstrom S: Harvard Encyclopedia of American Ethnic Groups. Cambridge, Mass. Belknap Press of Harvard University, 1980, p vii.

Bibliography

- Bates B: A Guide to the Physical Examination and History, 5th ed. Philadelphia, JB Lippincott, 1991.
- Bernstein L: Interviewing: A Guide for Health Professionals, 3rd ed. New York, Appleton-Century-Crofts, 1980.

- Enelow A, Swisher S: Interviewing and Patient Care, 3rd ed. New York, Oxford University Press, 1985.
- Guckian J (ed): The Clinical Interview and Physical Examination. Philadelphia, JB Lippincott, 1987.
- Henderson G: Physician-Patient Communication. Springfield, Ill, Charles C Thomas, 1981.
- Sherilyn-Cormier L, Cormier W, Weissen RL: Interviewing and Helping Skills for Health Professionals. Montery, Calif, Wadsworth Health Sciences Division, 1984.
- Stevenson I: The Diagnostic Interview, 2nd ed. New York, Harper & Row, 1971.

Chapter 33

Documentation

▷ David Asprey

Goals and Objectives

Goal: To provide clinicians with the necessary knowledge and understanding of documenting clinical procedures.

Objectives: The student will be able to . . .

▶ Describe the purpose of documenting clinical procedures.

▶ Discuss the importance of documenting clinical procedures in the medical record.

▶ List the components of a standard clinical procedure note.

Background and History

The medical record is a repository of information that is compiled by many individuals regarding a single patient. The information includes history and physical examination findings, data, interpretation of data, and descriptions of medical acts that were performed. The record serves many different audiences, which may include the clinician, other health professionals involved in the patient's care, the patient, supervisors, clinical investigators, and administrators.

Many of the clinical procedures discussed in this text will warrant or require the clinician involved in performing the procedure to prepare and record a clinical note for the medical record that documents and describes the performance and findings of the procedure. Performing the procedure without documenting it in the clinical note can result in loss of critical information affecting patient care or the ability of the health care system to receive reimbursement for the care provided. Documentation of the procedure in the medical record can serve several purposes. These purposes include the following:

- *Memory aid:* The medical record originally served as a vehicle for recording information that may otherwise be forgotten about the patient's ongoing conditions. However, the patient's complete medical database is a combination of the clinician's written and thought processes. Documentation of the clinical procedure and its findings can serve to assist the clinician in recalling important findings, techniques used, or complications encountered while performing the procedure.
- *Communication tool:* The medical record will also function to communicate information about the procedure performed and its findings to other clinicians and health professionals. Because medicine is a team function, many others will access the information recorded in a patient's medical record as they provide care to the patient. Because many others will utilize this same medical record, it becomes important to follow convention in the manner in which this information is recorded.
- *Quality assessment tool:* Individuals and organizations involved in providing patient care need to monitor the quality of the care provided. A key component of this process involves medical record review by peers. The medical record will be assessed for thoroughness, accuracy, and documentation of essential elements of the procedure.
- *Risk reduction aid:* One of the best defenses against malpractice litigation is a detailed, concise, and accurate medical record that demonstrates the rational and systematic approach the clinician used in performing the procedure. The medical record will serve as a legal document and may be used in court as evidence.
- *Reimbursement aid:* Most third-party payers require chart review in assessing reimbursement or reimbursement levels. In performing clinical procedures, it is essential to document all aspects of the history, physical examination, indications, and findings to support the charges

for which reimbursement is being requested. The medical record is used to verify that procedures were indicated and performed. In view of this, it becomes critical to document carefully all the associated activities involved with performing the procedure. The perspective that the third-party payer will use is: *If it is not recorded, it was not done.*

- *Evaluation tool:* Documentation of clinical procedures may be used in evaluation. Virtually all medical systems have a mechanism of quality control that includes evaluation of all clinicians' charts by peer review or quality control boards. Student write-ups are evaluated, and performance is monitored by faculty and staff.

- *Research tool:* The medical record also serves as a data source for clinical research in some cases. Retrospective chart reviews are commonly used in clinical epidemiology studies. Data must be carefully and accurately recorded for it to be useful in research studies.

Other Points for Consideration in Recording Clinical Procedures

- *Record all the pertinent data*: Both positive and negative findings from your examination or procedure findings may contribute directly to your assessment and differential diagnosis. Any diagnosis made or problem identified should be clearly spelled out in the record. When other aspects of the history or physical examination suggest that an abnormality might exist or that it should be ruled out, be sure to include this information, even if the abnormality is absent or the finding is negative. Another clinician should be able to read your account and be able to determine how you came to your conclusion.

- *Data not recorded are data lost:* Regardless of how vividly you may recall the detailed information associated with your patient and the procedure performed today, it is highly improbable that you will remember it clearly in a few weeks or a few months. Unless you record the presence and absence of findings and the specific steps completed in performing the procedure, you are at risk of being unable to answer questions regarding the activities associated with that procedure. The fact that something is not present in the medical record does not mean that it was not done or not observed (absence of evidence is not evidence of absence), but it does allow for this to be an equally plausible explanation.

- *Be objective*: The clinician recording the data in the medical record needs to take great care to ensure that only objective information is recorded. Statements that can be interpreted as judgmental or condescending have no place in the medical record. Although it is important to remain objective, this should not be misconstrued to mean that clinical impressions should not be recorded, rather, there should be a rational basis for your conclusions or impressions.

- *Consider the use of diagrams*: Diagrams can sometimes provide a better description than words alone. Diagrams used to identify topographic locations of lesions or techniques used in performing a procedure or to illustrate clinical findings can be powerful tools. Clinicians who learn to use diagrams can help improve the accuracy of their record and improve their efficiency. Clinical procedures often have findings that warrant the use of a diagram to document findings or techniques used in the procedure.
- *Avoid the use of nonstandard abbreviations:* Although abbreviations may useful in some limited instances to provide a measure of efficiency in making entries into the medical record, they have considerable potential for error and confusion on the part of those who read and interpret them. This same principle is true of acronyms and symbols; exercise caution in electing to use any of these tools in a medical record. **When in doubt, spell it out.**
- *Make sure the record is legible:* If your record is not legible to others, it will not serve its purpose well as a communication tool, nor will it serve you well as a legal document. Follow the conventional rules used in making entries into the medical record.

Clinical Procedure Notes

Entries made into the medical record specifically regarding clinical procedures performed constitute a unique format. Although they may be incorporated into a subjective, objective assessment and plan (SOAP) note format in some instances, the more significant procedures will often warrant a separate entry specific to the procedure performed. Each time that an entry is made into the medical record regarding a clinical procedure, a conventional format should be used to help ensure that the essential and important aspects of the procedure are included and to aid others who access the record in finding the important information. One such format is listed in the following section. A sample note is presented in Figure 33–1.

Clinical Procedure Note Format

If the clinician performing the procedure determines that a separate note is warranted, the format proposed in this section may be used to record the essential information.

1. Demographic data (patient name and identification number, age, date, time, and location)
2. Name or description of procedure performed
3. Primary indication or indications for performing the procedure

Demographic data:
  Name: Mary Smith, ID# 123-45-6789, **Age**: 48 years, **Date**: 08/09/01, **Time**: 1:45 pm,
  Location: Procedure room W139, outpatient clinic.

Procedure performed:
  Incision and drainage of abscess in perirectal area

Primary indications for performing the procedure:
  Treatment of localized skin infection and relief from associated pain

Contraindications:
  None, patient reports no known allergies

Consent:
  Informed consent was obtained and form signed and filed in medical record before
  performing the procedure.

Personnel:
  Procedure was performed by Jane Doe, PA, with assistance from Sara Shoe, RN.

Anesthesia:
  A regional field block was performed using 8 mL of 1% lidocaine without
  epinephrine.

Description of the procedure performed:
  The patient was positioned in a dorsal recumbent position and the skin of the
  perianal area was cleansed using povidone-iodine (Betadine). A regional field
  block was performed with 1% lidocaine. The patient was then draped, and an
  elliptic incision was performed parallel to the skin tension lines in the skin overlying the abscess. The abscess was explored with a sterile cotton-tipped applicator,
  and cultures were obtained and sent to the laboratory. A sterile, blunt hemostat was
  then used to disrupt loculations in the skin comprising the abscess with blunt
  dissection technique. The area was massaged to facilitate the expression of purulent
  material from the depths of the abscess. The wound was irrigated with 300 mL of
  normal saline solution. The wound was then packed with iodoform gauze. The wound
  was covered lightly with an absorbent bandage.

Findings:
  The abscess margins were approximately 1.5 cm deep × 2.0 cm wide. Moderate
  amounts of purulent material were expressed from the abscess with no unusual odor
  noted. Multiple loculations were present within the abscess, and they were disrupted
  with blunt dissection. The depths of the abscess were explored with no evidence of
  rectal fissure formation, and the abscess appeared to be limited to the subcutaneous
  fat layer of the skin. No foreign bodies or matter were noted in the abscess.

Description of any important physical examination findings, after the procedure:
  No evidence of rectal fissure formation was noted on reexamination of the abscess
  after drainage.

Complications, including blood loss side effects and adverse reactions:
  No complications were encountered. Estimated blood loss was 5 mL.

Instructions and follow-up plans:
  The patient was instructed about the proper technique to pack the abscess with
  iodoform gauze and bandage the wound. Patient was advised to repack the wound
  twice daily. Patient was educated regarding signs of advancing infection and
  instructed to contact our office or return to the clinic if they occur. A prescription for
  Tylenol No.3—to be taken 1 to 2 tablets PO every 6 hours during the next 48 hours
  "total of 16 tablets"— for pain relief was given. The patient was advised not to drive or
  operate equipment while taking this medication. Patient was advised to schedule
  a return appointment in 10 days.

Time procedure completed and condition of patient:
  The procedure was completed in 20 minutes, and the patient was released to travel
  home with her spouse in good condition.

Figure 33–1. Sample procedure note.

4. Contraindications, including potential allergies to medications that may be used in performing the procedure
5. Consent (if obtained)—indicate that informed consent was obtained and that forms were signed and filed in medical record before performing the procedure
6. Personnel—indicate the clinician who performed the procedure and any attendants who assisted with the procedure
7. Description of any important physical examination findings before performing the procedure
8. Anesthesia (specific agent, quantity used, and route administered) if applicable
9. Description of the procedure performed (include description of equipment used and any variations to the technique); diagrams may be useful in documenting the location of lesions, and so on
10. Description of the relevant findings associated with the procedure, including abnormal structures, pending laboratory tests, or specimen samples sent for examination; diagrams may be useful in recording pertinent findings
11. Description of any important physical examination findings after the procedure
12. Complications, including blood loss, side effects, and adverse reactions
13. Instructions and follow-up plans
14. Time that procedure was completed and the condition of patient at that time

Conclusion

Documentation of the clinical procedure in the medical record is an essential component of any complete procedure. Exercising care to be certain that the entry into the medical record follows a conventional format and is thorough will help avoid potential problems associated with incomplete entries.

Bibliography

- Anderson BH, Rahr RR: Patient record. In Ballweg R, Stolberg S, Sullivan EM (eds): Physician Assistant: A Guide to Clinical Practice, 2nd ed. Philadelphia, WB Saunders, 1999.
- Bates B: A Guide to Physical Examination and History Taking, 6th ed. Philadelphia, JB Lippincott, 1995.
- Coulehan JL, Block MR: The Medical Interview: Mastering Skills for Clinical Practice, 3rd ed. Philadelphia, FA Davis, 1997.

Index

Note: Page numbers followed by f refer to figures; page numbers followed by t refer to tables.